Praise for **Master You**

"We know more about diabetes than ever in history, yet disease rates are not declining appreciably, while costs to manage the disease continue to soar. In *Master Your Diabetes*, Dr. Morstein draws from the best of conventional and integrative therapies to provide diabetic patients an easy-to-implement program to regain their health."

—ROBB WOLF, author of *Wired to Eat* and *The Paleo Solution*

"This book is as complete a compendium on diabetes management as I have ever read. What is more, it tells the truth: 'To be blunt, no person with T2DM should ever wind up on insulin if they follow the protocol established by an integrative physician.' Type 2 diabetes is both preventable and in a majority of cases can be put into remission. This book is an ideal reference to understand how and why."

—TIMOTHY NOAKES, MD, PhD, emeritus professor, University of Cape Town, South Africa; founder, The Noakes Foundation

"In *Master Your Diabetes*, Dr. Mona Morstein covers the topic of holistic diabetes management in exceptional detail, providing real-world guidance for creating a low-carb lifestyle based on anti-inflammatory, organic, nutrient-dense foods and supportive lifestyle measures to improve blood sugar control and reduce disease risk. This comprehensive, well-written, and evidence-based book is ideal for medical and nutrition professionals, those with diabetes or prediabetes, and anyone interested in improving their overall health and vitality through healthy, low-carb living."

—FRANZISKA SPRITZLER, RD, CDE

"Dr. Morstein has developed a comprehensive and unique approach to the treatment of diabetes; the information she provides is priceless."

—DR. JARED ZEFF, ND, LAc

"Dr. Morstein is certainly one of the world's top experts in the integrative management of diabetes. This book is a must-have resource for both clinicians and for people diagnosed with diabetes."

—LISE ALSCHULER, ND, FABNO, executive director, TAP Integrative

MASTER YOUR DIABETES

MASTER YOUR DIABETES

A Comprehensive, Integrative Approach for Both Type 1 and Type 2 Diabetes

Dr. Mona Morstein, ND, DHANP

Chelsea Green Publishing
White River Junction, Vermont

Project Manager: Patricia Stone
Project Editor: Michael Metivier
Copy Editor: Deborah Heimann
Proofreader: Rachel Shields
Indexer: Ruth Satterlee
Designer: Melissa Jacobson
Page Composition: Abrah Griggs

Printed in the United States of America
First printing September 2017.
10 9 8 7 6 5 4 3 2 1   17 18 19 20 21

Our Commitment to Green Publishing

Chelsea Green sees publishing as a tool for cultural change and ecological stewardship. We strive to align our book manufacturing practices with our editorial mission and to reduce the impact of our business enterprise in the environment. We print our books and catalogs on chlorine-free recycled paper, using vegetable-based inks whenever possible. This book may cost slightly more because it was printed on paper that contains recycled fiber, and we hope you'll agree that it's worth it. Chelsea Green is a member of the Green Press Initiative (www.greenpressinitiative.org), a nonprofit coalition of publishers, manufacturers, and authors working to protect the world's endangered forests and conserve natural resources. *Master Your Diabetes* was printed on paper supplied by Thomson-Shore that contains 100% postconsumer recycled fiber.

Library of Congress Cataloging-in-Publication Data
Names: Morstein, Mona, 1961- author.
Title: Master your diabetes : a comprehensive, integrative approach for both type 1 and type 2 diabetes / Dr. Mona Morstein, ND, DHANP.
Description: White River Junction, Vermont : Chelsea Green Publishing, [2017] | Includes bibliographical references and index.
Identifiers: LCCN 2017017295 | ISBN 9781603587372 (paperback) | ISBN 9781603587389 (ebook)
Subjects: LCSH: Diabetes—Alternative treatment. | Non-insulin-dependent Diabetes—Alternative treatment. | Diet therapy. | BISAC: HEALTH & FITNESS / Diseases / Diabetes. | HEALTH & FITNESS / Naturopathy. | HEALTH & FITNESS / Nutrition.
Classification: LCC RC660.4 .M68 2017 | DDC 616.4/62—dc23
LC record available at https://lccn.loc.gov/2017017295

Chelsea Green Publishing
85 North Main Street, Suite 120
White River Junction, VT 05001
(802) 295-6300
www.chelseagreen.com

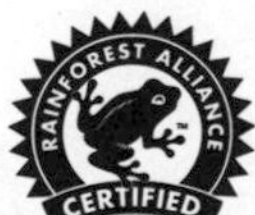

To everyone who has diabetes,
everyone who cares for someone with diabetes,
and every physician who has diabetic patients—
may we all come together to successfully
treat this condition, and even better,
eradicate it worldwide.

Contents

Acknowledgments

Writing this book has been a long process, with starts and stops over quite a few years. It's amazingly exciting that it is finally done.

I would like to thank all the ancestors of naturopathic medicine, over the last three hundred years, who helped form this beautiful and encompassing field of medicine, designed to create open-minded physicians who stringently believe a patient can indeed heal and achieve maximized health.

As we all know, life proceeds in curious ways, and if we take each troublesome situation, remove our egos, and learn from it, the capacity for self-growth is exponential. The very first diabetic patient I saw as a physician made me realize my significant deficiencies in treating that condition, and was the motivation for me to engage in serious study from then on, leading me to become a diabetes expert. I lost touch with that patient long ago, and I hope he is doing well.

My studies took me to the clinic of Dr. Richard Bernstein, the author of *Dr. Bernstein's Diabetic Solution*, the initial key book on successfully treating diabetes. Dr. Bernstein is a Type 1 diabetic patient, diabetologist, and a brilliant originator. He brought both the low-carb diet and innovative insulin dosing to diabetic patients and physicians who, like me, immediately saw the truth in his directions. Dr. Bernstein allowed me to shadow him in his Marmaroneck, New York, clinic, and was always welcoming when I called with questions throughout the years. He allowed me to quote him to promote my "Insulin Intensive Seminar," and I consider myself a healthy branch off his foundational tree.

I am very thankful to Chelsea Green for accepting my book for publication. If you have read books, you have seen authors thank their editors on their acknowledgment pages. I am deeply compelled to do the exact same. My editor, Michael Metivier, has been admirably patient (and at times understandably frustrated) with me. I am endlessly grateful for him working with me, taking my manuscript, and making it so much incredibly better.

In one short, broad, and deeply heartfelt statement, I would like to thank my family, friends, colleagues, and patients for their support and encouragement over the years.

Last, I would like to offer thanks to Hashem. Viewing my life in twenty-twenty hindsight, I am sure G-d has clearly offered His invisible yet evident guidance throughout my life to get me to this point. I am thankful for the many lifelong kindnesses Hashem has bestowed upon me.

— INTRODUCTION —

Diabetes: Victim or Victor?

Diabetes is typically considered a progressive disease. Once diagnosed, patients tend to require more and more medicine to control glucose levels, and many eventually develop a diabetic complication. After many years of increasing disability, they suffer premature death, typically six to twelve years earlier than people without diabetes. A bleak outlook indeed, and it simply doesn't have to be that way! This book is designed to give you the information you need to become the *victor* in your relationship with diabetes, rather than a victim. It can empower you in the knowledge that you can fully control the condition, even reversing Type 2 diabetes, and prevent diabetes' harmful effects or even reverse damage that has already occurred. The goal is for you to continue living a full, active, enjoyable, and long life.

As a diabetic patient, you may have found yourself frustrated by standard health care. You may not have received good nutritional advice, or *any* nutritional advice. You may have experienced too-short office visits, your labs may continue to show poor glucose control, and it may be that the only treatment you have been offered is more and more medications to help bring your sugars down.

Most conventional doctors are good people who care about their patients, but their medical training has mostly emphasized using medications to palliate chronic conditions. These types of doctors may also be leery of integrative treatments, such as specialized diets, lifestyle analysis, and supplements, which they haven't been trained for and which are not always cleared by randomized controlled double-blind studies. I've been to many "conventional care" diabetic conferences over the years. At a typical conference,

> **KEY TREATMENT NOTE**
>
> If you are not seeing an integrative physician, and the following are true, then of course, stay with that physician: You are happy with your physician; you feel you have time in your visits to have all your questions answered; your care is comprehensive; your glucose control is excellent; and you have no complications. However, if any of the above-mentioned aspects of your diabetic care are not positive, you may wish to consider changing the kind of medical treatment you receive.

the majority of the lectures are on medications and how to use them with patients. It's rare to find any discussions on nutrition, and I have never heard a lecture on using food to effectively control diabetes. At the last diabetic conference I attended, the meals served to attendees consisted of pastries for breakfast, large cookies for morning snacks, pizza for lunch, and ice cream for afternoon snacks. It was as though the conference organizers were helping create the very diabetic patients they were running a conference to treat!

However, there are other physicians to consider when you have diabetes: physicians who have specialized training in nutritional biochemistry and methods that work *with* the body to help it heal. Naturopathic physicians are one type, but there are other medical professionals who have what are called "integrative" (also known as "functional") medical practices.

What is "integrative" medicine? Integrative medicine combines the best of conventional medicine with alternative philosophic ways of looking at the body and the processes of health and disease. As a general rule, physicians using integrative medicine are educated equally as well as or beyond standard primary care physicians. Integrative practitioners look at the whole body, mind, and spirit, together, when creating their treatment plans for patients; focus on the physician-patient relationship; and tend to spend more office time with patients. Integrative medicine makes use of many healing modalities aside from prescription drugs, such as nutrition; exercise counseling; sleep hygiene; stress management; environmental detoxification; healing the intestines and the gut's microbiome; using supplements such as vitamins, minerals, nutraceuticals, and botanical medicines; hydrotherapy; homeopathy; acupuncture; and other modalities. There are many different integrative healing modalities, and many can be useful for patients with diabetes.

The focus of the integrative physician is not to palliate diabetic symptoms with escalating amounts of medications; it is to use other means to control a diabetic patient's blood glucose so that they:

- Have the control of a nondiabetic person
- Need minimal (if any) medication
- Do not suffer problematic glucose highs and lows
- Heal from or do not develop diabetic complications
- Have energy and health to live their life completely and fully

This book is designed to educate people who have diabetes and physicians who treat the condition. Its intent is to promote mutually respectful teamwork, so patients will feel heard and physicians can coordinate a comprehensive protocol that patients value and integrate into their life, thus experiencing positive results.

I am a naturopathic physician, and I have been educating my patients on this type of successful, comprehensive diabetic program for over twenty-five years. Naturopathic medicine is a composite of time-honored medical approaches that have benefited people for thousands of years. Ancient Greek physician Hippocrates said around 400 BCE, "Let food be your medicine and

Disclaimer

In this book, I will be mentioning specific labs or products from companies that I use to help patients get better. I am not in any way, financially or otherwise, associated with these companies, except my own diabetes specialty supplement, "Diamend." I mention the products because they work. In the event that I do have a relationship, I will disclose it.

your medicine be food." While regular medicine has evolved to promote pharmaceuticals and surgery as the main therapeutics, naturopathic medicine has evolved to choose an overlapping series of therapeutic options.

Formally, naturopathic medicine came into existence at the end of the 1800s, when John Lust coined the term for a field of medicine that included the concepts of diet, botanical medicine, physical medicine, and hydrotherapy (water therapy). Although the popularity of naturopathic medicine waned during the 1900s due to lack of funding and the discovery of antibiotics, today naturopathic medicine is a thriving and well-established profession with increasing public demand.

Naturopathic physicians (ND or NMD) are licensed physicians who specialize in integrative medicine without forgoing the skills and knowledge of diagnosis and treatment using standard, conventional tests and medicines. As a naturopathic physician, I conduct all of the normal physical exams and blood tests and also send patients for further testing such as x-rays, ultrasounds, and MRIs. I refer patients to specialists when necessary.

Naturopathic physicians also use alternative testing, such as food allergy tests, comprehensive stool analyses, liver detoxification tests, and others, to help uncover all obstacles that impair a patient's health and ability to heal. The ND's goals of treatment include:

- Safe, responsible care for each patient
- Helping patients avoid the need for prescription drugs or facilitating lower doses
- Helping patients avoid noncrisis surgery
- Reducing or stopping the use of antibiotics in acute conditions where they may have limited effectiveness and may promote antibiotic resistance, by using powerful natural agents to treat acute conditions
- Helping patients recover from and manage chronic conditions
- Teaching patients how to maintain their health once it has been restored

Further, there are six principles that guide NDs, giving us the foundational precepts for how we see, analyze, and treat our patients.

Finding a Naturopathic Physician

You can easily find a local naturopathic physician by entering your state (or province, for Canadians) and the words *naturopathic physician* into your internet browser's search engine. This will provide links to your state/province association, which will have its own, more focused search capacity. Or, you can go to www.naturopathic.org, the website of the American Association of Naturopathic Physicians, which enables you to conduct a search in all states. Please be aware that not all states license naturopathic physicians, so you want to ensure you go to a real ND, one who went to a four-year federal government–accredited naturopathic medical school, one who graduated, passed national boards, and has a state license.

Naturopathic medical schools are four-year postgraduate accredited medical institutions that combine the science of conventional medicine with the philosophy, science, wisdom, and effectiveness of integrative medicine. As of this writing, there are eight four-year post-graduate naturopathic medical schools in North America: Southwest College of Naturopathic Medicine (Tempe, Arizona), National University of Naturopathic Medicine (Portland, Oregon), Bastyr University (Seattle, Washington; and San Diego, California), University of Bridgeport (Bridgeport, Connecticut), National University of Health Sciences (Chicago, Illinois), Canadian College of Naturopathic Medicine (Toronto, Ontario), and Boucher Institute (Vancouver, British Columbia).

Due to the amount of information readily available on the internet, many patients feel they can treat themselves, but in reality, it's always best to find a physician who is an expert in your condition, to have someone to help guide you, examine you, prescribe for you, support you, and enable you to be in better control, feel much more energy, lose weight, need less medication, and heal and protect your body.

1. THE HEALING POWER OF NATURE

Naturopathic medicine observes that the body and mind have inherent wisdom as well as the capacity to heal. For example, when we cut our finger with a kitchen knife, we know that in about a week the finger will have healed perfectly, without us having to do anything aside from keeping the wound closed and protected. In more severe cases, a stitch might be needed to keep the wound closed, but the wound still repairs itself. Amazingly, this healing capacity is not limited to minor wounds. We know the body will naturally heal torn skin, broken bones, and pulled muscles. Powerful marketing by conventional medicine and drug companies through commercials and other advertisements has promoted societal fear, however, so many individuals may not be aware that their bodies can heal from many other, more serious illnesses. The truth is, people can heal from both acute and chronic conditions without the use of medications, conditions including strep throat, asthma, diverticulitis, migraines, ulcerative colitis, arthritis, and many others. Naturopathic physicians tap into this powerful healing ability through their care and use it to the patient's benefit.

2. REMOVE OBSTACLES TO CURE

Many factors prevent or inhibit the natural capacity to heal. Obstacles can exist on a physical level—for example, due to a nutrient deficiency or poor digestive functioning—or on mental, emotional, or spiritual levels. In any particular office visit, for example, depending on the needs of the patient, I might discuss diet, exercise, emotions related to relationship history, job fulfillment, life stresses, methods of stress reduction, exercise, and spiritual activity. By taking sufficient time to connect with patients in our office visits, and by doing appropriate testing, NDs often can uncover specific obstacles and work with the patient to remove them and move toward a cure.

3. FIRST, DO NO HARM

Ideally, NDs avoid using medicines that suppress or simply palliate symptoms, as these therapies can often, over time, worsen the patient's health, and they also may produce side effects. The therapies we use are designed to gently but effectively work *with* the body instead of covering up and suppressing symptoms. However, NDs, in states where they are licensed to, do indeed prescribe conventional medications when the patient requires them.

4. TREAT THE WHOLE PERSON

Treating the whole person naturally follows uncovering obstacles to cure. Once the blocks to health are uncovered, on any level, they will all be fully addressed in treatment. Only by understanding the entirety of the person, and not simply his or her disease, can true healing occur.

5. PREVENTION

In twenty-eight years of private practice I have had perhaps four or five patients come in healthy and simply request that I analyze their diet and supplement intake to help them prevent sickness and keep them healthy as they age. The rest of my patients have come to me only when they are ill or have a current condition. Prevention in that regard means helping a patient recover from his or her acute or chronic illness and then teaching the individual how to stay well and not have the condition return or how to keep the condition under excellent, and often drug-free, control. With my diabetes patients, once we get their blood sugars and other diabetes indicators under control, then prevention of the complications typically associated with diabetes is our focus. Prevention also means teaching parents how to eat better so their children are healthier, too. (If only integrative practitioners could enter schools and assist in setting up programs that comprehensively teach students how to be healthy before they become ill!)

6. DOCTOR AS EDUCATOR

This is the key to naturopathic medicine. Naturopathic physicians spend a lot of time with their patients, allowing the doctor to educate patients about their condition, what scientifically has been shown to cause or worsen the condition, and what scientifically has been demonstrated to improve or cure the condition. I have loads of handouts about how to implement suggested diets and instructions on the modalities I suggest. When we connect to patients at the heart and mind level, mixing compassion, nonjudgment, and support with the clinical skill to treat the condition, the patient learns their obstacles to cure, how they have been weakening or damaging their constitution and preventing healing, and how to remove the obstacles and stimulate their ability to heal. An educated patient is almost always an inspired, motivated, successful, and healthy patient!

I frequently use the term *comprehensive integrative medicine* in this book to describe medical professionals who view (and treat) patients in a different way, along the lines of the key concepts of naturopathic medicine. I focus specifically on naturopathic medicine, as that is my profession. However, different fields of medicine are producing medical professionals who think outside the box and work with patients in ways that allow a deeper

The Eight Essentials®

I am both the founder and the executive director of the Low Carb Diabetes Association (LCDA), a 501(c)3 tax-exempt education non-profit. Our mission statement defines us as committed to educating patients and their caregivers, medical practitioners, businesses, and the worldwide community about using comprehensive integrative medicine to prevent and successfully treat all types of diabetes, enabling patients to live long, healthy lives without diabetic complications and premature death.

We focus on teaching what we call "The Eight Essentials" of a comprehensive integrative protocol for prediabetes and diabetes:

1. Diet
2. Exercise
3. Sleep
4. Stress Management
5. Healing the Gut and Microbiome
6. Environmental Detoxification
7. Supplementation
8. Medications

These eight categories of treatment will help empower people to overcome the worldwide diabetes crisis and become victors over, understanding of the patient, giving them time to create broader and more far-reaching treatment protocols. It's exciting to note that there are now integrative doctors of medicine (MDs), of osteopathic medicine (DOs), and of chiropractic (DCs) and integrative nurse practitioners, physician assistants, nutritionists, and so forth. Many of these medical practitioners may also have a good foundational basis for integrative treatment of diabetes.

One of the problems with conventional care for diabetes that integrative practitioners seek to correct is how clinics are set up. In standard medical

not victims of, diabetes. There is no other nonprofit designed to educate diabetic patients, caregivers, and medical practitioners treating diabetic patients with leading-edge integrative information. Patients want to have the capacity to control, and maybe at times, in Type 2 diabetic patients, even reverse their diabetes. In Type 1 patients, superb control is the attainable goal. This nonprofit hopes to be the guiding light for this concept. The LCDA is the organization to turn to for newsletters, blogs, forums, interviews, webinars, podcasts, and conferences, all about the comprehensive integrative analysis and treatment of all types of diabetes. It is designed to be accessible and understandable for both lay people and medical practitioners.

Throughout this book, I will note in the treatment chapters which of The Eight Essentials is being addressed. All are covered extensively in this book. As the LCDA website develops, you will be able to find medical practitioners who are certified by the LCDA as integrative experts on treating diabetes.

The LCDA is the diabetes organization for the future. Preventing diabetes and treating it via effective comprehensive integrative care is what patients and family members want, and what the world needs. I hope you will join the LCDA and work with us to change the diabetic present and future. Basic membership is free! Please begin learning about diabetes from an integrative perspective at www.lowcarbdiabetes.org.

diabetic clinics, there's often a "team" approach: the physician sees the patient for the typical short visit, and then prescribes, changes, increases, or adds to his or her medicines, but usually doesn't know or ask about diet. Meanwhile, a registered dietician may give the patient some dietary advice based on the problematic American Diabetes Association guidelines, but cannot change the medications. There is usually not enough time for the conventional doctor to discuss specifics on exercise, sleep, or stress management, if they even inquire about those. As a result of this compartmentalized medical care, patients cannot easily succeed in controlling their glucose numbers, cannot escape feeling a victim to their diabetes, and cannot become victors.

In integrative medicine the entire patient is focused on, enhancing the doctor-patient relationship. Longer office visits mean more time is spent with the patient, where they are fully analyzed for all etiological factors affecting their health condition. Any medical practitioner from any field who practices integrative medicine and is a diabetic expert is, I feel, your best bet for getting your diabetes under excellent control.

When a patient sees an integrative physician, the first office visit tends to be quite long. My initial office visit lasts ninety minutes. In that time there's a thorough intake and physical exam. I make decisions about what lab work to perform and any necessary medical referrals. Patients are required to record their diet and blood sugars for a week as their homework. At the second office visit, generally a week later, I see the patient for another sixty to ninety minutes solely to institute the extensive treatment protocol, answer all questions, and explain each aspect of care. Subsequent follow-up visits last thirty to sixty minutes and are dedicated to problem solving and giving positive support.

For patients who fly in to see me, everything is organized beforehand—labs, diet diary, glucose graph—so the first and second visits are done together, maximizing the time and getting the treatment initiated right away.

KEY TREATMENT NOTE

Please do not change your diet, take any new supplements, engage in any lifestyle changes, or change your medication dosage without seeking the guidance and approval of your medical practitioner.

Doesn't it sound great to have an integrative medical practitioner treating you? The only potential drawback is that while naturopathic medicine is covered by insurance in some states, there are many states where it is not. Most insurance plans will cover standard labs done by a naturopathic physician, which can help with costs. Even though many costs are out of pocket for patients, many HSAs, Flex Plans, and some insurances do cover this type of care, so it's a good idea to check with your health insurance provider. Nevertheless, the care is excellent, your diabetes will wind up in the best control possible, and you will save a great deal of money in the long term by returning to and maintaining your health.

I hope you now have a better understanding of the foundational principles of naturopathic medicine and know more about how the entirety of integrative practitioners, no matter their medical field, work with patients. I encourage you to stay with your current physician if you are fully satisfied with him or her, but if not, I urge you to seek out a new type of practicing medicine through integrative care.

Now it's time to start learning about diabetes!

— CHAPTER ONE —

Different Types of Diabetes

Diabetes mellitus (DM), commonly referred to as diabetes, is now a worldwide epidemic, one our economy has spent billions of dollars to poorly treat, causing endless suffering to millions of patients. There are currently 29 million diabetic patients in the United States (9 percent of the population), while an estimated 87 million Americans have prediabetes, which means nearly one out of every three people in the United States is either a prediabetic or diabetic patient, including one out of every four seniors over the age of sixty-five. Type 2 diabetes (T2DM), which used to be found only in adults, is now, sadly, increasingly common in children and adolescents between the ages of ten and nineteen, and in higher percentages in African American, Mexican American, Native American, and Asian American communities. The CDC estimates that by 2050, half of all Americans will be diabetic patients. Worldwide, an astounding 350 million people have been diagnosed with diabetes, nearly 10 percent of all adults. By 2035, estimates are that nearly 600 million people will be a diabetic patient, and nearly 500 million people will be prediabetic; that's nearly 1 billion people. However, diabetes in and of itself causes no problems if it is well controlled. It is only uncontrolled diabetes that damages the body and leads to so many problems. Fully controlling diabetes is the goal of this book.

Before we define the different types of diabetes, it is important that we learn about the pancreas, the key organ most associated with diabetes. (Although the liver and fat cells are intricately involved as well, these will be discussed in later chapters.) The pancreas is a long, narrow organ that lies behind the stomach in the left upper quadrant of our abdomen. The pancreas has both an exocrine and endocrine system. The exocrine system produces digestive enzymes and releases them down the pancreatic duct into the duodenum, the first section of the small intestine, where the stomach dumps food after processing it. This is an essential part of digesting our food and making it available for absorption through our intestinal tracts. These cells of the pancreas are not the part affected by diabetes (except in some patients whose disease has been very poorly controlled for many years; then these cells may become damaged and insufficiently produce enzymes). The pancreas's endocrine system makes and releases hormones into the bloodstream that affect cells throughout the body. Our discussion of diabetes focuses on those cells.

The Pancreas and Its Hormones

There are four pancreatic endocrine cell types, known as *islet* cells: beta, alpha, delta, and gamma. Beta cells produce two hormones, insulin and amylin; alpha cells secrete glucagon; delta cells secrete somatostatin; and gamma cells produce an unknown protein.

Beta Cells: Insulin

The function of insulin in our bodies is to direct our cells to take in and use glucose. Glucose is formed in our bodies mostly from the carbohydrates we eat, with a small amount formed from ingested proteins. Insulin is sometimes called the "fat-building hormone." It has several actions in the body, all designed to help the body store energy and to prevent cells from metabolically burning, meaning both blood sugar and blood fats are drawn into body cells when insulin is secreted. Insulin stimulates cholesterol production, and elevates serum triglycerides, also known as fatty acids.

ACTIONS OF INSULIN

- Stimulates muscle fibers to take up glucose and store it as glycogen (a type of starch)
- Stimulates muscle fibers to take up amino acids and store them as proteins

- Stimulates liver cells to take up glucose and store it as glycogen
- Inhibits the liver from breaking down glycogen stores
- Inhibits the liver from undergoing gluconeogenesis—that is, prevents the liver from converting amino acids and glycerol into glucose
- Stimulates the liver to produce cholesterol and fatty acids
- Stimulates fat cells to take up glucose and store it as fat
- Acts on the hypothalamus to reduce appetite

Beta Cells: Amylin

Amylin is the other hormone found in our pancreatic beta cells. When we eat, insulin is released to lower blood sugars, followed by the secretion of glucagon by alpha cells to raise them. Next, amylin comes out to moderate glucagon's response to help keep blood sugar levels from rising too much. Glucose regulation is a complicated, complex body process! When beta cell damage occurs, amylin levels decrease just like insulin levels do, leaving glucagon unopposed. Amylin also helps slow digestion, which keeps blood sugar levels lower, and it's one of the helpful hormones, like insulin and somatostatin, that helps control our appetites so we do not overeat. We lose lots of benefits when the beta cells are damaged!

ACTIONS OF AMYLIN

- Inhibits the secretion of glucagon
- Slows the emptying of the stomach
- Initiates a signal of satiety that is sent to the brain

Alpha Cells: Glucagon

As noted, our body's balancing of blood sugar is extremely intricate and interactive. Once we eat something, and our blood sugars begin to rise, we release insulin to lower them. Insulin is an extremely strong hormone, and even though it has a short life span in our blood, it can cause significant lowering of our glucose if unchecked. To prevent hypoglycemia, the body, upon sensing the stomach being stretched when food enters it, releases glucagon, which is designed to elevate the blood sugar.

Since glucagon comes from alpha cells, these hormones are not injured with diabetes. Thus, even when the diabetic patient cannot make insulin and amylin, due to beta cell damage, the pancreas can still make glucagon, and it does so after the person eats. Excess glucagon secretion after eating can be a glucose problem especially for T2DM patients, and it can have a significant impact on after-meal glucose elevations.

Glucagon is such a magnificent elevator of blood sugar that when a person with diabetes is having a serious hypoglycemic event, and honey or other sugars are not raising their blood sugar levels sufficiently, we can inject glucagon directly into the person. This injection causes the liver to immediately release blood sugar through the breakdown of glycogen stores and can help save a person's life.

ACTIONS OF GLUCAGON

- Stimulates the liver to break down glycogen into glucose and release it into the blood
- Stimulates the liver to break down amino acids and glycerol into glucose and release it into the blood
- Stimulates the muscles to convert stored starches and proteins into blood sugar
- Stimulates the kidneys to break down proteins into blood sugar
- Reduces cholesterol production

Delta Cells: Somatostatin

Also secreted by the pancreas, the hormone somatostatin has several actions, but essentially these are related to reducing the rate at which food is absorbed by the gut, which naturally slows the rise of blood sugar.

ACTIONS OF SOMATOSTATIN

- Inhibits stomach secretion of gastrin, which aids the stomach in producing its own digestive juices
- Inhibits the duodenum release of secretin, a hormone, and cholecystokinin (CCK), a gastrointestinal hormone. Secretin directs the pancreas to put bicarbonate into the gut to lower the acidity of food the

stomach just dumped into it. CCK promotes digestion by stimulating the gallbladder and pancreas, and sends satiety signals to the brain.

- Inhibits the pancreatic release of glucagon

Gamma Cells: Gamma Polypeptide

Basically, this protein seems to reduce appetite.

Understanding the organs and hormones related to diabetes is important. All of the interactions listed above are vital to keeping a person's blood sugar in the healthy range of 70–120 mg/dL consistently throughout their entire life, twenty-four hours a day, seven days a week.

Now that we know a little about the pancreas, we can discuss the different types of diabetes, and how they develop in the body.

Type I Diabetes

Only about 5–10 percent of patients with diabetes have Type 1 diabetes (T1DM), which is an autoimmune disease whereby a person's own immune system attacks their pancreatic beta cells, destroying enough of them that they cannot produce enough insulin to live. Patients with Type 2 diabetes (T2DM), which is discussed in chapter 2, can produce insulin (at least at first), but their body cells do not respond normally to the hormone and do not absorb glucose as they should. Type 1 used to be called insulin dependent diabetes mellitus (IDDM), but that term is no longer used. The correct term is T1DM, as some people with T2DM will also become insulin dependent. T1DM tends to come on suddenly and has a small genetic association, meaning a person is at low but noticeable risk of developing it if either or both of their parents have it. If one parent has T1DM, a child has a 10 percent risk of getting it. If both parents have T1DM, a child has a 40 percent risk of getting diabetes. Most people develop T1DM out of the blue, with no previous family history.

By the time a person presents with the disease, 85 percent of the beta cells have already been lost. Although we used to think that the pancreatic cells were irrevocably dead, we now know this is not true. And, we can work with T1DM patients to keep their sugars in perfect control, preventing the progression of the disease and the complications that develop as a result.

Risk Factors for Developing Type I Diabetes

In 2004, the National Institutes of Health (NIH) established the TEDDY trial, an ongoing trial with the goal of identifying which of multiple risk factors are truly key etiological factors for initiating the development of T1DM in children. The NIH is studying the following possible factors: health of the mother during pregnancy, early infections of the child, differences in food introduction timing, vitamin deficiencies, immunizations and timing of them, lack of early infections, drinking water purity, exposure to pets and other allergens, excessive weight gain, and emotional stress.

Genetic Trait for Diabetes, Tested through Blood Work

T1DM is associated with certain genes. These genes can be passed down in the family, but in T1DM this happens with less frequency than we see in T2DM. Approximately 90 percent of people with T1DM have one or both of the genes labeled HLA-DQA1, HLA-DQB1, and HLA-DRB1 (also known as HLA-DR3/4). These genes are only found in 20 percent of the typical population. Genetic HLA variations occur; some increase the risk of developing T1DM up to 40 percent and some are actually protective against the disease. Genetically, Caucasian/White people have the highest rate of T1DM, and we have seen family groupings of T1DM throughout generations and between siblings and cousins.

Here are some specifics:

- If an immediate family member (parent, sibling, child) has T1DM, one's risk of developing T1DM is ten to twenty times higher than the general population. In fact, this risk can be even higher depending on which family member has T1DM and at what age they developed it.
- If one child has T1DM, all brothers and sisters have around a one in ten chance of developing it by age fifty.
- If the mother has T1DM, the risk of a child developing T1DM is lower than if the father has T1DM. If the father has T1DM, the chance

of a child developing it is one in ten. If the mother has T1DM, and delivered the child when she was younger than twenty-five years old, the chance is one in twenty-five. If the mother was over twenty-five years old when she delivered the child, the chance drops to one in one hundred, which is the same as the average American's risk.

- If one parent developed T1DM before they were eleven years old, there is a higher risk for one of their children to develop T1DM than if the parent was older than age eleven at T1DM onset.

If a child develops T1DM, it is helpful to test their siblings for T1DM genes and antibodies that occur against the beta cells. If the results are positive, but the sibling does not yet clinically show diabetes, there might be ways to help prevent the direct onset of T1DM. I will discuss them below in the prevention section.

Dietary Factors

There are many studies investigating whether the early introduction of gluten or dairy into an infant's diet might cause the child to develop illness or autoimmune problems, and nothing is absolute. Children who were never introduced to gluten have still developed T1DM, and many children who eat gluten every day will not develop T1DM.

Certainly, the introduction of actual dairy or gluten food (or any food) before the infant is four months old is associated the development of poor health later in life. Babies should not be fed any food other than breast milk or formula for at least the first four months of their lives. Most integrative medical practitioners prefer mothers to breastfeed exclusively for the first six months of the newborn's life.

Ideally, mothers should use their own breast milk to nourish their babies. When introducing foods that can produce allergic reactions, caregivers should do so gradually, such as a few tablespoons of those foods a week. Multiple studies show this approach reduces the body's reaction to those proteins and reduces the onset of skin rashes, asthma, and other conditions oftentimes associated with those foods.

Gluten is associated with celiac disease, T1DM, thyroid disease (Hashimoto's and/or Grave's), and many other health conditions. Approximately 8–16 percent of T1DM patients have celiac disease. If a child is found to have celiac disease and gluten is fully removed from the diet, that child's risk of subsequently developing T1DM reduces to pretty much zero. I believe this is such a powerful tool of prevention that performing a celiac screening by the time a child is one to two years old should be part of every pediatrician's protocol.

There are many studies related to dairy and T1DM. Avoidance of cow's milk may be helpful particularly if the milk supply is from A1 as opposed to A2 milk-producing cows. A1 milk contains a histamine molecule in the milk peptides, which produces a higher allergic effect than A2 milk, which contains a proline molecule, instead. Studies show an increase in T1DM in countries that drink primarily A1 milk. Most milk consumed in the United States comes from A1 cows, and it is very difficult, if not impossible, to find A2 milk in this country. For children who are antibody positive for T1DM, consumption of cow's milk has increased the risk of developing T1DM. In a Finnish study, children were weaned to either a 100 percent hydrolyzed milk formula, or a mix of cow's milk and 20 percent hydrolyzed milk formula. Over a decade, both groups saw children develop T1DM, but there were more with T1DM in the milk/hydrolyzed group than in the fully hydrolyzed group.

Unfortunately, using soy milk as an alternative to dairy carries with it its own controversies. One study in China, for example, showed that babies drinking soy milk had a higher rate of T1DM development than babies not drinking soy milk. However, it should be noted that although the results of dietary studies often make intuitive sense, they are not universally conclusive; no particular food affects every child in the same way, especially in terms of developing T1DM.

More and more research points to the need for mothers to feed their babies breast milk for overall infant health, and there is a weak association between breastfeeding and a reduction in T1DM onset in the child. If for some reason breastfeeding isn't possible, then using a specialized elemental formula such as Nutrimagen or Alimentum may be the next best option, as this seems to reduce T1DM onset when compared with cow or soy milk formula. If you're a mother or mother to be, please make a point of calling your local La Leche League, an organization designed to help women breastfeed their babies. This is important especially for mothers who are having trouble making milk or who desire to (or have to) go back to work sooner than six months. There are also breast milk "banks" from which mothers can buy breast milk if they are unable to breastfeed. The Human Milk Banking Association of North America is a good place to start.

Viral Infection

There is a lot of research currently being conducted on whether viruses may provoke the immune system to attack beta cells. Some upper viral illnesses, for example, are associated with promoting T1DM onset; apparently, when they stimulate the immune system to fight the infection, the immune system then gets confused and begins attacking the beta cells as well. I would say 20–30 percent of my T1DM patients remember having some sort of viral illness in the immediate weeks or months before their T1DM diagnosis. But many other factors have to be in place for a typical illness to initiate T1DM, such as those discussed in this section. See the section on gut dysbiosis later in this chapter for a discussion of enteroviruses.

Xenobiotics (Environmental Toxins)

Xenobiotics are foreign chemicals that are not naturally produced by or expected to be found in humans. Another term commonly used is *POPs*—persistent organic pollutants. Both are technical terms for chemicals commonly used in the environment, such as herbicides and pesticides.

Over eighty thousand chemicals are now used in the United States for myriad purposes, and between one thousand and two thousand new chemicals are introduced every year. Shockingly, the US government does not require chemical companies to prove these chemicals are sufficiently safe even on their own, let alone when combined with other substances in the environment. In a sampling by the Centers for Disease Control and Prevention (CDC), almost 100 percent of pregnant women had measurable levels of many toxic chemicals in their bodies: PCBs, organochlorine pesticides, PFCs, phenols, PDBEs, phthalates, polycyclic aromatic hydrocarbons, and perchlorate. Xenobiotics may be one reason why T1DM diabetes is increasing all over the world, as the use of environmental chemicals is increasing.

Leading-edge research is trying to determine if toxins in the environment can promote the autoimmunity of T1DMs. Ironically, scientists know chemicals can cause T1DM because they use specific chemicals on lab rats that end up acquiring T1DM. Scientists know many chemicals can destroy beta cells and may also increase the development of autoimmunity against beta cells. Toxins such as n-nitroso compounds, air pollution, and POPs are associated specifically as being risk factors for T1DM development. See the website www.diabetesandenvironment.org for more research on the links between environmental toxins and diabetes.

While it's too early to have definitive proof, there is enough evidence that confirms we should avoid using and consuming many industrial chemicals in our homes by striving to eat "greener" food and making healthier lifestyle choices by using more natural cleaners, paints and finishes, flooring, toiletries, and more.

Vaccinations

On the one hand, a large meta-analysis study showed there was no association between immunizations and the development of T1DM. On the other hand, however, there is lingering concern that mass vaccinations in childhood may be associated with an increased risk for developing T1DM. Barthelow Classen, MD, has done extensive analyses on that subject and has shown that in New Zealand and Finland, mass vaccinations significantly increased the rate of T1DM onset in children. Some physicians in the integrative medical community believe that injecting live, weakened viruses as vaccinations does seem to have a suspicious connection to T1DM. The MMR (measles, mumps, and rubella) vaccine seems particularly concerning.

However, there are no definitive studies as yet that connect vaccinations with T1DM. And vaccines may be used in curative ways, as well. The US Food and Drug Administration (FDA) has approved a study injecting T1DM adults with a vaccine from bacillus Calmette-Guérin (BCG) to see if it leads to reversal of their diabetes.

I am not wholly an antivaccination advocate, although I do feel not all current recommended vaccines are necessary or even helpful. Whether to vaccinate at all, or to only choose some vaccines, on what type of schedule, is something parents must decide in discussion with their pediatrician and integrative physician. If vaccinations are given, supporting the immune system can be helpful before, during, and after the injections. Dosing a child with vitamin D_3, B vitamins, glycerin Echinacea or elderberry, vitamin C, and giving some *Silybum marianum* (milk thistle) to help support liver detoxification of vaccine ingredients may be helpful to reduce the risk of any vaccination reaction.

Drinking Water Quality

Although this topic is closely related to the xenobiotic concerns noted earlier, it's worth a quick note. In chemistry, pH is a measure of the acidity or alkalinity of a solution. A pH of 7.0 is neutral, less than 7.0 is considered acidic, and over 7.0 is considered alkaline. Our blood's normal pH is approximately 7.34, slightly alkaline. A compelling study showed that in households where tap water was acidic (pH 6.2–6.9), there was a fourfold higher risk of T1DM than in households where the water was more alkaline (pH ≥7.7).

Another study found that tap water low in zinc was associated with increased risk for T1DM. Zinc is needed to produce and secrete insulin from the pancreas and also to assist the pancreas in triggering the insulin receptors on the cell walls.

In general, healthy water means filtered water. Most tap water contains some level of pollutants, including chlorine. Spring water, carbon-filtered water, and reverse osmosis purified water are considered safe. For people using reverse osmosis, I suggest adding in extra minerals, as minerals are also extracted during the reverse osmosis process. I do not feel anyone should drink distilled water or "alkaline" water. I would also check the pH of one's drinking water and ensure it is not acidic.

Nutrient Deficiencies

Another risk factor in developing diabetes is nutrient deficiency, especially of vitamin D_3 and omega-3 oils, which help the body suppress the development of autoimmunity. The Finnish people, who historically have had the highest per capita occurrence of T1DM in the world, have conducted some interesting studies around this topic. One study showed that giving infants vitamin D_3 and omega-3 oils significantly reduced the onset of T1DM in those children as they aged. The levels of both vitamin D_3 and omega-3 oils can be tested via a serum blood draw. These nutrients are very safe; even newborns can be dosed 1,000–2,000 international units (IU) of vitamin D_3 a day. The American Academy of Pediatrics agrees that all newborns should receive at least 400 IU of vitamin D_3. And nursing mothers can take high doses of omega-3 oils so that those nutrients can be fed to their babies through their breast milk.

Psychosocial Factors—Stress in Child or Family

While "stress" is associated with causing or aggravating many conditions in life, it has not been scientifically proven to be an etiological factor in developing T1DM. In fact, the authors of one paper analyzed many studies and found that stress was not an important factor for the onset of T1DM. However, poorly handled stress can certainly be a notable detriment to diabetic control, and it is fairly common for a person with diabetes, particularly T1DM, to experience "burnout." I will be reviewing more about stress and burnout in chapter 9.

Gut Dysbiosis

The term *microbiome* refers to the vast collection of microorganisms that live in our intestinal tract and other parts of the body, and includes bacteria, viruses, archaea, fungi, and protozoa. Typically, a person's microbiome is established by the time they are two years old, and it can have between five hundred and one thousand species, although thirty to forty of these comprise the vast majority. The gut is the largest housing of our microbiome; there are 1.3 times as many microorganisms in your small and large intestines as there are other cells in the rest of your body! Sixty percent of the dry mass of your stool is composed of cells from your microbiome.

It is becoming well known that one's microbiome can determine health or sickness. A healthy microbiome helps us absorb nutrients, creates some nutrients, reduces the formation and absorption of toxins into our bodies, prevents pathogens from colonizing, produces antimicrobial agents and food for our colon cells, supports our immune system, and reduces autoimmunity reactions.

However, if one's gut develops *dysbiosis*—the term used when the microbiome is out of balance—this can lead to autoimmune reactions elsewhere, including in the pancreas. Part of the process may have to do with what is known as *leaky gut*, increased intestinal permeability in the gut lining that causes inflammation and overstimulation and concurrent loss of regulation of the intestinal and systemic immune system. Leaky gut refers to passageways between small intestine cells called "tight junctions." Certain proteins—zonulin, occluding, and claudins—regulate how wide or narrow the tight junctions are. Elevated zonulin can be a sign of intestinal permeability.

Early studies indicate that children with T1DM have different gut microbiomes than children who do not have diabetes. Children with T1DM may have less diverse and less stable microbiota. This may lead to increased gut permeability, small intestine inflammation, and immune dysregulation.

Some fascinating recent studies have shown that the manifestation of T1DM is preceded by a "prediabetic" period that may last several years. That is, the person has positive circulation of autoantibodies against beta cells. Increased intestinal permeability is associated with T1DM prediabetes. Elevated zonulin has been found in T1DM patients matched against nondiabetic people of the same age. Zonulin was also detected in 70 percent of T1DM prediabetic patients, preceding the onset of clinical T1DM diabetes by around three and a half years.

Many enteroviruses—viruses in the small intestine—are associated with T1DM, such as coxsackie B virus. Coxsackie B virus has been found in beta cells in newly diagnosed T1DM patients, in children who develop T1DM but not in their nondiabetic siblings, and also in mothers of children who developed T1DM. Other culprits may include rotavirus, mumps virus, or cytomegalovirus. These may activate the immune system and cause it to mistakenly attack beta cells.

Unfortunately, we cannot measure small gut bacteria except in a condition called small intestine bacterial overgrowth (SIBO), but T1DM with neuropathy is associated with being a risk factor for causing SIBO, not the other way around. We can analyze colonic bacteria, fungi, and parasites, however, as well as colonic inflammation, pancreatic digestive capacity, and short-chain fatty acid production (the food for the colon cells and beneficial bacteria). But what is happening in the colon has little or nothing to do with the small intestinal microbiome and intestinal permeability.

I have performed comprehensive stool analyses on individuals with T1DM. Sometimes the colonic flora is indeed imbalanced, although this colonic flora is not reflective of the small intestine. Treating imbalances, even if a pathogenic bacteria was involved, has not "cured" the T1DM or even done much to help with glucose control. Therefore, checking stool cultures on all children with T1DM doesn't seem necessary *unless* significant digestion problems are also occurring. Checking for zonulin would be more helpful.

Conclusion

While there are many potential causes of T1DM under investigation, and some compelling possibilities yet to explore, we currently don't know why any particular child develops T1DM. For parents, this means that when their child is diagnosed with T1DM, they should never feel guilt or remorse for what they may or may not have done.

Presentation of Type I Diabetes

The child presenting with T1DM cannot produce insulin; thus, glucose is not admitted into their body cells and is instead urinated out. Symptoms appear suddenly, usually coming on strong within a few days or weeks, and include:

Weight loss. The body type of the child who generally develops T1DM is lean. Their body loses weight because it is burning fat, since it cannot burn glucose.

Constant hunger. Because the person is not processing glucose into energy, and is instead excreting it into the urine, hunger is constant.

Frequent urination. Blood sugar that is not burned is excreted by the body in the urine.

Frequent thirst and drinking. Because the person must urinate so often to get rid of blood sugar, they are constantly thirsty and drink frequently.

Sweet-smelling breath. When the body burns fat, it forms ketone bodies, which emit a sweet, fruity smell through the breath.

Poor wound healing. High blood sugar slows the capacity of the body to heal wounds.

Fungal infections. Fungi live on our skin and in our mouth, genitals, and intestines, but are normally kept well under control by our immune system. High blood sugars can cause these fungi to proliferate, and the child with T1DM may get thrush (overgrowth of fungi in the mouth) or fungal skin infections.

Of course, when these symptoms show up in a child, most parents see the doctor right away. The doctor then does blood work to substantiate the diagnosis of diabetes. The labs often show the following:

- Blood sugar is usually very high, well over 200 mg/dL. A child without diabetes never has blood sugar levels this high.
- The presence of islet cell antibodies (ICA), antibodies to the cells of the pancreas, indicates that an immune system attack on the pancreas is underway.
- Glutamic acid decarboxylase antibodies (GAD-65) are found in 75 percent of children with T1DM. These antibodies attack an enzyme in the beta cell and can persist for a long time.
- IA-2 (islet antigen 2) antibodies, or ICA-152, are found in 80 percent of children with T1DM, but do not persist long, and are rarely positive in people over the age of thirty. These antibodies attack a protein on the beta cell.
- Insulin autoantibodies (IAA) are found in 70 percent of children on onset of T1DM, and are generally higher in children than adults. These antibodies attack the insulin molecule.

Antibodies usually occur in autoimmune diabetes when the immune system is attacking the pancreas and causing destruction, typically to the extent that insulin can no longer be effectively made or secreted.

It is common for doctors to skip testing for antibodies with a newly diagnosed T1DM patient in the hospital. Testing for antibodies seems an unnecessary diagnostic test if a lean person walks into an emergency room with a blood sugar of 600 mg/dL after several days of feeling poor; at this point, the diagnosis of T1DM is immediately made without any further testing.

Usually around 90 percent of pediatric T1DM patients have at least one positive antibody. It is possible, but uncommon, for a T1DM patient to have all antibodies negative. The MODY type of genetic diabetes (see below) should be ruled out in these cases.

The following are diabetes-related antibodies:

Insulin autoantibodies (IAA). These antibodies attack insulin.

Beta cell antibodies. These antibodies attack different areas on the pancreatic beta cell:

Glutamic acid decarboxylase 65 (GAD-65). This antibody attacks an enzyme in the pancreatic beta cell. Although it can be high in pediatric T1DM, it is also the elevated antibody used to diagnose LADA in older patients (see below).

Zinc transporter 8 antibodies (ZnT8). This is an antibody discovered recently that has been studied to help identify adult-onset autoimmune diabetes, along with GAD-65.

Islet cell antibody. This antibody reacts against a protein in the beta cell.

Tyrosine phosphatase-like protein antibodies, AKA insulinoma-associated antibody (IA-2). This antibody attacks the tyrosine phosphatase protein.

The presence of antibodies can either help diagnose T1DM or predict who is at high risk; the more antibodies present, the higher the risk of developing T1DM if it has not already been diagnosed.

Upon diagnosis, serum tests for ketoacidosis will also be drawn. Although other lab results play a part, and are listed in the laboratory section, these tests are the ones that are specifically used when diagnosing T1DM.

Please be aware that when treating a child with new onset of T1DM, the intent should be the following:

- Avoid focusing on "curing" the child—it is extremely unlikely a child will be cured of their T1DM condition. I have heard of

Type 1B

Type 1B, or idiopathic Type 1, is an unusual type of T1DM that is antibody-negative, and typically seen in Caucasians. This type is not an autoimmune disease, but people with Type 1B do have an insulin deficiency. Their need for insulin may wax and wane over time, but most need to be treated as if they had the typical antibody-positive T1DM.

this happening, but only once or twice in twenty-five years of working with Type 1 pediatric patients. I find some parents do excessive integrative testing and experimentation on their child, trying anything they can to cure the disease, and as a result, the patient's childhood is lost. We need to ensure that when we look at a child, we see a beautiful being, whole and complete, innocent and full of potential to live a life replete with joy and success, rather than a poor, tragic child, a victim stuck with an awful and horrible disease.

- Initiate and extend the honeymoon period. For many newly diagnosed children with T1DM, the honeymoon period, where very little or even no insulin is required, can be extended for months and even years using integrative medicine. Around adolescence and puberty, when the output of hormones for sexual development drives insulin resistance even in T1DM patients, it is

KEY TREATMENT NOTE

Standard care generally allows individuals with T1DM to eat whatever they wish and cover their food with their insulin injections. This is never going to give good control and will create a constant problem of high and low glucose levels all day long. Integrative physicians do not agree that T1DM patients should eat whatever they wish and cover it with insulin. We feel a certain diet is required and as a result of the diet, less insulin use and better, more stable glucose numbers can be achieved.

One vital thing to remember is that better glucose numbers mean better energy, better mood, better focus and concentration, and a positive sense of esteem and confidence. They can also mean less depression, anxiety, and irritability. A huge percentage of teenagers with T1DM are significantly stressed out by managing their condition. When teens see that their glucose numbers, energy, and mood can be wonderfully improved and enhanced, this can help lower their stress and increase their self-esteem. Better glucose numbers are not just numbers on a lab report; good numbers affect the entirety of the person with diabetes and are a very attainable goal.

common for T1DM teens to require initiating or increasing doses of insulin.

- Reduce insulin through healthy lifestyle choices. The key goals for any type of diabetic patient, including those with T1DM, are to have excellent glucose levels and to require the least amount of insulin. Following The Eight Essentials can lead to these two vital goals being achieved in nearly all compliant patients.

Latent Autoimmune Diabetes of Adults (LADA: Type 1.5 Diabetes)

LADA is a recently recognized form of diabetes, whereby adults, generally over thirty-five years old, develop an autoimmune reaction that harms their pancreatic beta cells. Onset of LADA can occur with equal speed to that of pediatric T1DM, but in some cases it happens at a slower rate. So the presentation signs and symptoms can be exactly like T1DM in those for whom the condition comes on aggressively. However, patients with milder presentations may be misdiagnosed as T2DM even though they often are lean and exercise regularly, because the onset occurs in adults and because not all physicians are aware of LADA or know how to diagnose it. In fact, statistics suggest that up to 20 percent of patients diagnosed with T2DM actually have LADA instead. I have properly rediagnosed as LADA dozens of misdiagnosed T2DM patients in my career.

LADA patients may respond to a wide spectrum of treatments after diagnosis. Some LADA patients need insulin right away and some do not, or at least not a full dosing of it.

The drug treatments for LADA and T2DM are different; inappropriate T2DM medications prescribed to a LADA patient can cause increased

KEY TREATMENT NOTE

If you are a lean adult patient diagnosed with T2DM, you should urge your physician to measure your GAD-65 antibody, to see if you actually have LADA. A positive GAD-65 antibody is an indication of LADA.

damage to the LADA patient's pancreas and may make them insulin dependent more quickly.

The simplest way to discern T2DM from LADA is to test the GAD-65 autoantibody. If it is positive, a LADA diagnosis can be made.

Gestational Diabetes

This type of diabetes occurs in women who were not previously diabetic but who become pregnant, gain too much weight, and develop insulin resistance and elevated glucose levels. Gestational diabetes will be comprehensively discussed in chapter 11.

Mature Onset Diabetes of the Young (MODY) and Neonatal Diabetes

Mature onset diabetes of the young (MODY) is a category of diabetes that results from one of six genetic defects in making insulin, secreting insulin from the pancreas, or responding to insulin on cell receptors. Some MODY individuals will need to be on insulin and some will do fine with an oral medication. MODY is a rare form of diabetes, but statistics say that up to 5 percent of diabetes patients may have MODY.

Although MODY is not associated with any particular body type, there are some clues to help discern if MODY should be in the differential diagnosis of what is assumed to be T1DM or T2DM:

- The patient has an extensive family history of diabetes—for instance, the patient's great-grandfather had it, as well as their grandfather and father.
- The lean pediatric patient is negative for all Type 1 antibodies.
- Three years after diagnosis, the patient is still producing normal levels of insulin.
- The patient has no signs or symptoms of insulin resistance, such as being overweight, hypertension, or elevated lipid panels.
- Oftentimes, the patient's glucose levels are never excessively high.

- The diabetes is usually discovered in adolescence or early adulthood (but may not be diagnosed until adulthood).
- The patient has mild symptoms of diabetes and it is usually diagnosed during routine blood tests.

Neonatal diabetes is even more rare than MODY. This usually occurs in newborns and young infants, and diagnosis is usually made in the first six months of life.

— CHAPTER TWO —

Type 2 Diabetes

Type 2 diabetes (T2DM) is a complex condition, and as such it requires an entire chapter to discuss its causes and how to evaluate it. Historically, T2DM was seen only in adults, but tragically, it is now seen in children and teenagers as well, though it comes on gradually and is one of the most preventable diseases that exist in the world today.

T2DM is highly associated with a genetic tendency in families. Between 90 percent and 95 percent of patients with diabetes have Type 2.

Signs and symptoms of T2DM may include being abdominally overweight, slow-healing wounds, thrush and other fungal infections, a family history of T2DM, fatigue and low energy, and various blood work labs that are positive for diabetes.

T2DM is a disease of insulin resistance. There are many etiological reasons insulin resistance develops in people. T2DM patients do not become diabetic overnight. It is a long process with several progressive stages. The earlier we can catch the disease, the simpler the treatment. If we can help heal people in the prediabetes stage, before they actually become fully diabetic, that is best. But, unfortunately, many patients progress to T2DM.

Let's imagine a common scenario: You're young, you're active, but you eat badly—junk food, French fries, soda pop, and nothing for breakfast because you're too rushed. Your basic metabolism keeps you lean, however, and you don't care or notice how you feel. But then, at around age thirty, your metabolism begins to slow down a little and it is suddenly easier to gain weight. You don't have as much energy as you once did, and you have to struggle through the day. In addition, your cravings for sweets become a problem that won't go away and your mood may be unstable.

Such was the case for one of my patients, Anita. As Anita aged she kept gaining weight. She was addicted to caffeine and her coffee was nicely sweetened. Her diet included some vegetables and a little fruit, but she also ate a lot of potatoes, breads, muffins, and other carbohydrates. When Anita came to me at age thirty-eight, she was forty pounds overweight. She wanted to lose weight, get her energy back, and feel great again. With medical tests and a physical exam, I was able to diagnose her with insulin resistance: prediabetes. This can be a scary diagnosis for many patients, and it was for Anita. While assuring her she was not yet diabetic, and never *had* to become diabetic, I supported her motivation to get healthy and follow a new regimen.

Insulin Resistance

Insulin, as noted in the last chapter, is a hormone secreted by beta cells in our pancreas. We secrete insulin when the glucose and amino acid levels in our blood rise, which we break down from carbohydrates and proteins. Insulin

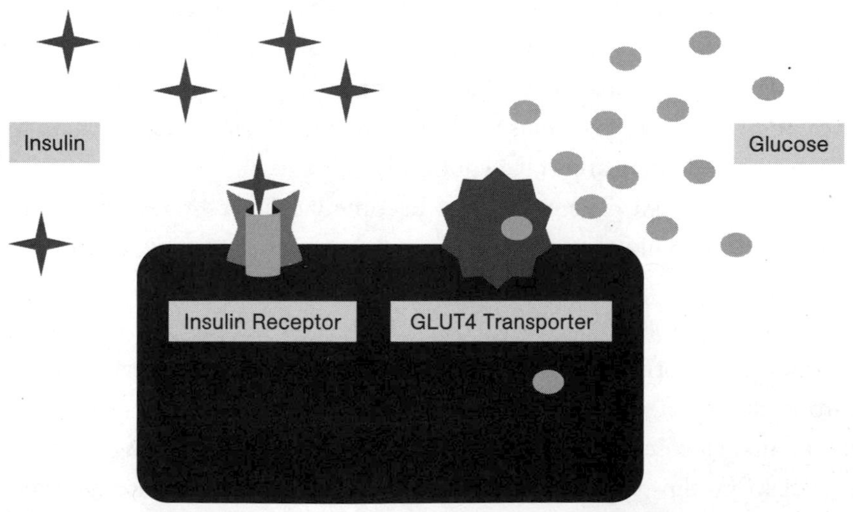

Figure 2.1. Insulin resistance.

travels to various cells, particularly our fat, liver, and muscle cells, and lands on a receptor. The receptor, which acts like a switch, signals a molecule called glucose transporter 4 (GLUT4) to move to the cell wall and take glucose from the bloodstream into the cell. The glucose is then transformed into fat or starch, and is stored. This is why insulin is known as the "fat-building hormone." When blood sugar drops, the pancreas stops insulin production and the body can break down the starch or fat to use for energy.

When people who have T2DM become overweight, and their abdominal fat cells are already packed full of fat, their fat cells can decide to prevent glucose from entering the cells, as they do not need to turn more glucose into more fat. As a result, their insulin receptors lose their responsiveness. When insulin lands on a receptor, the cell does not automatically absorb glucose from the blood. In conventional medicine, this is called "beta cell failure." In the early days and years following the diagnosis of T2DM, however, I do not find the pancreas "in failure" when patients are treated properly and comprehensively. During this early phase, patients will be able to avoid going on insulin and their insulin levels will be fine. It's typically only after many years of poor control that the pancreas of a person with T2DM can indeed "fail" and not make enough insulin, necessitating an insulin prescription. This failure is due to damage the high glucose levels have caused to the beta cells over the years.

Whether you're a T2DM patient with insulin resistance consisting of higher levels of insulin produced by your pancreas (early on) or are a T2DM patient given insulin injections to fight high glucose numbers, you have too much insulin floating around in your body.

Ironically, T1DM patients can also become insulin resistant. The average nondiabetic, non-insulin-resistant person makes around 30 to 40 units of insulin a day to process the entirety of his or her food. However, if a T1DM patient injects more than 40 units a day to correct his glucose numbers, he is essentially self-inducing a form of insulin resistance. This is usually from eating a high-carbohydrate diet. A T1DM patient can also become insulin resistant when her natural glucose numbers become elevated (higher than 170 mg/dL or so).

T2DM insulin resistance is associated with metabolic syndrome, which was first described as an array of medical signs that were grouped together by Dr. Gerald Reaven at Stanford University in the late 1970s. It is now a highly recognized T2DM concurrent condition.

There are several components to metabolic syndrome, according to the International Diabetes Federation, including central fat distribution (abdominal obesity, measured by waist circumference); raised triglyceride levels (greater than 150 mg/dL); lowered high density cholesterol (HDL, or "good cholesterol") levels (less than 40 mg/dL in males and less than 50 mg/dL in females); elevated blood pressure (greater than 130/84 mmHg); and raised fasting plasma glucose (greater than 100 mg/dL).

Obesity, insulin, and high blood sugar work in numerous biochemical ways to increase the blood pressure for some patients and also to release free fatty acids into the blood that raise triglyceride levels.

So, when a person comes to me with T2DM, it is typical for the person to also be overweight or obese, have high blood pressure, and have problems with their cholesterol and triglycerides. The majority of T2DM patients wind up on hypertension medications and often statin drugs for their cholesterol as well. All of these conditions can be completely reversed with comprehensive integrative care.

Factors Involved in Insulin Resistance

There are many reasons that a person may become insulin resistant, putting themselves at risk for developing T2DM.

The First Risk Factor: Genetics and Ethnicity

Unlike T1DM, which has a minor familial genetic connection, T2DM has an established genetic inheritance. A genetic risk factor essentially means that a person is more likely to develop a condition that his or her relatives had, especially if other factors are involved. Many medical conditions are genetically associated, including arthritis, autoimmune diseases, cardiovascular disease, cancers, and T2DM.

Identical twins have a 70 percent concordance of developing T2DM, meaning that if one develops T2DM, it's very likely the other twin will as well. If one parent has T2DM, there is a 40 percent risk of their offspring developing the disease, and if both parents have diabetes, there is a 70 percent risk of their children developing T2DM. That's a pretty high risk! Most people in the United States have at least one relative with T2DM.

Luckily, genetics does not mean a person is guaranteed to develop diabetes; eating well and having a positive, active, healthy lifestyle can absolutely prevent the occurrence of the condition. We are not victims of our genetics just by being alive. We have the capacity to keep diabetes at bay, and if we do develop diabetes, we can teach our children how to prevent the disease.

Some ethnicities have a higher risk of developing T2DM. Latinos, Native Americans, Inuits, and Native Hawaiians and other Pacific Islanders have the highest rates of diabetes in their populations compared to other groups. Diabetes is nearly 20 percent more prevalent in Asian Americans, 66 percent more prevalent in Latinos, and 77 percent more prevalent in African Americans compared to non-Latino Whites. In addition to a higher risk for developing the disease, minorities also have a higher risk of developing serious complications. For example, African Americans are two to four times more likely than Caucasians to suffer from diabetic-induced renal failure, blindness, or amputation. In addition, non-Caucasians in general are two to four times more likely than Caucasians to die from diabetes.

Therefore, it's vital to ensure that the best form of diabetic treatment is available to people of all races and ethnicities. Treating all who need care is the only way can we effectively control this condition, among all populations, and bring this epidemic to an end.

The Second Risk Factor: Overeating

Overeating is one of the biggest risk factors for developing diabetes. Overeating can easily cause someone to become overweight or, even worse, obese.

In 1950 obesity and diabetes were not as common as they are today. From 1950 to 2010, obesity rates increased 214 percent, and now two out of three people in the United States are overweight (66 percent of the population), and one out of three people are obese (33 percent of the population).

The 2015 Statistical Pocketbook from the Food and Agricultural Organization (FAO) of the United Nations showed how many calories people in different countries consume. Globally, the average caloric intake in 1961 was 2,196 kcal per day. By 2011 it had reached 2,870 kcal per day. The FAO reported that in 2015 the average intake of calories per person per day in the United States was 3,750 kcal per day; there were over sixty countries in 2015 where the average person's daily caloric intake was 3,000 kcal per day or higher.

Based on US Department of Agriculture (USDA) guidelines, adult women need around 1,600–2,400 kcal per day (depending on age, height, weight, and activity); adult men need around 2,000–2,800 kcal per day (depending on age, height, weight, and activity). Thus, it's obvious that many people around the world are significantly overeating, no doubt contributing to increasing worldwide rates of obesity.

One of the factors contributing to overeating is portion size; in the United States, where people regularly eat out instead of at home, portion sizes in restaurants have doubled or tripled over the last two decades. In 1950, the average burger patty was 3.9 ounces (oz.), twenty years ago it was 8 oz., and now it's 12 oz. A serving of French fries has increased from 2.4 oz. to 6.7 oz. A sugary soda used to come in a 7 oz. cup (90 calories) and is now 20 oz. on average, with some stores selling soda pop in 42 oz. cups (580 calories)!

Snacking is now a huge problem as well. While parents used to tell children not to snack, as it would ruin their appetites for meals, many people now eat frequently throughout the day. The USDA reports that from 1977 to 1978, 41 percent of Americans didn't snack at all. Today, 90 percent of Americans snack daily, eating an average of 2.2 snacks a day. Snack foods are available for purchase at work, gas stations, supermarkets, coffee shops—everywhere. Snacks can often provide up to 25 percent of daily caloric intake, mostly consisting of alcohols, carbohydrates, and sugars.

The Third Risk Factor: Central Obesity

When we discuss obesity and T2DM, we are mainly focusing on abdominal obesity, also known as truncal obesity and visceral fat. This is fat that is stored in the abdominal cavity around organs like the liver, pancreas, and intestines. This type of fat is worse for promoting insulin resistance than subcutaneous fat, which lies under the skin, or female fat around the hips and thighs. It is likely you have excess abdominal fat if your waist is more than 37 inches if you are male, and more than 35 inches if you are female. Simply put, abdominal obesity causes insulin resistance, which causes more abdominal obesity. And, insulin resistance causes abdominal obesity, which causes worsening insulin resistance. It's a vicious cycle.

Fat cells, also known as adipocytes, used to be considered mere storage receptacles, but now we know they are active, living cells that produce many substances and hormones. Fat cells play a key role in metabolic, endocrine, and inflammatory signals designed to balance energy use and storage. Many of the substances made by adipose tissue become imbalanced or impaired when abdominal obesity and insulin resistance occur.

Some of the main protein substances secreted by adipocytes include:

PPARG. Peroxisome proliferator-activated receptor gamma is a protein that regulates the expression of genes that affect blood glucose control, reduce insulin resistance, affect the levels of fatty acids in the blood and production of fat cells, and also may reduce the risk of cardiovascular disease. In the past, researchers developed drugs called thiazolidinediones that increased the activity of PPARG, reducing insulin resistance, but these drugs caused serious complications, including weight gain, and were removed from the market. In the United States they were recently reintroduced, but physicians still shy away from them. You can read more about them in chapter 5.

Leptin. This protein signals a person to eat less food while expending more energy. Obese people tend to secrete increased levels of leptin but also develop leptin resistance, which means their cells do not respond to the leptin they secrete. As a result, patients develop an increased appetite. Combined with a high calorie diet and lack of exercise, this can easily lead to even more weight gain.

Adiponectin. This protein is believed to play a vital role in modulating glucose and lipid metabolism in tissues that are insulin sensitive. In obese patients with insulin resistance, adiponectin levels are decreased. Adiponectin levels are lower in diabetic patients with coronary artery disease than in diabetic patients without coronary artery disease, leading researchers to believe the protein may have antiatherogenic properties; that is, adiponectin may reduce the formation of plaques in arteries.

Plasminogen activator inhibitor type 1 (PAI-1). This protein inhibits plasminogen activators, which are substances that break down clots formed in the blood. PAI-1 prevents clot breakdown, is increased with obesity, and is reduced with weight loss. Elevated circulating levels of PAI-1 predict the development of T2DM. It is linked to insulin resistance and also to blood clots and liver damage.

Interleukin-6 (IL-6). This inflammatory regulator has increased secretion from fat cells in obese patients. Its pro-inflammatory action has been shown in multiple studies to be clearly associated with causing insulin resistance and T2DM.

Tumor necrosis factor-alpha (TNF-a). This is a protein secreted by enlarged fat cells that, when elevated, induces insulin resistance and is pro-inflammatory throughout the body. TNF-a is also associated with promoting inflammation in fatty livers. Obesity-induced chronic inflammation as seen with elevated secretions of TNF-a and IL-6 by fat cells is a key component in the development of insulin resistance, metabolic syndrome, and T2DM. Pro-inflammatory chemicals can cause insulin resistance in adipocytes, but also in the liver and muscle cells. Chronic inflammation is also associated with increased risk of cardiovascular disease, Alzheimer's disease, and cancer—all conditions that T2DM patients experience more frequently than those who do not have T2DM. Reducing body inflammation is extremely helpful in prevention of diabetes and in treatment of diabetes and prevention and healing of diabetic complications.

During the night, abdominal fat cells release lots of free fatty acids, which travel directly to the liver through the portal venous system. As the liver is flooded with these fats, it becomes insulin resistant and begins to store extra fats, becoming a "fatty liver." A fatty liver is a very serious problem, and is discussed fully in chapter 14. As the liver becomes insulin resistant, however, it secretes a lot more glucose into the bloodstream; the fact that this process happens during the night is one reason fasting glucose numbers can be so high in the morning. Until that abdominal fat has been lost, insulin resistance will be a problem through the substances the fat produces.

The Fourth Risk Factor: Nutritional Deficiencies

The body's blood sugar–regulating metabolism requires many nutrients to work smoothly and healthily. Many people are deficient in these same nutrients. The CDC's "Second Nutrition Report" showed that in the United States, the most common nutrient deficiencies are vitamin B_6, iron, vitamin D_3, vitamin C, and vitamin B_{12}. The *Journal of Nutrition* reported that Americans are also not getting enough omega-3 fatty acids from their foods. Nutrient deficiencies are a real phenomenon in the food-rich United States.

Unfortunately, our food simply does not contain the same nutrients as it did one hundred years ago. As reported by the Organic Center, if we wish to eat well and obtain the recommended nutrients, we must be aware that conventionally raised foods may contain fewer antioxidants (substances that protect against oxidative damage), vitamins, and minerals than organic food. Whether conventional or organic however, people who develop insulin resistance typically do not eat enough fruits and vegetables, but rather eat a great deal of the processed food and beverages that are rampant in our society and that contain few, if any, nutrients.

The nutrients that are particularly needed by cells to have insulin work and prevent insulin resistance include zinc, chromium, magnesium, potassium, vanadium, essential fatty acids including omega-3 and omega-6 oils, and alpha-lipoic acid. Zinc is needed in the beta cells of the pancreas to make and secrete insulin; it is also needed on the cell wall to stimulate the receptor to take glucose in from the bloodstream. Chromium is needed to aid insulin in landing on its receptor and staying there, activating the cell to absorb glucose. The cell wall requires magnesium and potassium to be able to absorb glucose from the serum. Vanadium helps insulin work better at the cell wall. Lastly, essential fatty acids such as omega-3 fish oils and omega-6 GLA oils (evening primrose, borage oil, black currant oil) keep the cell wall healthy, so their receptors work well, and potentiate insulin's action. R-alpha-lipoic acid helps enhance glucose absorption into cells.

Nutrients are required to run our body processes; two of the main purposes of eating are to acquire both the calories needed to feed our bodies' energy to run and the micronutrients that allow enzymes in our body to work efficiently. If you want to make energy through our main energy-producing cycle, you need iron. If you want to make serotonin so you feel content and happy, you need vitamin B_6. If you want to make adrenal hormones like testosterone, you need vitamin C, folic acid, and pantothenic acid. If you want to make thyroid hormone to boost your metabolism, you need zinc, copper, selenium, and the amino acid tyrosine. For people getting most of their dietary intake from bad fats, refined carbohydrates, and fast foods, which lack most of these nutrients, it is obvious how their lack of nutrients can have drastic effects on so many areas of their bodies and minds.

Nutrients also affect how our brains function, and help make up the neurotransmitter chemicals that keep us happy, alert, satiated, content, and joyful. If we are nutrient deficient, then we might struggle to keep our moods happy, and subsequently fall prey to "comfort food" eating: unhealthy foods high in carbohydrates, sugar, and fat. Ensuring good nutrition and nutrient intake is vital for both physical and mental/emotional health.

Micronutrient deficiencies are common in Americans, even with the prevalence of huge supermarkets full of food. When individuals do not have the micronutrients their bodies need to work well and efficiently, insulin resistance and other problems can develop.

In summary, nutrient deficiencies contribute to diabetes in the following ways:

- Cause lower energy and lower motivation to work out
- Cause irritability, depression, anxiety, and need to seek comfort in food
- Increase the risk of developing insulin resistance
- Cause problematic food cravings leading to weight gain
- Prevent antioxidative protection of the body from higher glucose or insulin, causing damage to tissues
- Lead to reliance on caffeine for energy, which interferes with sleep, increasing risk of weight gain and carbohydrate craving
- Lower metabolism and ability to burn fat
- Negatively affect the functioning of organs and regeneration of healthy tissue. For example, liver detoxification requires many micronutrients, of which a lack can lead to increased risk of developing T2DM and T1DM

A keen integrative physician can uncover nutrient deficiencies through a comprehensive office intake, by analyzing a patient's diet diary, and via lab work, testing red blood cells, serum, or urine or feces, depending on the lab and the nutrients investigated. Correcting nutrient deficiencies can be easy, however, by improving the diet and through nutrient supplementation.

The Sixth Risk Factor: Lack of Exercise

Another key risk factor is lack of exercise. A typical housewife around one hundred years ago expended an estimated 3,000 calories each day keeping her house clean, doing laundry, cooking, and so forth. Think of how hard it must have been to haul coal upstairs to the apartment, as my grandmother did, to cook dinner!

Today, household chores are not nearly as strenuous for most people in this country. We don't walk; we drive cars. Most of us don't plow our own fields with oxen to sow our own crops, either. These days, many kids do not play outside with each other, but instead sit inside on their computers or watch upwards of seven hours a day of television. In all aspects of life, our natural caloric expenditure has plummeted.

In several studies, lack of exercise has been shown to be a greater factor in the development of obesity than overeating, and a main factor in the development of insulin resistance. But even thirty minutes of effective exercise a day can be enough to prevent weight gain in otherwise sedentary adults. Plus, exercise increases endorphins, chemicals that improve our mood, boost our self-esteem, and give us more energy.

The Low Carb Diabetes Association uses the motto *Be Fit. Be Strong*. While strolling on a treadmill for thirty minutes is not necessarily effective in reducing insulin resistance and lowering one's weight, there are effective exercise regimens that use measurable patient analyses to ensure treatment goals are being attained. The problem is that exercise can often be the modality of healing that patients are least interested in committing to and engaging in regularly, yet it is absolutely one of the most important aspects of reversing and controlling diabetes. Therefore, an integrative medicine physician should spend considerable time counseling patients about exercise, something that will be discussed in further detail in chapter 9.

The Seventh Risk Factor: Hormone Imbalances

Cortisol, categorized as an adrenal glucocorticosteroid, is one of the main hormones produced by the body in reaction to both perceived and actual stress. The adrenals are a main organ for cortisol production. There are many stimulants to cortisol secretion, including fasting; exercising; anxiety; anger; lack of sleep; feeling "stressed out" from work, relationships, or other life troubles; and too many carbohydrates in the abdominally obese person's diet.

Cortisol has been studied for years and is known to signal the liver to move fat from storage areas into abdominal fat cells; signal the liver to secrete glucose; encourage the body's use of protein for energy; help fat cells grow and mature; and produce triglycerides and blood sugar, initiating insulin resistance and, as a result, promoting abdominal obesity and high blood pressure.

Elevated cortisol at night can interfere with sleep, and good sleep is needed for energy, mood, and appetite control. Elevated cortisol can interfere with one's calmness and happiness, while low cortisol can cause significant fatigue, which in turn diminishes one's motivation to exercise and even presents risk of depression.

High levels of cortisol also interfere with thyroid hormone production, lowering one's basic metabolism and making it easier for less food to cause more weight gain. Lowered thyroid functioning also keeps levels of fats higher in the bloodstream, which also promotes insulin resistance. High levels of cortisol are catabolic and can wear down the lining of the intestinal tract and of the upper respiratory system. To make things more complicated, low cortisol levels can also interfere with good metabolism. Cortisol is required for our bioactive thyroid hormone to activate our cellular thyroid receptors, signaling our cells to burn more energy. If someone has low cortisol levels, then it can be harder for that person to lose weight.

Cortisol also helps regulate our inflammatory response; if it is too high (or too low) for too long, this can negatively affect the body and produce more inflammation, which aggravates insulin resistance, causes pain, and promotes diabetic complications.

Cortisol can be tested accurately through saliva and treated naturally whether it is too high or too low. The saliva test measures four salivary samples taken during one full day and night. Dehydroepiandrosterone (DHEA), another glucocorticosteroid, which is beneficial at balancing the effects of cortisol, is also tested. DHEA promotes anabolism (the building of tissues) and has an anti-inflammatory effect in the body, lowering problematic chemicals such as IL-6, noted above to promote insulin resistance. Also, DHEA can be transformed into sex hormones such as estrogen and testosterone.

Thyroid activity should also be tested in patients with suspected or confirmed insulin resistance. The patient does not have to be fasting but the blood should be drawn before 11:00 a.m., as thyroid secretion of hormones peaks in the morning. In chapter 4 I will discuss all the thyroid labs that should be checked.

Testosterone is another hormone with an interesting connection to insulin. In men, low testosterone levels produce weight gain and loss of muscle and bone mass. Studies have shown that giving men testosterone helps them lose weight, gain muscle mass, and have better control of their blood sugars. Men with insulin resistance and a "beer belly" often not only have low testosterone levels, but also have increased levels of estrogen. Low "T" and elevated estrogen can cause problems both physically and emotionally for men. Men with T2DM who are on statin drugs are at particular risk for developing low testosterone, as statins lower cholesterol, and cholesterol is the core around which all our body hormones are made. All adult male T2DM patients on a statin drug should have their testosterone tested, though it doesn't hurt to test all men, whether they are on a statin or not.

In women who experience insulin resistance, we see high levels of testosterone or DHEA (the androgen hormones) or both, and lower estrogen levels. The common medical problem polycystic ovarian syndrome (PCOS) is an outcome of these imbalances, and many women with PCOS, a disease driven by insulin resistance, are overweight or obese.

Postmenopausal women tend to gain weight in the abdomen more easily than younger women. This is because they have less ovarian estrogen production; estrogen directs fat to be deposited on the hips and buttocks, creating the pear shaped body typical of women, and also prevents the development of insulin resistance. When estrogen stops being produced, women will gain weight much more easily in their abdomen, creating the apple body shape and increasing their risk for insulin resistance. Excess testosterone given to postmenopausal women may actually cause abdominal fat and insulin resistance. Lower doses are fine, however. I have seen women mistakenly prescribed high dose testosterone shots by their integrative physician gain weight, all in their abdomen, and even develop fatty liver.

Bioidentical hormones are synthetic or natural hormones transformed in a laboratory to be exactly the same as human hormones. Giving bioidentical estrogen and progesterone hormones to postmenopausal women is safe, if necessary, and can reduce insulin resistance. That does not mean that every women must go on bioidentical estrogen after menopause, but if a woman is having significant menopausal symptoms, such as hot flashes, adding estrogen is safe and recommended. For postmenopausal women who are struggling to keep weight off or whose glucose or insulin serum values are rising, adding estrogen may be helpful. Always combine estrogen with progesterone, even if the woman does not have a uterus. Adding low dose testosterone is safe, as well, if indicated.

A hormone carrier protein called sex hormone binding globulin (SHBG), which carries both testosterone and estrogen, is lower in individuals with insulin resistance. When we have less SHBG, the hormones are more active and wreak more havoc on our bodies. In fact, one study showed that a good way to check if a pregnant woman is at risk for developing diabetes during her pregnancy is to test for SHBG in the first trimester. If it is low, then she is at high risk. This is very helpful, because usually we do not diagnose diabetes in pregnant women until the third trimester, using an oral glucose tolerance test. By testing for SHBG, we can work to prevent pregnant women from ever becoming diabetic.

Many hormones are thrown out of balance for many reasons. Imbalanced hormones can help initiate obesity and insulin resistance, and in turn insulin resistance and obesity can help create hormone imbalances. A good naturopathic or integrative physician should fully evaluate the hormone levels in both prediabetic and diabetic patients.

The Eighth Risk Factor: Increased Saturated Fat and Increased Refined Carbohydrates

Many countries in Asia, including Japan, are experiencing a rapid increase in obesity, insulin resistance, and diabetes, though their traditional diets have been composed of 70 percent carbohydrates, mostly white rice, for hundreds of years. Why now are they developing these problems? The answer is saturated fat, largely imported from American fast-food restaurants in the form of what we call "agri-industry" meat.

Historically, humans ate wild game, or raised their own beef, pork, poultry, or lamb fed on unspoiled grasses or insects their entire lives before being slaughtered. Half the fat of animals raised in pristine environments, eating their natural food, consists of essential fatty acids, which reduce insulin resistance. Today, a cow may be raised for many months on ranchland, but is then sent to a concentrated animal feeding operation (CAFO) and given estrogens, antibiotics, and genetically modified corn. This increases its fat content ("marbling"), which is transformed almost completely into saturated fat, losing nearly all the omega-3 fat it once contained. Saturated fat in moderation is not bad for you, but when it is so out of balance in your diet, it can definitely promote insulin resistance. Saturated fats are found in other foods as well, including dairy, eggs, lard, nuts, and seeds, and in cooking oils used for deep-frying. Studies show that replacing saturated fat with monounsaturated and polyunsaturated fats significantly reduced the onset of diabetes. Reducing saturated fat intake is very healthful and very important in getting T2DM under control.

Trans fats, present in partially hydrogenated oils, vegetable fats, and shortening, act like saturated fats in the body and are also a problem. In 2006, the FDA began requiring companies to list trans fats on their nutrition labels and has since ordered companies to remove all trans fats from their food by June 2018. Unfortunately, many companies removing trans fats are replacing them with fully hydrogenated oils and interesterified oils. In a 2017 study, interesterified oils were shown to increase blood glucose levels 20 percent in nondiabetic people.

Refined carbohydrates, such as high fructose corn syrup, are also associated with insulin resistance. One researcher, Dr. Liu, analyzed the American diet over a span of decades and found high fructose corn syrup and decreased fiber intake to be leading factors in the development of diabetes. According to the Health and Human Services of the US government, the average American ate only 2 pounds of sugar a year two hundred years ago. Today the average Americans eats 152 pounds of sugar a year! This statistic should help everyone understand why so many people are overweight and diabetic.

Many words on ingredient labels, both obvious and obscure, mean sugar: glucose, dextrose, brown sugar, sucrose, corn syrup, high fructose corn syrup, corn syrup solids, dehydrated cane juice, organic cane juice crystals, raw cane juice crystals, evaporated cane juice, invert sugar, raw sugar, turbinado sugar, Sucanat, agave, and honey.

Refined sugar does a number of problematic things to the human body, including the following:

- Adds extra calories but provides no nutrients
- Feeds problematic microorganisms in the gut, increasing the risk for systemic insulin resistance
- Causes cravings for more refined sugar

- Increases anxiety and depression
- Increases inflammation, like TNF-a, that promotes insulin resistance
- Makes the musculoskeletal system achy and painful, reducing the drive to exercise
- Lowers energy
- Increases blood pressure (even more than salt does)
- Decreases the liver's ability to detoxify
- Lowers the immune system

While overeating in general is a risk factor for diabetes, overeating saturated fats and refined sugars specifically can create a serious health problem.

The Ninth Risk Factor: Dysbiosis

As noted in the discussion of T1DM risk factors, gut inflammation, leaky gut, and dysbiosis are associated with promoting autoimmunity. Gut health is also associated with T2DM risk factors.

Gut bacteria help dictate how much energy a person absorbs from their diet. Obese people have been found to have different proportions of bacteria in their intestines than lean people. The changes make the obese person more likely to have intestinal permeability, allowing more absorption of gut toxins, and leading to an increase in systemic inflammation, causing insulin resistance. Obese people have enzymes in their microbiome that allow for the better breakdown of generally indigestible carbohydrates; that is, the obese microbiome harvests more energy from food. These processes are made worse on a diet high in fats and high fructose.

A good naturopathic or integrative physician will investigate all patients' gut histories to determine the priority of focusing on the microbiome. Most diabetic patients should have some intestinal support.

The Tenth Risk Factor: Gestational Diabetes

The mother-fetus connection is very strong, especially with regard to the health of the mom related to the future health of her child. Mothers who become diabetic during their pregnancy give birth to a child who has a much higher risk of becoming overweight and developing diabetes. Being exposed to higher levels of glucose in the uterus sets the child up for becoming overweight and diabetic at a younger age. The good news is that breastfeeding, feeding your child a healthy diet, getting exercising, having regular doctor visits, and, most importantly, parents who set a great example, are all ways to overcome the problematic uterine environmental impact on the child.

The Eleventh Risk Factor: Chronic Hepatitis C

Chronic hepatitis C affects 3 percent of the world's population and around 3.2 million Americans. Chronic hepatitis C can cause the liver to become progressively fattier, develop fibrosis (scar tissue), and eventually lead to cirrhosis.

There are several reasons why hepatitis C may increase the risk of developing T2DM. For one, hepatitis C increases some of the same pro-inflammatory chemicals also produced by abdominal fat, like TNF-a or IL-6, that cause insulin resistance in the body. Further, liver fibrosis can cause the liver to become insulin resistant, which in turn can initiate T2DM. Lastly, hepatitis-C-induced fatty liver can cause the liver to increase glucose production and promote development of fibrosis. Getting diabetes under control relies on getting hepatitis C under control, as well.

The Twelfth Risk Factor: Environmental Toxicity

Our society is polluted. As noted in the T1DM risk factors, persistent organic pollutants (POPs) are very common chemicals, and they include pesticides and herbicides used on farms and inside and outside our homes. POPs are called "persistent" because they resist biodegradation and are ultimately stored in our fatty tissue.

Environmental toxins highly associated with T2DM include phthalates, bisphenol A, and polychlorinated biphenyls (PCBs). Populations with a high occurrence of diabetes, such as Canadian Aboriginals, have extremely high levels of organochlorine pesticides: dichlorodiphenyldichloroethylene (DDE), PCBs, and polychlorinated diphenyl ethers (PBDEs), which are thought to come from eating high levels of fish polluted with those toxins.

To date there have been forty-one human studies on diabetes and POPs that have shown an interdependent relationship between contamination with POPs and the development of diabetes. One groundbreaking study in 2006 showed that people with the highest contamination of POPs in their body tissues were nearly 38 percent more likely to develop diabetes than those in the lower level of contamination. This same study showed that being obese did not increase the risk of T2DM in people with very low levels of POPs.

Another excellent (and frightening!) study published in *Diabetes Care* in 2014 compared two groups of people: One group was overweight with glucose dysglycemia, and the other group was normal weight with normal sugars. Those who were overweight had a higher level of POPs than those who were of normal weight. This adds credence to a study in Sweden showing that higher body levels of POPs predicted the development of T2DM.

The World Health Organization has stated that heavy metals, such as arsenic and lead, can induce insulin resistance at the cellular level and significantly increase the risk of T2DM.

The total list of POPs causing metabolic syndrome, insulin resistance, and diabetes is immense and troubling, as is the fact that they can be spread from mother to baby both in utero and through breast milk. Additionally, losing weight can actually increase the release of toxins from metabolized fat cells and increase serum levels. This may be a reason some people plateau with weight loss, as those released chemicals can cause insulin resistance. It is important to ensure good detoxification pathways are open in the body when weight loss is occurring. Any integrative physician should have knowledge and guidance on avoiding environmental toxins in your work, home, and life.

We will discuss many aspects of diagnosing, preventing, and detoxifying from environmental toxins in chapter 9.

The Thirteenth Risk Factor: Lack of Sleep and Sleep Apnea

In the busy world of stress and overworking, it's very common for people to get insufficient sleep. Getting less than five hours of sleep a night has been shown to increase one's risk of developing obesity by 235 percent (!), and not getting six to nine hours of sleep each night significantly increases one's risk for insulin resistance. Insufficient sleep throws off hormones that regulate our appetites and our cravings for carbohydrates.

Those hormones are:

Leptin. This hormone is made from our adipose tissue that helps control our appetite so we eat less food. If you do not get enough sleep, levels of this hormone are decreased, resulting in the loss of appetite control.

Ghrelin. This hormone, made in our stomach and small intestine, increases our appetite and increases our desire to eat carbohydrates. If you do not get enough sleep, this hormone is increased, so you'll crave more food, especially carbohydrates.

Cortisol. As mentioned, cortisol is not really related to sleep, but if one is not getting enough sleep, this stresses the body, causing the adrenals to produce more cortisol. Cortisol leads to higher glucose production and may cause a higher risk of insulin resistance.

In addition to lack of sleep, a condition called obstructive sleep apnea (OSA) is also associated with reduced glucose control and increased risk of cardiovascular disease. T2DM can cause OSA, and OSA can cause T2DM. If a patient has any signs or symptoms of sleep apnea, he needs to have a sleep study to confirm or rule out the diagnosis. If an overweight or obese patient states she snores, that is enough for me to send her for an official sleep study, as snoring is the first and main symptom of OSA. Tiredness during the day is another. Treatment of sleep apnea will help patients lose weight, get their glucose under control, and decrease their risk of heart disease.

These are the most common and implicated risk factors for developing T2DM. In later chapters, these factors will be discussed further, along with comprehensive treatment recommendations.

— CHAPTER THREE —

Physical Exams

Physical exams are vital for an initial analysis of the status of a diabetic patient and for following up on how they are doing physically, once treatment has begun. There are exams that a physician should regularly be doing with patients, exams patients should have done at least once per year, and exams patients should be doing themselves on a daily basis.

Regular In-Office Physical Exams

Vitals—blood pressure, pulse, respiratory rate, and temperature—should be measured each time you visit your physician.

Body Weight and Fat Measurements

There are several ways to measure a patient's fat status, and I do these measurements with all overweight or obese diabetic patients: body weight, waist circumference, body mass index (BMI), waist/hip ratio (WHR), waist/height ratio (WHtR), and calipers. Some physicians also do body impedance analysis, an electrical way to measure body fat. With lean or normal weight T1DM patients, just getting their basic weight is sufficient. These weight measurements are repeated appropriately during follow-up visits.

Weight

I measure weight on a scale that is also designed to measure lean muscle, water percentage, and bone mass. Using this type of scale in combination with the

BMI, WHR, and calipers, I can be assured that my patients' weight loss is due to fat loss (what we want) and not from muscle or bone (what we don't want).

Waist Circumference

The ideal waist measurement for the average woman should be 32 inches or less; stricter standards recommend 30 inches or less. Likewise, the average man's waist should be 38 inches or less, with stricter standards setting the bar at 35 inches.

Body Mass Index (BMI)

To determine your BMI, measure your height in inches and multiply that number by itself (squaring it). Then divide your weight in pounds by your height squared. Lastly, multiply that number by 703 to get your BMI. For example, a woman who is five feet three inches tall (63 inches) and weighs 180 pounds has a BMI of 31, which is considered obese:

$$63 \times 63 = 3969$$
$$180 \div 3969 = 0.045$$
$$0.045 \times 703 = 31$$

There are many BMI calculator websites and phone apps where one can easily enter one's height and weight and receive the BMI instantly, including from the CDC.

For most people, a BMI of less than 18.5 is considered underweight; the BMI for normal weight ranges from 18.5 to 24.9. You are considered overweight if your BMI is between 25 and 29.9, and obese if your BMI is over 30. You are considered grossly or morbidly obese if your BMI is over 40. Asian people are genetically so lean that there is a separate BMI calculator for them. There is also a pediatric BMI calculator for those under eighteen years old.

BMI readings can be inaccurate in some situations, particularly if the person is very muscular. Muscular people may have higher-than-average weight for their height, but this is due to developed muscles, not fat. However, it is very rare for an in-shape, muscular patient to present with T2DM; if one does have diabetes, I would recommend testing to determine if they have LADA instead. Otherwise, for our overweight and obese patients, BMI can be considered an accurate medical reading.

Waist/Hip Ratio

Waist/hip ratio is calculated by dividing your waist measurement in inches (taken at your belly button) by your hip measurement (widest area around buttocks) in inches. According to the World Health Organization, women should have a waist/hip ratio equal to or less than 0.85, while men should have a waist/hip ratio equal to or less than 0.9. Higher scores for both genders indicate obesity.

Waist/Height Ratio

Waist/height ratio is an important tool to measure the degree of central fat distribution. Waist/height ratio corresponds better to metabolic risk than

Table 3.1. Waist/Height Ratios for Men

Ratio	Categorization
< 0.35 or < 35	Underweight/Abnormally slim
0.35–0.43 or 35–43	Extremely slim
0.43–0.46 or 43–46	Slender and healthy
0.46–0.53 or 46–53	Healthy, normal weight
0.53–0.58 or 53–58	Overweight
0.58–0.63 or 58–63	Extremely overweight/obese
> 0.63 or 63	Highly obese

Table 3.2. Waist/Height Ratios for Women

Ratio	Categorization
< 0.35 or 35	Underweight/Abnormally slim
0.35–0.42 or 35–42	Extremely slim
0.42–0.46 or 42–46	Slender and healthy
0.46–0.49 or 46–49	Healthy, normal weight
0.49–0.54 or 49–54	Overweight
0.54–0.58 or 54–58	Extremely overweight/obese
> 0.58 or 58	Highly obese

BMI, and in a 2010 study an increased waist/height ratio was a stronger predictor of cardiovascular risk and mortality than a BMI.

Waist/height ratio is calculated by dividing waist size by height and is used to measure the distribution of body fat. If your waist measurement is less than half your height, you're likely not at risk for obesity-related disease. That would mean your waist/height ratio is 0.50/50 or less. Different online calculators list ratios either as 0.35 or 35, but the numbers mean the same (see tables 3.1 and 3.2 for how different ratios are categorized).

Waist/height ratio is a quick, easy, and accurate way to calculate and monitor abdominal adiposity in patients.

Calipers for Percentage Body Fat

Lastly, I also measure patients for percentage body fat via skinfold calipers. A skinfold caliper is a device that easily measures the thickness of a fold in one's skin, grabbing the underlying fat. Doing this in several locations is a very accurate way of measuring the total body fat in one's body. There is a certain trick to getting the correct measurement, and knowing when to read the calipers, but a physician who has experience regularly analyzing this can be skillful at measuring and assessing the scores.

Table 3.3. Body Fat Percentage Measurement Chart for Men

18-20	2.0	3.9	6.2	8.5	10.5	12.5	14.3	16.0	17.5	18.9	20.2	21.3	22.3	23.1	23.8	24.3	24.9
21-25	2.5	4.9	7.3	9.5	11.6	13.6	15.4	17.0	18.6	20.0	21.2	22.3	23.3	24.2	24.9	25.4	25.8
26-30	3.5	6.0	8.4	10.6	12.7	14.6	16.4	18.1	19.6	21.0	22.3	23.4	24.4	25.2	25.9	26.5	26.9
31-35	4.5	7.1	9.4	11.7	13.7	15.7	17.5	19.2	20.7	22.1	23.4	24.5	25.5	26.3	27.0	27.5	28.0
36-40	5.6	8.1	10.5	12.7	14.8	16.8	18.6	20.2	21.8	23.2	24.4	25.6	26.5	27.4	28.1	28.6	29.0
41-45	6.7	9.2	11.5	13.8	15.9	17.8	19.6	21.3	22.8	24.7	25.5	26.6	27.6	28.4	29.1	29.7	30.1
46-50	7.7	10.2	12.6	14.8	16.9	18.9	20.7	22.4	23.9	25.3	26.6	27.7	28.7	29.5	30.2	30.7	31.2
51-55	8.8	11.0	13.7	15.9	18.0	20.0	21.8	23.4	25.0	26.4	27.6	28.7	29.7	30.6	31.2	31.8	32.2
56 +	9.9	12.4	14.7	17.0	19.1	21.0	22.8	24.5	26.0	27.4	28.7	29.8	30.8	31.6	32.3	32.9	33.3
AGE	**LEAN**				**IDEAL**				**AVERAGE**					**ABOVE AVERAGE**			

I measure the front of a patient's upper arm, the back of the upper arm, the area underneath one scapula on the back, and the lower left aspect of the abdomen. By adding up these caliper numbers, I get a measure of the amount of body fat in my patient's body.

There are many different charts measuring caliper body fat levels, but research conducted by Jackson and Pollock resulted in well-known and accepted body fat charts to show what percentages are considered lean, ideal, average, and above average for men and women (see tables 3.3 and 3.4, respectively).

Obviously, women are designed to have a little more body fat than men. It's good to set up weight goals that include a patient's ideal or average body fat percentage.

Bioelectrical Impedance Analysis

BIA is a helpful tool to include with BMI measurement for those who are undergoing weight loss. Electrical pulses can define how much fat exists in a body. Although some machines can be expensive, I use a Weight Watchers scale in my office, which seems to be a very accurate way of measuring body fat if the person is not pregnant, has an empty bladder, is well hydrated,

Table 3.4. Body Fat Percentage Measurement Chart for Women

18-20	11.3	13.5	15.7	17.7	19.7	21.5	23.2	24.8	26.3	27.7	29.0	30.2	31.3	32.3	33.3	33.9	34.6
21-25	11.9	14.2	16.3	18.4	20.3	22.1	23.8	25.5	27.0	28.4	29.6	30.8	31.9	32.9	33.8	34.5	35.2
26-30	12.5	14.8	16.9	19.0	20.9	22.7	24.5	26.1	27.6	29.0	30.3	31.5	32.5	33.5	34.4	35.2	35.8
31-35	13.2	15.4	17.6	19.6	21.5	23.4	25.1	26.7	28.2	29.6	30.9	32.1	33.2	34.1	35.0	35.8	36.4
36-40	13.8	16.0	18.2	20.2	22.2	24.0	25.7	27.3	28.8	30.2	31.5	32.7	33.8	34.8	35.6	36.4	37.0
41-45	14.4	16.7	18.8	20.8	22.8	24.6	26.3	27.9	29.4	30.8	32.1	33.3	34.4	35.4	36.3	37.0	37.7
46-50	15.0	17.3	19.4	21.5	23.4	25.2	26.9	28.6	30.1	31.5	32.8	34.0	35.0	36.0	36.9	37.6	38.3
51-55	15.6	17.9	20.0	22.1	24.0	25.9	27.6	29.2	30.7	32.1	33.4	34.6	35.6	36.6	37.5	38.3	38.9
56 +	16.3	18.5	20.7	22.7	24.6	26.5	28.2	29.8	31.3	32.7	34.0	35.2	36.3	37.2	38.1	38.9	39.5
AGE	LEAN					IDEAL				AVERAGE				ABOVE AVERAGE			

and is barefoot. With patients who need to undergo weight loss, a Weight Watchers or Tanita scale is an effective way in office to ensure weight loss is fat and not muscle or bone.

Grip Strength

Weak grip strength is a leading risk indicator for developing T2DM. Grip strength is a key sign of innate muscle development, and having fewer muscles makes one more likely to gain weight and develop insulin resistance. I have a Jamar grip dynamometer in my office with which I measure patients' grip strength. It is a simple test, done in seconds. If a patient's grip strength is not at the average or above for their gender and age, that is very concerning to me, and initiating strength-building exercise then becomes very important. Without building muscle strength, in susceptible patients, it will be difficult to prevent T2DM or help reverse it if it already exists.

Foot Analysis

At least once a year, if not every visit (depending on how often you see your physician and if you have any diabetic nerve damage), you should have a very good foot exam that checks for any vascular, visual, skin, bone, or muscle changes.

The exam should include an inspection of your shoes, making sure they protect your feet and don't rub against any skin; checking two pulses in your foot, one behind your inner anklebone and one on top of your foot; checking for edema or rashes; and checking for calluses, sores, ulcers, bunions or hammertoes, fungal infections, muscle contractions, Charcot's foot (see diabetic neuropathy complications in chapter 14), or any other abnormality. Your physician should also do a sensory test of your nerves using a 5.07 mm 10 g monofilament on several toes and the ball of your foot. If your physician does not have a formal monofilament, it is equally effective for them to do an Ipswich Touch Test, by lightly placing an index finger on your first, third, and fifth toes for two seconds, waiting for you to respond "yes" if you feel the finger. During either sensory test the patient's eyes are completely closed. Even when a patient does not report early symptoms of neuropathy, it is fairly common that I am able to discover the development of mild neuropathy when they are unable to feel where the monofilament is on their toes or feet.

A physician will oftentimes do a vibratory test by placing a 128 Hz tuning fork on the bony prominence of the back of the big toe, proximal to the nail bed. This test is also done with closed eyes. Some physicians may also do a pinprick sensation proximal to your toenails and check your ankle reflexes. It's also good to check to see if you have flat feet or arched feet, which can cause irritation in shoes and increase the risk of ulcers.

Your physician should ask if you suffer any "rest pain," whereby your toes are crampy and aching only at night, or if you have "charley horses" in your calves when you walk, as these indicate peripheral artery disease may be occurring.

Ophthalmic (Eye) Exam

Some physicians may wish to do an in-office ocular examination of the retina and blood vessels in your eyes. This should not take the place of a diabetic patient seeing an optometrist or ophthalmologist at least once per year and getting a complete diabetic eye exam, as discussed in the following section.

Yearly Exams Every Patient Should Get

In addition to regular exams, patients should receive the following yearly exams to ensure they are being proactive and preventive, and so they can catch the development of a complication as early as possible.

Complete Eye Exam

A complete yearly eye exam includes assessment of general vision, as well as checks for cataracts and glaucoma. I also feel it is a necessity for my patients to receive a dilated eye exam by an optometrist who specializes in analyzing diabetic eyes or by an ophthalmologist. In fact, I refuse to set up a treatment plan with patients if they have not had a dilated eye exam within the previous six months. Any diabetic retinopathy (eye damage) should be uncovered before a comprehensive treatment plan is developed with a naturopathic physician. Diabetic eye diseases are covered further in chapter 14.

EKG and Stress Test

A patient does not need an EKG and stress test every year, but if someone has not been exercising for many years (or their whole life) and is overweight, has probable hypertension, and now is motivated to start exercising, a quick check with a cardiologist to ensure it is safe to begin an exercise regimen is a responsible referral.

Podiatrist Visit

Even though a diabetic patient should check their feet every day, as mentioned in the following section, or at least several days a week, seeing a podiatrist for a yearly analysis of one's feet, or more frequently for regular care, makes good sense.

Dental Exam

A diabetic patient should get a good dental cleaning and exam one to four times a year, depending on what one's dentist suggests based on one's oral exams.

Daily Exams a Patient Should Do

It is very helpful and positive for a diabetic patient to establish certain daily habits.

Checking Your Feet

All diabetic patients should check their feet every day and ensure they look healthy. You should ensure the shoes you wore that day fit your feet well and did not cause blisters, callouses, or irritation. You can prevent ulcers or sores from developing by catching skin changes early and going to a physician right away for prompt treatment.

Complications in the feet may arise more easily as a result of the decreased blood supply and decreased sensation in the feet that accompany diabetes. In addition to having your feet inspected regularly by a physician or podiatrist, here are a few guidelines to follow for the care of your feet. Please check both your feet daily, as per this list. If your vision is impaired, have a family member or friend inspect them.

- Check for signs of sores, redness, cracks, blisters, or other irritations. It is important to inspect between your toes as well. The use of a mirror can aid in seeing the bottom of the feet.
- Cut nails straight across.
- Exercise daily.
- Do not apply hot water bottles, heating pads, or very hot water to your feet.
- Do not apply strong antiseptics or chemicals to your feet.
- Feet should be washed daily with warm water and mild soap. Pat dry after washing.
- To avoid foot injury, never walk barefoot, especially outdoors.
- Wear properly fitted cotton socks, avoiding socks with seams.
- Do not wear shoes without socks.
- Shoes should fit properly at the time of purchase.
- Do not wear sandals with thongs between the toes.
- Inspect the inside of your shoes daily for foreign objects, nails, points, and torn linings.

Notify your physician if any of the following occur:

- Cuts or scrapes that do not heal
- Redness or swelling spreading along the foot
- Ingrown, infected toenails
- Any kind of injury to the foot
- Discoloration of the foot
- Loss of sensation in the foot

By following smart foot care habits (and controlling glucose levels), you can help avoid serious foot complications.

Caring for Your Teeth

Researchers are learning more and more about the connection between diabetes and dental health, notably gum disease.

Gum disease has two stages: gingivitis and periodontal disease. Gingivitis occurs when bacteria attach to your teeth and develop into a hard yellow film called plaque, which when hardened further is called tartar. If this is not cleaned off, it can cause damage to the gums, which make them redden, swell, and bleed. When that occurs and is not promptly reversed, it can progress to periodontitis, where the gums begin to pull away from the teeth. Recession of gums can then form pockets in the gum, where bacteria can thrive and spread infection down into the roots of the teeth. Around 50 percent of American adults have periodontitis; the percentage increases to around 70 percent in adults over sixty-five years old. Periodontitis puts people at a very high risk of losing both oral bone and teeth.

Chronic periodontitis causes severe inflammation in one's mouth, and that can cause inflammation in the whole body, leading to insulin resistance and increasing one's risk for cardiovascular disease. Here is the catch-22—oral inflammation causes systemic insulin resistance, which in and of itself causes inflammation, which worsens insulin resistance—you get the idea! Thus, periodontal disease can increase one's risk of developing T2DM, but having T2DM, especially if it is not well controlled, equally increases one's risk of developing periodontal disease. In fact, the 2008 NHANES (National Health and Nutrition Examination Survey) study showed that people with periodontal disease are *twice as likely* to develop diabetes as people who do not have the oral condition.

Gum disease also can chronically raise glucose levels and can significantly increase one's risk for developing, and dying from, kidney disease—patients with gum disease have up to three times more risk than those without gum disease.

The good news is that treating your gum disease may help your diabetes. Several studies have shown that getting one's gum disease treated can significantly lower glucose levels long-term, even months after "deep cleaning," a dental procedure used to get into dental pockets and clean out the bacteria.

Focusing on healthy teeth and gums is highly recommended for prevention and better control of diabetes.

So, what should you do?

- Strive to control your blood sugars!
- Brush your teeth at least twice daily, preferably with an electric toothbrush using ultrasound technology, for a full two minutes,

and then floss at least once per day, ideally twice a day. Using a Waterpik is equally good, and using toothpicks after meals is also beneficial.

- Use antibacterial mouthwash, either an herbal product or a typical one such as Listerine. Methyl salicylate is an ingredient in mouthwashes that can reduce plaque and gum disease by 75 percent.
- Suck on xylitol candies—xylitol, a safe sweetener for patients with diabetes, helps kill strep mutants, one of the main bacteria in the mouth that causes gum disease. I have a bowl of Dr. John's kosher xylitol sucking candies in my waiting room, and I encourage diabetic patients to order some for after meals, especially if they cannot brush or floss then. I like the kosher ones because the non-kosher xylitol candies from Dr. John's have artificial food colorings and flavors, but the kosher candies do not.
- Stop smoking.
- See your dentist as directed, but at least twice a year. Ideally, for patients with diabetes, seeing a dentist for a good cleaning is best three to four times a year.
- If your gums are sore or bleeding, make an immediate visit to your dentist.

Self-Monitoring of Blood Glucose

Self-monitoring of blood glucose (SMBG) is a vital component of monitoring diabetes. Pediatric T1DM patients can record glucose numbers up to ten times a day, for example (Medicare pays for two checks a day). While I recommend this to show patients their improvement and as an educational tool, one study has shown that SMBG can be depressing for some patients. If a patient's protocol is unable to help them attain their glucose level goals, and each glucose finger stick shows that their glucose numbers are too high, it can indeed be depressing. However, patients on a comprehensive integrative program tend to see their glucose numbers come down, so checking glucose becomes a positive task. It can also be educational, as the patient learns which foods maintain good glucose control and which do not.

I strongly encourage my patients to keep a diet diary and glucose graph and bring them to each visit. Without those tools, I cannot make the best treatment decisions on diet, supplements, exercise, medications, and other modalities.

Diet Diary

The diet diary, an example of which is in appendix B, relies on honesty and accuracy. It is not a tool of judgment, but a tool of education. Through a diet diary a well-trained, nutritionally focused physician can learn how the foods you are eating are affecting your glucose and your body organs and glands; what nutrients you are and are not ingesting; which foods you eat are pro-inflammatory and anti-inflammatory; which foods might cause negative reactions or sensitivities; and about your portion sizes. A physician can interpret food labels for you and teach you how food is helping or harming your health and your control of diabetes.

Filling out the diet diary enables your physician to interpret your initial diet and help you gently transition to a better one.

To keep a good diet diary you should do the following:

- Record everything you eat and drink for breakfast, lunch, supper, and snacks, including amounts.
- List the brand names of purchased foods.
- List the exact ingredients included in any home-prepared meals. For example, do not write "salad and casserole" but instead include all the veggies and amounts of veggies in the salad and the salad dressing and all the ingredients in the casserole. Or, bring in recipes.
- Record insulin injected before or after the meal—which type and how many units—if you are dosing insulin.
- List any physical, mental, or emotional symptoms you felt during the day and the times the symptoms occurred.
- Record your bowel movements and if they were regular, constipated, or diarrhea. A good daily bowel movement is necessary for full body health.

When starting out, my new patients keep a diet diary for a full week. After the second treatment visit, patients can choose to keep a diet diary for only the three days before each visit. I have been known to send patients home if they did not keep the diet diary or if they forgot it at home. It is that vital for me to see.

I suggest patients create an alert alarm days before their next scheduled office visit to start doing their diet diary. You can set up an alarm on your computer, cell phone, or tablet. Or, if you're low-tech, just write down the day you need to start your diet diary and put it up on your fridge. If you do not want to carry the paper diet diary paper with you, you can also do a diet diary on your phone with apps like Doctor's Diet Diary or Myfitnesspal, or on your computer, so you can easily email it to your doctor.

Glucose Graph

The glucose graph was initially developed by Dr. Richard Bernstein as a way to record blood sugars for his patients, but I adapted it and use it in a different way than he does to record valuable data. This form is in appendix C.

The glucose graph includes fields to record your glucose upon fasting/waking, after breakfast, before and after lunch, before and after supper, at bedtime, and also before, during, and after exercise. Your physician should instruct you when to record your glucose levels, but this is a typical methodology to use. Please note that for the purposes of this graph, "after meals" means one and a half hours after meals, which gives us a better view of the peak of your glucose rise after eating than measuring two hours after meals does.

When to record your glucose levels as a diabetic patient:

- If you are not on any insulin: upon fasting/waking, after breakfast, after lunch, and after supper.
- If you are only on long-acting insulin: upon fasting/waking, after breakfast, after lunch, after supper, and at bedtime.
- If you are on meal and long-acting insulin: upon fasting/waking, after breakfast, before and after lunch, before and after supper, and at bedtime.

Patients should also check if their glucose levels have a tendency to either lower or rise when they exercise. Some patients need to check their glucose levels in the middle of the night, for example if their nighttime insulin is increased or if they tend to have low levels during sleep.

KEY TREATMENT NOTE

Patients should check in the middle of the night (around 3 a.m.) for two or three nights after every single elevation dose change in long-acting insulin at night, to catch any low glucose level that might occur with the increase in insulin. If after two or three nights there is no low level, the patient can return to sleeping through the night.

Once your glucose levels are well controlled and stable, it is not necessary to check your glucose the maximum times listed above each day. Which checks you can avoid can be discussed with your physician, but we typically want at least a fasting glucose and a check after your bigger or more carbohydrate-heavy meal. Bedtime is common to analyze daily, too, if insulin is injected at night.

A medical practitioner who analyzes the diet and glucose graphs helps ensure the best treatment for the patient, especially if the patient is also taking medications. By analyzing this information, I know both how my patients are eating and how their glucose numbers are affected. This can be used to support and praise a patient eating on target who has improved or already has excellent glucose numbers, or to troubleshoot, encourage, and motivate a patient who is not yet following the program. It can also be used to see how all The Eight Essentials are working in tandem in the patient to get glucose numbers down to normal.

Glucose Meters

Since I am discussing the importance of recording your glucose levels, it seems pertinent to discuss glucose meters.

All diabetic patients need to have a glucose meter that can test their glucose levels. Glucose meters are not very expensive; your insurance should cover them, and there are coupons available for free ones. This is because glucose meter companies make their money on the test strips. I recommend getting a new glucose meter every three to five years. Check with your insurance company as to which ones they cover.

Most glucose meters do not need to be "coded" anymore, which is a great convenience, and you want to ensure your meter does not require coding. (If it does require coding, you have to code each new batch of glucose test strips to the meter instead of just opening up and using each batch.)

Name-brand glucose meters include Accu-Chek, OneTouch, Bayer, and FreeStyle. These will have the most expensive test strips—easily a dollar (or more!) per strip; however, most insurances will cover the cost of both the meter and test strips. For people paying out of pocket, less expensive generic meters can be purchased at most pharmacies. Often each strip for a generic brand only costs 30–40 cents.

It's important to make sure your meter is of good quality. You can test a meter's accuracy by checking your blood sugar twice, fifteen minutes apart; if the numbers are more than 20 mg/dL off, the meter is not accurate. That does not necessarily mean it is accurate if the numbers are 15 mg/dL off, either, but 20 mg/dL is the established threshold of accuracy. Obviously, the closer the two numbers are, the better!

There are two glucose meters available that also measure blood ketones: Nova Max Plus and Precision Xtra. These are for T1DM patients. The vast majority of T1DM patients do not need to have meters that measure both glucose and ketones, but for those who have had many struggles with highs and lows, particularly with high glucose numbers, one of these meters might be beneficial to purchase. Bayer has come out with the first glucose meter with a USB port, so you can connect your meter to your computer and print out test results. It is called the Ascensia Contour or Contour NEXT USB meter. That is a nifty innovation, and I imagine other such meters will follow.

Along with a glucose meter and test strips, you also need lancets. You need to match the lancets to the type of lancing device used with your meter. It is not uncommon for many diabetic patients to put a new lancet in the meter in the morning and use it all day long for their glucose tests. That is fine as long as you do not share your lancet with anyone else, but remember that the more you use any needle, the duller (and more painful) it can get. The lancet devices rated the least painful are Bayer and Accu-Chek brands. If you wish to change your lancet with each glucose test, they are very inexpensive to buy.

Another lancet worth mentioning is the Genteel Lancet. Slightly larger than other lancets, the Genteel Lancet uses vibration, depth control, and a vacuum to reduce the pain of drawing blood both from fingers and in alternate sites. The vibration numbs the nerves, the depth ensures the needle reaches a capillary but not nerves, and the vacuum draws up enough blood to test in between two and eight seconds. It is a more involved process, but one that is easily learned, and for those patients who struggle with measuring their glucose many times a day it can be a real winner, especially for pediatric patients.

Lancet devices have various depths, typically using the lowest depth setting for children, and higher depth settings for adults. Historically, lancet devices have always been used on the tip of a finger, one of the most sensitive areas of our body. Now, most meters allow patients to do "alternate site testing," which means drawing blood from other areas, usually the forearm, upper arm, thumb pad, palm/sides of palm, calf, thigh, or abdomen. However, most people use the forearm, palm, or thigh.

The benefit of alternate site testing for many people is that they experience less pain when testing their glucose level. This is helpful especially for those who have to test their glucose level many times throughout the day. However, there are also cons to alternate site testing, because the glucose level from those areas will be about fifteen minutes behind the glucose level in your fingertips; it's not a good idea to use alternate sites if your glucose numbers are dropping or rising dramatically and you want to know where the glucose number is *right now*. In those cases you should use your fingertips. You should also not test alternate sites if you feel "low" or are about to go driving, if you have what is called "hypoglycemic unawareness," if you are exercising, right after insulin injections, or if you are ill and feverish. However, during the typical day, or after a meal, alternate site testing is a valid way to test your glucose level.

Here is the methodology for using alternate site testing:

1. Use the clear tip that came with your glucose meter and a fresh lancet that is sharp.
2. Use a deep depth setting in most circumstances.
3. Massage the area you are going to use.
4. After you inject the lancet, do not remove the device until you see there is enough blood for a test.
5. When there is enough blood, remove the device and use your glucose strip as normal.

— CHAPTER FOUR —

Lab Work

Integrative physicians use many different tests to analyze a person whom we are first diagnosing with diabetes and then to keep checking to ensure improvement is occurring and glucose numbers are getting under control. And there are other labs we measure when checking for general health guidelines. It is important for your blood work to be fully analyzed when you have diabetes.

Glucose

When testing for diabetes, glucose levels are measured while fasting, one and a half to two hours after eating, and at random.

When fasting, glucose levels should be between 75 and 85 mg/dL. Results of 100 to 125 mg/dL indicate the patient is prediabetic, while levels equal to or higher than 126 mg/dL are considered a diagnosis for diabetes.

Healthy postprandial (two hours after eating) levels are below 120 mg/dL; between 140 and 199 mg/dL are prediabetic; and levels equal to or higher than 200 mg/dL are a diagnosis for diabetes.

NOTE: Internationally, other countries use mmol/L instead of the American mg/dL for their glucose levels in lab work. When American glucose numbers are listed, Canadians can divide by 18 to get the mmol/L equivalent.

Medically, it is recommended that random levels should be tested at least two times for formal diagnosis unless the glucose is significantly elevated, such as at a level higher than 250 mg/dL, in which case a patient can be diagnosed right then and there as diabetic. In reality, if a person is walking around with glucose equal to or higher than 200 mg/dL at any time, I will diagnose them as having diabetes.

Table 4.1. A1C Levels and Their eAG Equivalents

A1C	eAG	A1C	eAG	A1C	eAG	A1C	eAG	A1C	eAG
4.0	68	6.0	125	8.0	183	10.0	240	12.0	298
4.1	71	6.1	128	8.1	186	10.1	243	12.1	301
4.2	74	6.2	131	8.2	189	10.2	246	12.2	303
4.3	77	6.3	134	8.3	192	10.3	249	12.3	306
4.4	80	6.4	137	8.4	194	10.4	252	12.4	309
4.5	82	6.5	140	8.5	197	10.5	255	12.5	312
4.6	85	6.6	143	8.6	200	10.6	258	12.6	315
4.7	88	6.7	146	8.7	203	10.7	260	12.7	318
4.8	91	6.8	148	8.8	206	10.8	263	12.8	321
4.9	94	6.9	151	8.9	209	10.9	266	12.9	324
5.0	97	7.0	154	9.0	212	11.0	269	13.0	326
5.1	100	7.1	157	9.1	214	11.1	272	13.1	329
5.2	103	7.2	160	9.2	217	11.2	275	13.2	332
5.3	105	7.3	163	9.3	220	11.3	278	13.3	335
5.4	108	7.4	166	9.4	223	11.4	280	13.4	338
5.5	111	7.5	169	9.5	226	11.5	283	13.5	341
5.6	114	7.6	171	9.6	229	11.6	286	13.6	344
5.7	117	7.7	174	9.7	232	11.7	289	13.8	346
5.8	120	7.8	177	9.8	235	11.8	292	13.8	349
5.9	123	7.9	180	9.9	237	11.9	295	13.9	352

For managing a patient who is already diagnosed with diabetes, goals are as follows: For fasting glucose, values should ideally be between 70 and 100 mg/dL, and for postprandial glucose, values should ideally be lower than 120 mg/dL.

Glycosylated Hemoglobin A1C (HbA1C or just A1C for short)

This lab value measures the percentage of hemoglobin proteins on red blood cells covered by glucose. The hemoglobin A1C score is the key monitoring tool for glucose regulation. It measures where the glucose levels in the patient have been on average, twenty-four hours a day, for the last three months, as that is the typical life span of a red blood cell.

What is a normal A1C? The normal, nondiabetic A1C percentage is 4.6–5.1 percent; that is, in a person without diabetes, on average, only about 5 percent of their red blood cells are covered in sugar. The A1C is then translated into the eAG, or estimated average glucose. An A1C of 5.0 percent has an eAG of 100 mg/dL. That means that a person without diabetes or insulin resistance has their blood sugar level sink, for example, to 80 mg/dL when they wake up in the morning, and has their blood sugar level rise to 120 mg/dL after meals. 80–120 mg/dL averages out to 100 mg/dL; the A1C of 5 percent (in general medical usage we often do not use the percent mark). Table 4.1 shows A1C levels and their eAG equivalents.

Since the A1C is the average, that means that if your A1C is 7.5 percent, and the eAG is 169, half your glucose numbers are below 169 and half are above.

One problem with A1C values is interpretation. A patient may have an A1C of 6.0 percent (eAG 126 mg/dL), for example, if the patient's glucose levels are in any of the following ranges:

40–212 mg/dL
80–160 mg/dL
100–145 mg/dL

The A1C is a helpful diagnostic and monitoring tool, but it has limitations in the analysis. A person may have a low A1C because they have a lot

Table 4.2. Glucose Status Based on A1C Levels

A1C Percentage	Definition
< 5.7	Normal
5.7–6.4	Prediabetic
≥ 6.5	Diabetic

of hypoglycemic episodes, dragging their A1Cs down, but not because of good, safe, stable glucose control. If your blood sugars go dangerously low frequently, your A1C will be low, but that is not a safe or pleasant way to be a diabetic patient.

In one study, A1C was analyzed to see if it was more reflective of fasting glucose or postprandial glucose. The conclusions were that if the A1C is less than 7.3, it seems to indicate more postprandial glucose, but if the A1C is more than 10.2, it seems split, with around 70 percent related to fasting glucose numbers and around 30 percent related to postprandial glucose. So, it's not wholly clear what particular types of glucose readings A1C defines.

How does this all apply in clinical medicine? Table 4.2 shows in a simple way that physicians typically analyze a patient's glucose status based on their A1C levels.

The American Diabetes Association allows diagnosing a patient with diabetes solely off an A1C that is higher than or equal to 6.5 percent. The two organizations representing endocrinologists disagree. The American Association of Clinical Endocrinologists (AACE) and the American College of Endocrinology (ACE) both recommend ensuring glucose levels are drawn for verification. I agree with the endocrinologists.

There is another huge concern using those definitions. Many patients who fall within a prediabetic level are not aggressively and medically treated as developing a potentially life-threatening condition; often I've heard prediabetic patients report that they were told their glucose levels would be addressed once they became a diabetic, and that they were doing fine until

Table 4.3. Target A1C Ranges according to ADA and AACE

	Accepted A1C Percentage Range Adults	Ideal A1C Percentage Range Adults	Accepted A1C Percentage Range Pediatrics
ADA	< 7.0	< 6.5 (without hypoglycemia)	< 7.5
AACE	< 6.5	< 6.5	< 6.5

their A1C reached 6.5 percent. All prediabetic patients should be treated with a comprehensive integrative protocol to reverse their condition and ensure they never develop full diabetes! Unfortunately, as I will discuss further in this chapter, damage to the human body begins with an A1C higher than 5.5 percent, which is 0.2 points below even being diagnosed as a prediabetic.

What about after one is diagnosed as a diabetic patient? What is the best A1C score to achieve? Table 4.3 shows recommended diabetic glucose goals.

The AACE's 2015 recommendations also suggest that a less stringent A1C goal of 7–8 percent should be considered for patients with a history of severe low blood sugar, limited life expectancy, advanced renal or cardiovascular disease, who are dealing with other medical conditions, or who have long-standing diabetes in which the A1C goal has been difficult to attain, as long as the patient is not suffering from overt symptoms of high blood glucose. Pregnant women should have an A1C that is lower than 6.0 percent.

There are some real problems with these conventional recommendations. First, of course, they are based mostly on eating higher carbohydrate diets and using medications for the main treatment. As a result, it can indeed be difficult to decrease glucose levels substantially and have lower A1C values. And, in reality, the majority of people with diabetes in the United States do not have very good control of their glucose.

What are the real A1C values of Americans with diabetes? Table 4.4 shows A1C values for Americans from 2003 to 2006, the latest records accumulated by the CDC.

This means that in the most recent analysis of A1Cs in diabetic patients in the United States, only 23 percent of patients had an A1C value less than

Table 4.4. A1C Values by Percentage of the Population with Diabetes

A1C Value (%)	Population (%)
< 6.0	23
6.0–6.9	34
7.0–7.9	20
8.0–9.0	10
> 9.0	13

Source: http://www.cdc.gov/diabetes/statistics/a1c/a1c_dist.htm

6.0 percent, still a high number compared to nondiabetic people, while 43 percent of patients, nearly half of all diabetic patients, had A1Cs of 7.0 percent or higher, setting them up to develop diabetic complications. Conventional treatment of diabetes does not seem very effective overall if you go by these numbers.

The key information to know is that A1Cs have to be much lower than even the ADA or AACE organizations recommend in order to best protect diabetic patients from damaging their bodies and developing complications. If a person without diabetes has an A1C of 4.8–5.1 percent and does not develop diabetic complications, it makes sense to strive to have patients with diabetes have A1C scores as low as patients without diabetes.

Recent studies have shown that an A1C higher than 5.5 percent begins to cause damage to the human body. Brohall, Oden, et al., reported on research in their paper "Glucose Control and Vascular Complications in Veterans with Type 2 Diabetes," which showed that having an A1C between 5.5 percent and 6.4 percent caused damaged to the vascular endothelium—the lining of the blood vessels; so, even prediabetic A1Cs can cause damage to the body. Another study confirmed that an A1C above 5.5 percent increases risk of developing diabetic retinopathy, and a third showed an A1C higher than 6.0 percent increased the risk of diabetic nephropathy. Other studies have shown that there is damage to the body when glucose levels go above 140 mg/dL.

Lowering A1C to as close to a nondiabetic's level as possible is imperative. It is good if the patient has lower than 6.0 percent, excellent if lower than 5.5 percent, and ideal if around 5.0 percent. Science supports that lower A1Cs mean considerable reductions in comorbidity complications of diabetes. I am delighted when a diabetic patient of mine has an A1C between 5.0 percent and 5.5 percent, and even less than 6.0 percent is good.

While some physicians desire their patients to be under 5.0 percent, that is a very strict level that the vast majority of patients with diabetes will not be able to achieve consistently. A few physicians who have a much stricter belief in normal blood sugars believe that a nondiabetic A1C is 4.2–4.6 percent, and glucose values should be between 72–86 mg/dL. I find this too strict and do not believe nondiabetic patients walk around with numbers that low all the time; at least, I have not seen it in my practice, or even in myself!

If patients can achieve A1Cs lower than 5.0 percent, that's fine, and some of my patients do, but I have not seen studies showing that having an A1C of 4.8 percent is less damaging than one of 5.2 percent. I also don't want patients to feel like failures when they have achieved a wonderful A1C of 5.3 percent, say, but their physician demands they achieve even a lower A1C. I believe that patients with A1Cs between 5.0 percent and 6.0 percent who are eating well and taking protective supplements can do fine, and that is what I have seen over the last twenty-five years.

So, putting all these studies together, why do the ADA and AACE organizations set guidelines for A1Cs to be significantly higher? Unfortunately, a study called ACCORD that was published a few years ago showed that using aggressive diabetes treatment with older patients who had cardiac disease caused significant congestive heart failure and death. Why did many people die in the ACCORD study? In my opinion, the answer is pretty clear. In this study, numerous medications were prescribed to seniors to push their glucose levels down into good control, that is, in order to have their A1Cs under 6.5 percent. However, the problem is they used metformin, thiazolidinediones, sulfonylureas, and insulin in the study, all drugs that cause weight gain and edema (all of these are discussed in chapter 5).

As a result, as you might imagine, the seniors with diabetes in the aggressive control group had a tendency to develop edema, gain weight, and, as they were older and already had heart disease, they developed congestive heart failure and many of them died. The study was ended early due to the deaths.

As a result of that study, many of my patients are told by their physicians that an A1C lower than 6.5 percent is bad for their hearts. I've even had physicians tell patients to eat more carbohydrates and raise their A1C when their A1C was lower than 6.0 percent! That is a *very unhelpful* recommendation to patients with diabetes.

Another reason standard care physicians, particularly endocrinologists, would prefer patients to have higher rather than lower A1Cs is due to malpractice risks. It takes a lot of time and focus to work with patients with diabetes, especially those on insulin or on oral medications that can more easily cause hypoglycemia. Most of those physicians do not have the time to deal with patients, given they are supposed to see thirty to forty patients a day. Also, conventional care based on A1C allows patients to have higher glucose and higher A1Cs, as the development of devastating diabetic complications is considered to be a natural part of the disease. Thus, if a patient is on medications but their diabetes is poorly controlled, they have a high A1C, and the physician is treating the patient along American Diabetes Association guidelines, they are protected from malpractice suits. If the physician got more aggressive and wanted to have lower A1Cs than standard care suggests, and the patient had a serious low, the physician would be at risk for a lawsuit. In standard care, being "more aggressive" would mean using stronger doses of medications and more medications, not comprehensive integrative care. So, naturally, but sadly, physicians run their practices worried that pushing A1Cs down to normal physiological levels, allowing patients to establish excellent control, may cause legal difficulties.

Luckily, there are physicians with integrative protocols who spend more time with patients to allow much better control and much lower A1Cs. It is very important for every patient to know what an A1C is and what it means. It is best to have a physician who will go over all your blood work with you, explaining clearly all your lab results, and who is open to developing a more comprehensive treatment regimen than simply prescribing more and more medications.

Having a low A1C, into the range of people who do not have diabetes, is the goal of diabetes treatment, without the level being reached via frequent hypoglycemic events. Please ensure your physician is in agreement with this target, as having the support of your physician will make your progress and control so much easier to reach.

Analyzing A1Cs can be a little inaccurate due to lab inaccuracies. Labs have a 0.5 variance, which means that if your A1C comes back at 6.0 percent, it may in reality be anywhere from 5.5 percent to 6.5 percent.

It's important to note that some populations may have natural discrepancies with A1C readings. The normal hemoglobin in our bodies is hemoglobin A, or HbA. Some people, particularly African Americans and those of

Mediterranean descent, can have hemoglobin variants—their bodies make other forms of hemoglobin. Those variants include HbC, HbE, HbSC, and HbF, all of which may interfere with accurate readings of an A1C.

You should be concerned you may have a hemoglobinopathy if:

- You belong to an ethnic group that produces other A1Cs.
- Your A1C is different than expected.
- Your A1C does not match self-monitoring of glucose.
- Your A1C is greater than 15.
- Your A1C is radically different from a previous A1C result after there is a change in laboratory methodology.

Also, in general, iron anemia can artificially raise A1Cs, while heavy bleeding and kidney failure can artificially lower it. Liver disease can also affect A1Cs. If the A1C test may not be accurate for you, consider having a fructosamine test, also known as a glycated serum protein or glycated albumin. While fructosamine is a valid test, it does have two drawbacks. First, it only shows the average serum glucose for the last two to three weeks (unlike the A1C, which shows the last two to three months). Second, it is not standardized, so we cannot translate the fructosamine score into an average glucose number—we can only learn if your glucose as a general rule was low, normal, or high. I do not use the fructosamine test unless I am concerned there is hemoglobinopathy occurring in a patient.

A hemoglobin A1C can also increase normally as we age. If a senior who is over seventy years old has a slightly elevated A1C but is normal weight, has normal fasting and postprandial glucose, and has an acceptable diet, the A1C may be a sign of natural aging.

Your A1C should be drawn every three months until your A1C is low, stable, and consistent. If your diabetes is very well controlled and you are following your comprehensive protocol, then your A1C can be drawn every six months to yearly.

To summarize, the A1C is the key monitoring lab for understanding how well a patient is controlling their diabetes. Numerous studies show that an A1C over 5.5 percent indicates a patient is at risk of developing damage to their body from elevated glucose levels. It is important to work with a physician who agrees with you about lowering your A1C in a comprehensive regimen that does not depend solely on using medications.

KEY TREATMENT NOTE

Do you know your A1C? Is your A1C less than 6.0 percent? If your A1C is higher than 6.0 percent, or if it is in the 5 percent range but is low only due to frequent low blood sugar events, you might wish to investigate a more comprehensive treatment protocol for your diabetes.

Complete Blood Count (CBC)

This is part of a yearly blood work panel, showing your red blood cells and white immune cells—how many you have and what types are present. We can discern iron anemia, find clues about vitamin B_{12} and folic acid deficiency, and get indications about allergic reactions and infections. Since metformin, the number one prescribed oral medication for diabetes, has been shown in studies to be a significant risk factor for becoming deficient in vitamin B_{12} or folic acid, it is important to check labs to make sure this is not occurring.

However, if I really am concerned that a patient has low vitamin B_{12} or folic acid due to their symptom presentation, I will follow up with serum B_{12} and serum or red blood cell folate, methylmalonic acid, and homocysteine. With those four labs, a physician can have an excellent idea of vitamin B_{12} and folate status. However, your physician should not test only serum B_{12} and folic acid, as the results of these labs are incredibly inaccurate in diagnosing many cases of deficiency.

I draw a CBC once every year, and more frequently if there is a history of imbalance in order to ensure that the condition has resolved.

Comprehensive Metabolic Panel (CMP)

This panel shows us information on liver and kidney function, electrolytes, serum calcium, protein components, and glucose. Let's discuss some of this panel's individual components.

Kidney Panel

The kidneys are the body's blood filters. They contain around one million tiny filters, called glomeruli, which are made up of clusters of blood vessels. We can check kidney function by estimating how much blood the glomeruli filter in a minute. This kidney test should be drawn at least once per year.

Serum creatinine is a breakdown product of creatinine phosphate in the muscle and is usually broken down at a fairly steady rate. It is a very important lab reading for kidney function because it is excreted unchanged by the kidneys. Therefore, if creatinine elevates in the blood, this shows the kidneys are failing. Serum creatinine is used to create the glomerular filtration rate (eGFR). The eGFR is now generally included in all lab results of creatinine, giving more data on kidney health. Serum creatinine is paired on lab forms with blood urea nitrogen (BUN), and if both are elevated it is of serious concern.

Kidney disease is present when creatinine is elevated, BUN is elevated, and the eGFR is lower than 60 ml/min. However, seniors may have lowered eGFR due to age, so eGFR is not always a good reflection of kidney health on its own for someone sixty-five or older.

A physician can also do a twenty-four-hour urine collection to analyze creatinine, also called a creatinine clearance test. In this test the volume of blood plasma that is cleared of creatinine per twenty-four hours is analyzed. This test is not common, but it is not unusual either.

Your physician may likely refer you to a nephrologist, a kidney specialist, if kidney lab values are problematic or worsening.

While not part of the CMP, the random microalbuminuria test, which compares the amount of albumin in the urine to the concentration of creatinine, is the best, earliest test to uncover kidney disease; it is covered in detail in chapter 14.

Liver Panel

In analyzing liver health, we are particularly interested in these three lab values:

AST—aspartate aminotransferase
ALT—alanine aminotransferase
GGT—gamma-glutamyl transferase

In particular, when looking at liver labs, we are seeking to uncover if a liver has extra fat stored in it, a condition known as fatty liver. Since the majority of obese people have livers with excess fat stored in them, monitoring liver health is an important task for your physician, as a fatty liver is a serious diabetic complication.

GGT elevation signifies many possible situations, including an increased risk of cardiovascular disease and liver disease, and possibly alcoholism. However, in diabetic patients, it is most associated with fatty liver disease, and if your blood work shows elevated GGT with or without any other liver enzymes elevated, you should have an abdominal ultrasound to help diagnose a fatty liver. Fatty liver is a common reason GGT is elevated in T2DM patients.

If ALT and AST are elevated, either your physician or a gastroenterologist or a hepatologist (liver specialist) should do a further workup, especially if the ultrasound does not show a fatty liver. Elevated ALT and AST *with* fatty liver can mean you have nonalcoholic steatohepatitis, or NASH, which is when the fatty liver becomes inflamed and can cause serious damage over time if the inflammation is not reduced. I discuss fatty liver and NASH indepth in chapter 14.

Elevated ALT and AST can also indicate that a different liver disease is manifesting or that a medication or supplement is aggravating the liver.

I check liver enzymes at least once per year. However, if the liver enzymes are elevated, the specific medical reason needs to be discerned. If it is due to fatty liver, I draw liver enzymes every three to six months to monitor.

Lipid Panel

A basic lipid panel looks at cholesterol, triglycerides, HDL ("good" cholesterol), LDL ("bad" cholesterol), and chol/HDL ratio to uncover the risk of cardiovascular disease. We often see these results outside the normal reference ranges in patients with diabetes, which is another reason they may be at a higher risk for having a heart attack or stroke. Let's discuss these labs briefly.

Triglycerides (fatty acids). Normal is less than 100 mg/dL. Triglycerides (TG) are usually elevated in diabetic patients because this is usually more a reflection of carbohydrate intake than of fat intake. I've seen triglycerides drop from 688 to 88 in three months with just a change to a low carb diet. TG/HDL ratio is another way of assessing insulin resistance: TG/HDL ratio greater than 3 indicates insulin resistance.

HDL—high density lipoprotein ("good" cholesterol—takes cholesterol to the liver for processing). Normal is lower than 40 mg/dL. HDL is raised mostly by exercise, so it is typically low in patients with diabetes who do not have a solid exercise regimen.

LDL—low density lipoprotein ("bad" cholesterol—takes cholesterol from the liver into the blood where it can begin forming atherosclerotic plaques). Normal is lower than 100 mg/dL, or even lower than 70 mg/dL in some populations. LDL is typically elevated in patients with poorly controlled diabetes.

Cholesterol. Normal is lower than 200 mg/dL, or even lower than 170 mg/dL in some populations. Total cholesterol is usually high in patients with uncontrolled diabetes.

In the section on medications, I'll discuss cholesterol again when I discuss statin drugs.

I draw basic lipid labs at least once per year. If I am working to lower them substantially, I may draw them every three months. In addition, there are other more specific blood work tests for cardiovascular risk done by specialty labs. When I am really concerned about my patient's risk of cardiovascular disease due to family history, heart attack or stroke, poor lifestyle, high blood pressure, tobacco use, T2DM, abnormal lipid/cholesterol panel, or a patient desires to gather all the data they need to help them commit to and maintain a healthy protocol, I do an extensive panel through a specialty lab. The following are a few of the key specialty tests on that comprehensive panel:

LDL-p—particle number. Clinically, the number of LDL particles is more important than how much cholesterol it contains. The lower the particles, the less your risk of cardiovascular disease. The ideal goal for LDL-p is less than 1,000 nmol/L.

Apo-lipoprotein b. This lab is a good measure of circulating LDL-p concentration and a more reliable indicator of cardiovascular disease risk than basic LDL.

Lipoprotein a. Elevated lipoprotein a is a genetic risk for cardiovascular disease.

HDL density and size and LDL density and size. It's best to have many larger HDL particles, and few larger LDL particles, as both are associated with less cardiovascular disease.

APOE gene. There are three alleles (manifestations) of the APOE gene: E2/3/4. APOE2/E2 may increase the risk of early heart disease and is associated with increased triglycerides and a higher risk of premature vascular disease. APOE4/E4 or E4/E3, found in one out of four people, is associated with an increased risk of atherosclerosis and increased LDL-C cholesterol and triglycerides. APOE3/E3 is the most common gene presentation and is associated with normal lipid metabolism. Having an APOE4/E4 gene mutation and uncontrolled T2DM puts a person at significant risk for cardiovascular disease. Extra cardiac care should be added to the comprehensive protocol.

Essential fatty acids. Levels of omega-3 and omega-6 in cells.

Fibrinogen. Elevated levels show the patient is at a higher risk of developing a blood clot.

High sensitivity c-reactive protein (HS-CRP). HS-CRP is a nonspecific lab showing if there is inflammation or injury in the body. If there is no medical reason—such as a known inflammatory condition occurring—elevated HS-CRP is a notable factor for increased risk of cardiovascular disease.

Serum Ferritin

Serum ferritin is the most common lab result that shows a patient has fatty liver. Serum ferritin is stored iron; when it is elevated it can mean one of three things.

Hemochromatosis. This is a genetic disease found in around 2 percent of the population whereby the patient absorbs much more iron than normal. Iron is stored in the liver and other body organs and tissues. If you have high ferritin, your physician should right away do an iron panel to see if you have hemochromatosis. If you do, you will need to be referred to a hematologist, a physician who specializes in blood conditions, for regular blood draws.

Serious bacterial infection. Ferritin can be elevated if a serious bacterial infection exists somewhere in a person's body.

Acute phase marker. Ferritin is also elevated as "an acute phase marker"—that is, due to inflammation. It is very likely that if you are an abdominally overweight T2DM patient and your ferritin is elevated, you have fatty liver, which is inflammatory to the liver. Your physician, after ruling out hemochromatosis, should refer you for an abdominal ultrasound to see if fatty liver can be discerned, which it usually is. Elevated ferritin is more common than elevated GGT or other liver enzymes showing fatty liver is present.

If ferritin is low, it is the first indication in lab work, before it shows up in a CBC, that a patient is developing iron deficiency anemia. However, most of my T2DM patients have elevated ferritin.

It is always good to catch any developing condition as soon as possible. I am not sure why most conventional care physicians do not include ferritin in their usual blood work screens. I draw ferritin levels at least once a year. If ferritin is elevated, and the patient has fatty liver, I will draw ferritin every three months to see if the levels are reducing with our protocol and supplements. I'll redo the abdominal ultrasound after significant weight loss has occurred, to once again measure the presence of fat in the liver.

Fasting Insulin Levels

A "normal" fasting level is lower than or equal to 17 uIU/mL. Integrative medical practitioners do not agree with that reference range. I feel a fasting insulin level should be lower than 9 uIU/mL, and ideally it should be lower than 6 uIU/mL. Having a lower insulin level means you are more sensitive to insulin and so need to secrete only minimal amounts from your pancreas to process your meal and keep your glucose levels within normal limits.

Unfortunately, laboratory values of some tests are not strict enough to ensure patients are tightly controlled. It is surprising how some lab values are established by our main laboratories. I called a major United States lab one day to ask them why their postprandial (after eating) insulin lab value was considered "normal" if it was lower than 89 uIU/mL. In most medical studies I've read, the general guideline for illustrating insulin resistance at postprandial levels is 30–33 uIU/mL. The lab manager told me they established the lab value by simply testing fifty of their "normal" employees—by having them fast, drink Glucola (a pure glucose drink), and then measure their insulin levels two hours later—and the range they saw was up to 89 uIU/mL. That is how millions of patients are now being judged; by fifty "normal" people who worked at this laboratory!

So, in this book I will be focusing on where integrative physicians who have a strong clinical practice in diabetes desire labs to be in order to maximize patient health.

In summary, healthy, ideal fasting insulin levels are lower than 6 uIU/mL. Ideal postprandial insulin secretion levels are lower than 30 uIU/ml (the lower the better). With regard to diabetes, typical presentation of fasting insulin values are low to none for T1DM. With T2DM, values may be elevated at first, showing strong insulin resistance, but can become low or none over the years if the person is very poorly controlled, suffers pancreatic damage, fails to produce normal insulin levels, and develops a need for insulin injections.

As soon as someone injects insulin, whether their diabetes is Type 1, Type 2, or LADA, the person develops insulin antibodies, and that makes insulin tests inaccurate. That's when a physician should start drawing c-peptide.

Serum C-Peptide

Insulin is a curlicue shaped molecule, and it is composed of different peptides. C-peptide is the last peptide that comes off the molecule to make insulin. For every one molecule of insulin, there is a molecule of c-peptide.

A person can develop insulin antibodies, whether it is part of her T1DM or if she has ever injected insulin into herself, as noted above. Those antibodies attack and destroy insulin, so in those cases measuring insulin status may not be accurate. However, we never make antibodies to c-peptide, so c-peptide will always be an accurate guide for how much insulin your pancreas is making.

C-peptide below 1.0 ng/mL is a sign you'll likely need to start injecting background insulin, and near or lower than 0.5 ng/mL means you'll likely need full insulin dosing, both background and for meals. As with insulin, c-peptide may be elevated in some T2DM patients, because they are insulin resistant and have to produce excessive insulin in an attempt to lower their glucose levels.

When do we draw c-peptide? We do not draw c-peptide to diagnose diabetes. If you are a T2DM patient with elevated glucose numbers and you are not on insulin, or you are just on long-acting insulin, ask your physician to check your c-peptide numbers. Low c-peptide numbers may mean a T2DM patient needs to start insulin, or needs to add more insulin or add in mealtime insulin, if glucose is not under good control with a comprehensive protocol and it looks like the pancreas is failing to secrete effective amounts of insulin. If c-peptide is high, the patient is still very insulin resistant. If a T2DM patient on insulin has high c-peptide, there is a good chance that over time, with weight loss and following a comprehensive integrative protocol, they may decrease or even stop taking the insulin, as their pancreas is still very functional. We can never promise a T2DM patient that will happen, but it is a real possibility.

In established T1DM patients already on background and meal insulin, it is probably not helpful or necessary to check their c-peptide—usually c-peptive levels are very low—but many patients are interested in learning how their pancreas is functioning. In newly diagnosed T1DM patients, we can use c-peptide to keep an eye on honeymoon periods, and also at times we see c-peptide elevate, showing recovery of some pancreatic beta cells.

We can also measure c-peptide postprandially, after meals, which will tell us how much insulin the patient is producing after he eats. C-peptide can be a helpful tool for analyzing pancreatic beta cell function.

Fructosamine

Fructosamine is a glycated molecule of serum proteins, mostly albumin. I am not much of a fan of fructosamine for the drawbacks mentioned above in the A1C section. I only draw fructosamine if someone has a hemoglobinopathy, and therefore measuring the hemoglobin A1C is not accurate. I might also draw it if a patient needs positive feedback right away that my diabetic protocol is working for him; he needs to see results in weeks, not wait three months. The problem is, of course, it usually takes three months to show an amazing improvement in labs. As a result, I do not feel this test is overall a useful tool.

GlycoMark

GlycoMark is not yet a well-known test. As I've said, A1C can be high due to fasting or after-meal glucose. Sometimes it is hard to know what is most affecting A1C, and glucose variability can inhibit good control. The GlycoMark test is designed to help physicians determine if after-meal glucose regulation is good or not.

The GlycoMark test measures 1, 5-anhydroglucitol (1, 5-AG), which is found in foods including bread, rice, pork, beef, tea, and soy products. When serum glucose is well controlled, most 1, 5-AG is reabsorbed by the kidneys, and our serum levels stay in a high range. Nondiabetic patients have 1, 5-AG readings above 20 mg/mL.

The GlycoMark test measures the last two weeks of glucose control. It measures the average maximum glucose levels you've had, and usually that relates to after eating.

When hyperglycemia occurs, excess serum glucose prevents the renal reabsorption of 1, 5-AG, and so it is lost in the urine. Every time your glucose goes over 180 mg/dL, the body loses more 1, 5-AG. The GlycoMark test shows what types of elevated glucose levels you've had over the last two to three weeks. The peaks may be due to after-meal spikes, stress, sickness, low exercise, or, of course, not enough insulin, if you are injecting it (see table 4.5 for GlycoMark scores and their associated glucose values).

The lower the GlycoMark score, the higher the average daily peak glucose was for you during the last two weeks.

Table 4.5. GlycoMark Results and Associated Glucose Values

GlycoMark Score mg/mL	2	3	4	5	6	7	8	9	10	11	12	13
Glucose Value mg/dL	> 290	248	225	212	203	196	191	186	184	182	180	< 180

GlycoMark scores from 2 (or lower) to 6 mean that glucose spikes over 180 mg/dL occur daily or very frequently; scores between 7 and 9 mean that glucose spikes over 180 mg/dL occur frequently; between 10 and 13 mean that glucose spikes over 180 mg/dL occur occasionally; and scores over 13 mean that glucose spikes over 180 mg/dL occur rarely. To be honest, I'm not sure I agree with that rating system, as the glucose values do not quite play out accurately with my patients—that is, with their glucose graph recording and their A1Cs—but I do believe the GlycoMark test is helpful in showing the reality of glucose elevations.

If the A1C is high but GlycoMark is also high, the patient rarely has glycemic excursions over 180 mg/dL. I look at baseline insulin dosing and investigate the patient's diet and exercise regimen. If the A1C is high and GlycoMark is low, the patient has frequent glycemic excursions over 180 mg/dL. I check to see if the patient has been ill, has run out of medication, got a cortisone injection, or got off their treatment protocol. I ensure the patient has no advanced kidney or liver condition. And, I check to see if mealtime insulin is required.

The GlycoMark test is not affected by hemoglobinopathies or by other labs, such as triglycerides, glucose, uric acid, or creatinine. It can be used to help diagnose certain types of MODY. Here is what can affect the accuracy of the GlycoMark score:

- Advanced kidney disease
- Advanced liver cirrhosis (GlycoMark might be artificially low)
- Pregnancy (GlycoMark might be artificially low)
- Reduced food absorption (after gastrectomy or on the drug acarbose) (GlycoMark might be artificially low)
- Persistently positive urine glucose levels in some kidney conditions or patients on SGLT2 inhibitors (GlycoMark might be artificially low)
- Steroid use (GlycoMark might be artificially low)
- Hyperalimentation and some Chinese medications (*Polygala tenuifolia*, senega syrup) (GlycoMark might be artificially high)

I have spoken to the company and received studies from them showing that GlycoMark is an accurate test in pediatric patients, although the

KEY TREATMENT NOTE

I feel a GlycoMark test is helpful for analyzing recent glycemic control, especially after meals.

reference ranges listed on labs are standardized only for adults. I run the GlycoMark test whenever I run an A1C.

Vitamin D_3

Vitamin D_3 (serum 25, OH cholecalciferol) is a very important nutrient for everyone, diabetic patients included. It is synthesized in the skin when the skin is exposed to the sun, and it is also found in a few foods: oily fish and fortified foods such as milk, nondairy milk alternatives, orange juice, egg yolks, and cheeses. Vitamin D_3 is deficient in many people due to lack of exposure to sunlight, and people do not get a lot of vitamin D_3 from foods.

It is important to know a patient's serum vitamin D_3; I do not draw for 1, 25, OH-cholesterol—it is not the lab test of vitamin D_3 that's helpful.

The societal idea that the sun is a huge cancer-causing ball in the sky is something I have always disagreed with. Vitamin D_3 is, first of all, an extremely anticarcinogenic nutrient, and being deficient in it increases one's risk to develop many different types of cancer. The UV rays of the sun can indeed cause oxidative damage to our DNA, and that damage can cause changes that lead toward skin cancer, but the earth also produces a bounty of vegetables and fruits, full of *anti*oxidants, with the help of the sun's energy. If people avoid drinking soda pop and eating cookies and cakes, heavily grilled meats, ice cream, and so on during the summer (i.e., avoid doing more oxidative damage to their bodies), and instead go outside and get exposed to reasonable amounts of sunlight, eat numerous daily servings of fresh vegetables and fruits, and take some oral antioxidant supplements, their bodies can more effectively protect them from skin cancer. Typical sunscreens can contain problematic chemicals; sunscreens using topical antioxidants, such as vitamins C and E, and selenium, are shown to be protective and safe.

In the sunny months of spring and summer, light-skinned people need to be in the sun for only around twenty minutes between the hours of 10 a.m. and 2 p.m. to make all the vitamin D_3 they need; people with darker skin require longer to meet their daily need, from half an hour to a full hour. However, anyone with a family history of skin cancer should be cautious about their sun exposure.

Your level of vitamin D_3 should ideally be between 40 ng/mL and 80 ng/mL. Although some doctors feel it should be at the higher end of this range, I find it is very hard to get vitamin D_3 up to 70–80 ng/mL in most patients, and that there is no real clinical change or improvement from 40 to 80 ng/mL. In other words, I do not see glucose numbers dramatically changing with increases in vitamin D_3 when it is already in a good solid "normal" range. Nonetheless, you should not be deficient in this essential vitamin! Under 30 ng/mL is insufficient and under 20 ng/mL is deficient.

Some research suggests that vitamin D_3 may be lower if a person is in a very pro-inflammatory state, and that lower labs are more a reflection of the inflammation than an actual deficiency. Obese people tend to have lower levels as well. Right now, however, I treat low vitamin D_3 when the labs are evident.

With regard to diabetes, studies have shown that vitamin D_3 is useful in glucose homeostasis; it is needed to have insulin secreted from the pancreas and to have cells react to the insulin and be sensitive to it. Vitamin D_3 can lower fasting glucose and insulin levels and reduce insulin resistance. Vitamin D_3 protects the bones, can be anti-inflammatory, reduces autoimmunity, reduces risk of cancer, reduces depression, and has many other positive effects on bodily health.

People with lower levels of vitamin D_3 are at higher risk for developing T2DM. Vitamin D_3 may help pancreatic beta cells function better. When T1DM patients were given 4,000 IU of vitamin D_3 a day, they had improved glycemic control and lower A1C levels. T1DM patients with lower levels of vitamin D_3 were more likely to die of any cause than those patients who had higher serum vitamin D_3 levels. Vitamin D_3 can reduce the risk of infections, and infections in people with diabetes can be serious with increasing glucose levels.

During the late fall, winter, and early spring months, when sun exposure in northern latitudes is not sufficient to produce vitamin D_3, supplementation with vitamin D_3 makes sense. Vitamin D_3 should be dosed with vitamin K (to ensure the calcium gets into the bone, not the blood vessels or body tissues), vitamin A (which is needed by the vitamin D receptor to work), and calcium and magnesium. Your physician should not just give you high doses of vitamin D_3 alone. Discuss this with your physician if you are not getting a mixture of all the nutrients you should.

This test should be done at least once per year. If you are found to be deficient, the test should be redone in three months, also measuring serum calcium, to ensure you are back in the normal range, and your serum calcium levels are not dangerous. Hypercalcemia—elevated calcium—is more of a danger with elevated vitamin D_3 levels. After you have your levels back in normal range, you can check vitamin D_3 and serum calcium one to two times a year.

Uric Acid

Studies have shown that elevated uric acid, which is a risk factor for gout, is also a risk factor for cardiovascular disease in patients with diabetes, heart failure, or high blood pressure. This is a simple test to add on to a blood panel at least once per year to see if you are at higher risk for cardiovascular disease.

Uric acid can be elevated due to dietary intake of certain foods and beer, and is also excreted by candida fungal species in the gut. If your uric acid is elevated, check it every three months until levels return to normal.

Celiac Disease Panel

Celiac disease is found in 0.5–1.0 percent of the American population but 8–16 percent of T1DM patients. Around two million people have celiac disease in the United States. There is a well-known medical triangle of T1DM, thyroid disease, and celiac disease. This is vital for patients to know and it is standard to have thyroid and celiac disease monitored in all T1DM patients.

Celiac disease is an autoimmune reaction caused by eating gluten, a protein found in wheat, rye, and barley. If a person has celiac disease and eats one of those proteins, their immune system attacks the gluten and then attacks the lining of their small intestine, causing atrophy. This causes intestinal problems, systemic conditions, nutrient deficiencies, and sets the body up for more autoimmune reactions.

A newly diagnosed T1DM patient should be tested for both celiac disease and the genes to develop celiac disease. If they do not have the main genes, it is likely (though not definite) that they will not develop it, but if they do have the genes, and the celiac antibody test is negative, it means they might develop it but have not so far.

One key fact is that when a child is found to have celiac disease and gluten is removed from his diet, his subsequent risk for developing T1DM is pretty much nil. That is an astounding statistic and it means to me that *all* children, ideally even toddlers, should be screened for celiac disease at some point by their pediatrician. To test for celiac a person has to eat gluten grains daily for at least three weeks, and ideally four to six weeks.

The lab tests for celiac disease are as follows:

Genetic test. HLA DQ2 (DQA1 0501/0201/0302 and DQB1 0201/0202), DQ8 (DQA1 0301/2), and some labs measure HLA DQ7 (DQA1 0505). If you have any one of these, you have a gene for celiac disease.

Antibody tests.

- Deamidated gliadin, a specific protein in the overall category of gluten.
- Transglutaminase IgA, a protein found in the lining of the small intestine.
- Endomysial IgA, connective tissue that is wrapped around an intestinal muscle fiber; we test an antibody against it.
- Serum IgA levels. Some people do not genetically produce enough of the immunoglobulin called IgA. If this level is abnormally low, then the lab should redo the above antibody tests using the IgG immunoglobulin.

Thyroid Labs

The thyroid is a little gland that sits like a butterfly at the bottom of the trachea, right on top of the collarbone. It is the main organ that helps our body set its metabolism. It is important for all types of diabetes patients to measure thyroid labs at least once per year.

If the thyroid is not functioning well, it can increase glucose levels, decrease energy, cause water retention, and cause many other symptoms that can negatively affect getting diabetes under control.

Insulin resistance, which drives T2DM, can interfere with the production of thyroxine, the main hormone made by your thyroid. Also, elevated cortisol levels—a hormone made by the adrenals—can interfere with thyroid production, and decreased cortisol can inhibit the thyroid's effect of stimulating metabolism in your cells. Not all patients with slight elevations in thyroid stimulating hormone (TSH), with normal free T4 and free T3, called "subclinical hypothyroidism," need to be placed on thyroid hormone medication. Once a comprehensive protocol is begun, insulin resistance can significantly decrease and enable the thyroid to begin working normally again. I do not always place patients on thyroid medicine immediately; instead I often give them three months to show improvement in thyroid function following their regimen. I may add in a thyroid support product with nutrients and botanicals that can help the thyroid function better. If the thyroid levels are persistently problematic or grossly problematic from the beginning, I then feel dosing thyroid is a good idea.

KEY TREATMENT NOTE

Most integrative practitioners believe subfunctioning thyroid usually gets better when treated with natural desiccated thyroid (NDT) that contains T4, T3, and T2, instead of levothyroxine products, such as Synthroid, which contains only T4. However, some patients do fine with levothyroxine. If a patient has been on levothyroxine for years and her thyroid seems under great control, I won't change it to NDT. For NDT, I only recommend Nature-Throid, Westhroid, or WP Thyroid to patients. There is also synthetic T3, known as Cytomel, but this should be dosed rarely and carefully with patients.

Patients with T1DM have an increased risk of developing thyroid disease if they also have celiac disease, and especially if the celiac disease is undiagnosed.

Many physicians do not draw the right thyroid labs. The following is a full thyroid panel:

Thyroid stimulating hormone (TSH). This hormone is secreted by the pituitary to promote thyroid hormone production. A TSH should be below 2.0 uIU/mL.

Free T4/thyroxine (FT4). Thyroxine can be bound to a protein or free; only when it is free can the body make use of it. Free T4 can become free T3.

Free T3/triiodothyronine (FT3). Triiodothyronine can be bound to a protein or free; only when it is free can the body make use of it. Free T3 is the key thyroid hormone for energy production.

Total T4 or total T3. Some physicians also test for total T4 or total T3, but most integrative physicians do not.

T3 uptake or free T3 index. If your physician is still ordering T3 uptake, free T3 index, ask her to test for thyroid values that are not archaic and unhelpful. In 1992, I was instructed by my lab to stop ordering those!

Reverse T3. This is created to "throw out" thyroid hormone. It can be high when the body is under stress, although it does not define the type of stress. It can be high when a patient is low in selenium, which prevents the body from turning free T4 to free T3, and instead, reverse T3 is formed.

Thyroid antibodies.

- Thyroglobulin antibodies. This measures antibodies against thyroglobulin, the protein molecule from which thyroid hormones are made. It is often elevated in Hashimoto's thyroiditis, the main cause of hypothyroidism in the United States.
- Thyroid peroxidase antibodies. This measures antibodies against an enzyme that helps attach iodine to tyrosine residues on thyroglobulin. It is often elevated in Hashimoto's thyroiditis, the main cause of hypothyroidism in the United States.

- Thyroid stimulating immunoglobulin (TSI). This measures antibodies against the thyroid receptor of TSH. It is elevated in Graves' disease, that is, hyperthyroidism.

Thyroid labs should be measured yearly; they should be done earlier in the morning, ideally before 11 a.m., to match the natural physiologic rise of thyroid levels in our body.

Thyroid medicine must be taken on a stomach that has been completely empty of food, other medications, and supplements for at least an hour.

Prediabetes Evaluation

It's best to diagnose diabetes as early as possible. When I have a patient on the borderline of diabetic lab values, I may request they do the following lab test for measuring insulin resistance. I put this section on evaluation of prediabetes at the end, instead of the beginning, so you would be aware of lab values and be better able to understand the details.

We often measure insulin or c-peptide levels after people are fasting for twelve hours. In early diabetes, a fasting draw has allowed the body to work hard to reduce glucose and insulin for the long hours overnight and so may not really show that during the day and while eating, a person becomes diabetic, or very close. This is why I perform this lab test on patients on the borderline. This test should *never* be done on a patient already diagnosed with diabetes!

For this test, the patient fasts for twelve hours and then gets glucose and insulin levels drawn at a lab. In general, the standard lab then typically would have the patient drink 100 grams of straight glucose. I prefer to see how people react when they eat actual food. I have put together a meal that contains 100 grams of refined carbs and also contains a lot of saturated fat.

The patient goes to a local fast food restaurant (one hopes for the last time!), and orders the pancake meal and eats one pancake, on which one container of syrup is poured, eats a hashbrown, and drinks only water. If a meal full of refined sugar, refined grains, and a lot of saturated fat does not cause insulin resistance, nothing will! One and a half hours later the glucose and insulin are retested. Having both the fasting and postprandial glucose and insulin levels means I can determine if a patient is not insulin resistant, or if the patient is mildly, moderately, or severely insulin resistant.

Let me give you few examples of test results. As discussed above, a normal fasting insulin should be lower than 6 uIU/mL (and certainly lower than 9 uIU/mL), and postprandial insulin should be lower than 30 uIU/mL; fasting glucose should be lower than 90 mg/dL (and certainly lower than 100 mg/dL), and postprandial glucose should be lower than 120 mg/dL.

LAB EXAMPLE #1

Fasting glucose: 98 mg/dL
Postprandial glucose: 131 mg/dL
Fasting insulin: 11 uIU/mL
Postprandial insulin: 36 uIU/mL

This patient is very mildly insulin resistant. The lab numbers are only slightly above what are considered acceptable results.

LAB EXAMPLE #2

Fasting glucose: 106 mg/dL
Postprandial glucose: 153 mg/dL
Fasting insulin: 17 uIU/mL
Postprandial insulin: 60 uIU/mL

This patient is moderately insulin resistant—lab results are climbing clearly above reference ranges. Note that the insulin is 43 units higher after eating. That means it took more than an entire day's insulin output in a nondiabetic patient to maintain the glucose at still a high level of 153 mg/dL.

LAB EXAMPLE #3

Fasting glucose: 124 mg/dL
Postprandial glucose: 201 mg/dL
Fasting insulin: 34 uIU/mL
Postprandial insulin: 264 uIU/mL

This patient is about two weeks away from becoming a full diabetic. The postprandial glucose number, at 264 mg/dL, tipped the scale into diabetes, as a score over 200 mg/dL is diagnostic. And, again, note the insulin scores: This patient secreted 230 units of insulin—a week's worth of insulin in a nondiabetic—and still could not contain glucose levels at all.

By doing this test on patients who I am suspicious have insulin resistance and who I may not be getting a good analysis on due to the standard of using fasting glucose and insulin, I can really pinpoint how intensely a patient has to engage a diabetic prevention protocol. And, even though this book is on treating diabetes, it's certainly best to first prevent it from developing.

— CHAPTER FIVE —

Conventional Treatment of Diabetes

I've learned from patients who switch their medical care from conventional treatment to me that patients who have been treated with standard care eat what they wish; take numerous medications; have not received any guidance on how to exercise, how to lose weight, or how to incorporate stress management into their lives; and do not take the correct, if any, supplements at the correct doses. Furthermore, fifteen-minute office visits cannot lead to excellent care, and that's usually all the time a conventional physician has to see a patient. Integrative physicians schedule much more time with patients to ensure the entirety of good care is discussed and processed.

It is important to discuss the problems with how conventional care addresses diet (as recommended by the American Diabetes Association), and also to go over the pros and cons of the different types of medications used to treat T1DM and T2DM. By understanding current mainstream medical practices, it is easier to both see how and understand why integrative care has, in some ways, a significantly different approach.

Diet

Studies have shown that only 50 percent of patients with diabetes receive some form of dietary and nutritional counseling from their medical practitioner's office, and even fewer are referred to a nutritional professional. In one study of over eighteen thousand patients with diabetes, only 9 percent had at least one nutrition visit in a nine-year span, even though diet and exercise are the quickest, most effective ways to lower one's glucose, reduce or wean off of medications, heal and prevent diabetic complications, and achieve complete control of diabetes.

The most concise definition of a diabetic patient is someone who has lost the capacity to metabolize carbohydrates. Promoting a high-carbohydrate diet in these patients leads to poor control, overmedication, and the risk of diabetic complications. So, why isn't every diabetic patient guided to eat a low-carbohydrate diet?

More than one hundred years ago, Dr. Elliot Joslin, a renowned specialist in treating T1DM, worked successfully with patients for twenty-five years before insulin was isolated from dogs' pancreases and turned into an injectable medicine. Dr. Joslin recommended that his patients eat a low-carbohydrate diet consisting of no potatoes, no bread, and no sweets, and he made them exercise.

After insulin was invented and was used to treat diabetes, those patients lived long enough to die from something other than high blood sugars. In the 1940s and 1950s, patients with diabetes died of cardiovascular disease at a high rate. Autopsies of patients with diabetes showed that they had a great deal of atherosclerosis in their arteries, formed, as we know, from a buildup of cholesterol. The medical opinion at the time thus declared that patients with diabetes should avoid eating fats and too much meat, and instead eat more carbohydrates.

The American Diabetes Association (ADA), formed in 1940, is a wonderful organization committed to preventing diabetes and educating people about the disease. They are amazing advocates for all patients with diabetes. They support leading-edge research and are highly regarded as experts in diabetes. However, for a long time they have been working under the archaic idea that fat is the problem with patients with diabetes, when the new paradigm of cardiovascular disease shows that the situation is more complex.

Cardiovascular disease is now shown to be the result of inflammation and oxidative damage; as you've already seen, insulin, fat cells, and glucose are all pro-inflammatory and pro-oxidative in the body. There is little credible evidence now that fat intake is primarily responsible for cardiovascular disease, especially if the fats in question are healthy fats; even saturated fats have been acquitted of the accusations that they cause heart attacks and strokes.

Especially in patients with diabetes, eating a high-carbohydrate diet leads to insulin resistance, elevates cholesterol and triglycerides, produces more abdominal fat, produces inflammation, is pro-oxidative, and causes macro-vascular damage, all of which leads to cardiovascular disease.

On its website, the ADA recommends people consume 45–60 g of carbohydrates per meal, which at its maximum would be 180 g per day (if one did not snack and eat even more carbs). At 4 kcal per gram, that diet equals a total of 720 kcal per day of carbs. That is a lot of carbs! I believe the ADA's recommendation is terrible and even dangerous. A person will never be able to control their glucose levels with that type of intake, even with numerous hypoglycemic medications.

Because a high-carb, low-fat diet is the ADA's signature diet, patients with diabetes are commonly told by their registered dietician (if they are referred to one) to eat a big bowl of oatmeal for breakfast every day, which is high in whole grains and low in fat. Of course, almost always, diabetic patients see their glucose rise to over 200 mg/dL as a result, but this does not seem to matter to the nutritional counselors. Low fat and high carb is recommended by the ADA; therefore, it is considered the best diet.

What's worse is that historically the ADA was not adverse to patients with diabetes eating refined sugar. The ADA once conducted a study showing that serum glucose levels rose the same amount when a person ate refined sugar as when she ate bread. There are two conclusions to be made from that study: the ADA conclusion that a diabetic can eat both sugar and bread, just not at the same time, simply "exchanging carbs," and my conclusion that since both sugar and bread noticeably raise blood sugar, *both* should be avoided. I once ordered informative brochures from the ADA on the recommended diet for diabetic patients, and I was stunned to see the ADA write that, as part of their carbohydrate "exchange" system, if a person with diabetes wants to eat a piece of chocolate cake, they should simply eat fewer noodles at their main meal.

And yet, the ADA has come a long way. When Dr. Richard Kahn was the chief scientific officer of the ADA more than a decade ago, the ADA signed a three-year $1.5 million sponsorship deal with Cadbury-Schweppes. Dr. Kahn defended the deal by saying "There is not a shred of evidence that sugar, per se, has anything to do with diabetes." Now, on their website, the ADA clearly warns against drinking sugar-sweetened beverages and points out that "research has shown that drinking sugary drinks is linked to Type 2 diabetes." So at least they are now suggesting avoidance of sweetened beverages. Perhaps in the future they will take a stronger stand against all refined sugar and high-carbohydrate food.

A decade ago even the World Health Organization (WHO) came out with a statement suggesting that no more than 10 percent of daily calories should come from sugar. They supported their position by stating:

- Foods containing sugar can be lacking in essential micronutrients and can contain more calories than foods without sugar.
- Sugar is the main contributor to the global epidemic of obesity and the health consequences of diabetes.
- Sugar causes tooth decay.
- Sugar can cause weight gain.
- Children who drink sugary drinks are more likely to gain weight and become obese than children who do not.

This last point is very important. Studies done on various isoenergetic diets (diets containing the same number of calories) showed that the diet highest in sugar was the one on which children gained the most weight.

In 2015, WHO proposed new global sugar intake guidelines that state refined sugar intake should comprise less than 10 percent of daily energy intake and that less than 5 percent (6 teaspoons) of daily energy intake was ideal. The lower level maximum, at 6 teaspoons per day, is the equivalent of less than a full can of Coke. WHO has also stated an increasing concern that consumption of free sugars, particularly in the form of sugar-sweetened beverages, may result in both reduced intake of foods containing more nutritionally adequate calories and increased total caloric intake, leading to an unhealthy diet, weight gain, and increased risk of contracting noncommunicable diseases.

To help prevent the worldwide pandemic obesity crisis, the American Heart Association released a scientific statement recommending reduction in added sugar intake to no more than 100–150 kcal per day. One of the worst forms of dietary sugar is the sugar-sweetened beverage (SSB), which Americans have tripled their ingestion of since the 1970s. Even one SSB a day has been shown to increase obesity in children, and SSB intake is highly correlated to adult weight gain as well. However, there is more to a healthy diabetic diet than only avoiding sugar.

Displaying some wonderful evolution, in 2013 the ADA came out with new, progressive, and commendable nutritional guidelines. Although their website, as I noted, still promotes a high-carbohydrate diet, the new guidelines revealed that the ADA was no longer recommending a specific diet for all patients with diabetes to follow. The ADA realized that each patient with diabetes should be given dietary recommendations based on their needs, and as a result they included in their guidelines several different types of diets that have enough good research behind them to consider.

Mediterranean: significant plant foods from vegetables, fruits, grains, beans, nuts, and seeds; minimally processed, locally grown, and seasonal foods; rare refined sugars or honey; cheese and yogurt; four eggs per week; olive oil; red meat sparingly; wine at a low to moderate intake.

Vegetarian: no meat or poultry foods, but may eat dairy and eggs; vegetables, fruits, grains, and oils; beans, nuts, seeds, and soy.

Vegan: vegetables, fruits, grains, oils, beans, nuts, seeds, and soy.

Plant-based low-fat diet: vegetables, fruits, grains, and beans; a small amount of nuts, seeds, and oils.

Low carbohydrate: meat, poultry, fish, eggs, dairy, nuts, seeds, and soy; fats and oils; vegetables (avoiding potatoes, sweet potatoes, yams, and corn); some fruits (minimal berries); reduction or avoidance of grains.

DASH (Dietary Approaches to Stop Hypertension): lower salt; low fat or no fat; high grains; moderate vegetables; high fruit; lean meats, fish, and poultry; low to moderate nuts, seeds, and legumes.

The ADA guidelines also include nutrition recommendations. While some of these new guidelines are good, many will still cause problems for patients with diabetes.

On the helpful side, they recommend that diabetic patients receive nutritional counseling, work on portion control to encourage weight loss, and limit or avoid sugar-sweetened beverages; that diets reflect the cultural, religious, and economic differences of all patients; that patients substitute low-glycemic for high-glycemic foods, which may moderately improve glucose numbers; that patients eat more medium and polyunsaturated fatty acids, oilier omega-3-rich fish (but not bother with fish oil supplements) to prevent cardiovascular disease, and the same amount of saturated fats as the generation population. Also, they state that it's okay to use nonnutritive, noncaloric sweeteners in lieu of typical caloric sweeteners; to eat more plant stanols and steros if the patient has elevated lipids; drink alcohol in moderation, though it may cause hypoglycemia; that even though sugar and refined carbs both raise glucose levels, one should avoid eating sucrose, which displaces more nutrient-dense, healthier food; and that patients with diabetes should have a sodium intake equal to or less than 2,300 mg per day.

However, the guidelines also state that there is no ideal established protocol of carbohydrate, fat, and protein intake for a patient with diabetes; that patients with diabetes should eat the same fiber and grains as nondiabetic patients; and that "there is no clear evidence of benefit from vitamin or mineral supplementation in patients with diabetes who do not have underlying deficiencies." This is not only unhelpful and wrong but is contradictory; *Diabetes Care*, the medical journal sponsored by the ADA, has reported numerous benefits from many supplements, which are discussed further in chapter 10.

Overall, the ADA guidelines represent a huge step forward, and should be welcomed and applauded, but they don't go far enough yet. The low-carb diet is *the* diet for diabetes. Most integrative physicians realize this and counsel patients along these lines. I hope that in the future all organizations representing and advocating for diabetic patients will agree.

KEY TREATMENT NOTE

Diet is *the* key method of glucose control, aiding weight loss, helping to heal hypertension, avoiding and healing diabetic complications, and preventing the use of or reducing or removing the need for medications. It is important for patients to work with physicians who believe in the value of nutrition and who are knowledgeable about a low-carbohydrate therapeutic diet. To be honest, there is little to no chance for a person with diabetes to get their blood sugars under superb control by following the basic high-carbohydrate diet that is recommended in standard care.

Exercise

The standard government recommendation for exercise is moderate exercise thirty minutes a day, five days a week. If one does vigorous exercise, the recommendation is twenty minutes, three days a week. If one needs to lose weight, the recommendation is one hour of exercise, five days a week.

Those are good basic starting recommendations; however, unless a patient who has been given an exercise regimen is analyzed for cardiorespiratory fitness, strength, balance, and agility and there are noted significant improvements, there is no guarantee that their level of exercise will achieve the desired goals. Exercise is discussed further in chapter 9.

Weight Loss

To state the obvious—if you are an overweight or obese patient with diabetes, it is a good idea to lose weight. This might be difficult, however, if you eat 60 grams of carbohydrates at every meal and take diabetic medicines that increase your weight and interfere with weight loss as a result! On a comprehensive integrative protocol, weight usually tends to come off efficiently. If not, then there are other avenues to investigate, as we'll see in chapter 7.

Smoking

Conventional care recommends that you stop smoking. So do integrative physicians. So does everyone else!

KEY TREATMENT NOTE

As you can see from the above, diabetes is a complicated condition with many etiological factors that have an impact on your blood glucose. It is vital for you to have medical office visits that are long enough for you to learn about your condition and the best ways to treat it; fifteen-minute visits just cannot enable you to get the full care you deserve and require. Seek out a physician who spends between thirty and ninety minutes with you each office visit.

Conventional Prescription Drugs: The Eighth Essential (Medications)

I am not against medications as a general rule. Prescription drugs save lives at times, there's no doubt about it. I had to take antibiotics once when I had a terrible cellulitis infection—an infection in the fat layer under my skin—that was rapidly worsening, and I had a fever and lymph node enlargement. Sometimes people do need prescription medications to help heal a terrible infection or to help their bodies and minds treat a condition that otherwise might seriously harm them or be fatal. Of course, the problem is that drugs are currently overprescribed in America, cause over 100,000 deaths a year even when they are correctly prescribed, and cause up to 2.74 million hospitalizations a year for serious side effects.

Here is an overview of various medicines used with diabetes. In my opinion, some are good medications that can be helpful for patients, and others should simply be avoided.

Oral Hypoglycemic Agents (OHAs)

The main problem with oral medications for T2DM patients is that the only one that treats the cause of the disease—insulin resistance—also causes serious side effects and is essentially no longer prescribed. The other OHA medications do not treat insulin resistance. They help remove glucose from the serum, but not through eradicating insulin resistance; in fact, some of the medications *worsen* insulin resistance.

Several studies have been conducted that compare the results of lifestyle intervention to those of the drug metformin in treating diabetes. In one of them, lifestyle intervention, done solely through exercise, was shown to significantly reduce diabetes onset, more so than metformin, but it was more expensive because exercise entails buying home equipment, paying for gym membership, sneakers, Fitbits, and so forth. Considering that one can currently purchase metformin for only $4 per month, nearly any other treatment is going to be more expensive! In a second study, lifestyle intervention reduced an inflammatory marker more than metformin. A third, well-known study that is brought up frequently at lectures on oral diabetes medications compared the use of diet and lifestyle intervention with that of metformin to see which was more effective in preventing the onset of diabetes. The intensive diet and lifestyle modifications reduced diabetes onset by 58 percent, while using metformin reduced diabetes onset only 31 percent. We see over and over that changing lifestyle can have a huge impact on reducing inflammation and preventing diabetes.

However, oral medications do serve a purpose, and they should be initiated when glucose numbers still do not come down using a comprehensive integrative protocol, the A1C is greater than 5.5 percent, and the risk of developing diabetic complications is increasing; to enhance appetite control and support weight loss in patients; and for positive feedback for patients to see their glucose numbers reduced dramatically.

Medications tend to fail in this purpose when they are relied upon as the only way to control glucose. If one does not address all the etiologic reasons for high glucose, and a patient is only dosed with medications, more and more drugs are typically required. After three years on one OHA, for example, 50 percent of patients need to add a second drug. After five years on two OHAs, 75 percent of patients have progressed so far in their disease that they need to add a third OHA. When in a few years after that patients continue to worsen, they will be required to go on insulin. Relying solely on medications will cause many T2DM patients to be on insulin within three to seven years.

Both the ADA and the AACE have open guidelines for prescribing OHAs. The ADA guidelines suggest starting with metformin. If metformin alone doesn't work to reduce A1C within three months, there is no specific pathway for adding more medications; each physician can do as he or she wishes in adding another OHA, and then, if A1C is still uncontrolled in another three months, a third OHA, and then, if in another three months the A1C is still not controlled, basal insulin. Non-insulin injectables like GLP-1 are also an option.

The AACE guidelines divide treatment by how high the initial A1C is as follows:

- If A1C is lower than 7.5 percent, start with one OHA.
- If A1C is equal to or higher than 7.5 percent, start with two OHAs.
- If A1C is higher than 9.0 percent, either start with two or three OHAs or start with insulin.

I disagree with these guidelines, as I've seen A1Cs at initial diagnosis of diabetes come crashing down with naturopathic care. I had one patient (profiled in chapter 15) whose beginning A1C was 8.3 percent; after three months it was down to 5.2 percent using naturopathic care without any medications at all.

There are some integrative physicians who believe using any diabetic medications with patients is wrong or bad. I find this an unreasonable and potentially unsafe mindset. The key to being an excellent physician for patients with diabetes is realizing that high glucose numbers are the main problem. Any treatment used to keep the glucose and A1C numbers down is a good protocol. If we can control glucose numbers without medications, wonderful! Not every patient is fully compliant with the entire protocol and, if medications are required, then we need to prescribe them. We are lucky: we have accessible medications, when needed; we simply have to choose the best medication for each patient.

What's nice about the naturopathic treatment of diabetes is that we can at times get patients off their OHA, even if they started on two of them, while getting their A1Cs under better control than they were on the two drugs! That is not going to happen with every patient, but it does happen with many.

OHAs are used to treat prediabetes, T2DM, early Type 1.5 (LADA) diabetes, gestational diabetes, and MODY. There are several categories of these medications:

- Biguanides
- Sulfonylureas
- Meglitinides
- Thiazolidinediones
- Alpha-glucosidase inhibitors
- Dipeptidyl peptidase-4 (DPP-4) inhibitors
- Sodium-glucose co-transporter 2 inhibitors

The costs listed below for each OHA category are estimates for a patient paying out of pocket. With insurance, the cost should be entirely covered or have a much lower copay.

Biguanides

DRUG NAMES: Glucophage; Glucophage XR (brand name regular); Glumetza, Fortamet (brand name extended release); metformin HCL (generic regular); metformin ER (generic extended release)

BASIC INFO: Like many pharmaceutical drugs, this medicine originated from a plant. Goat's rue, used for hundreds of years for blood sugar regulation, was analyzed and found to contain guanides; drugs companies therefore began making biguanide drugs. The first generation of these medicines caused a problem called lactic acidosis, but that very rarely happens now with the newer biguanide metformin. This medicine can reduce the liver's production of glucose, reduces intestinal absorption of glucose, and enhances cells' uptake and metabolism of glucose. Metformin can allow weight loss in patients and does not cause weight gain, water retention, or hypoglycemia.

There is new interest in metformin as an anticancer treatment, as it reduces the amount of glucose available to cancer cells. Patients with diabetes on metformin had less incidences of cancer than patients with diabetes who were not on metformin. Metformin seems to reduce cancer cell growth and proliferation. Considering diabetic patients have an increased risk of developing cancer, being on metformin, science may show in the future, may help reduce the risk of cancer.

A recent meta-analysis of studies showed that metformin is safe for pregnant women and does not increase the risk of birth defects. It is also FDA approved for pediatric patients over ten years old.

SIDE EFFECTS: Gastrointestinal distress can occur in up to 33 percent of patients, including nausea, flatulence, and diarrhea. It is best to titrate this medication up slowly as a result.

KEY TREATMENT NOTE

If you are experiencing gastrointestinal distress on typical metformin, ask your physician to switch you to metformin ER, which the vast majority of patients can handle, even those who cannot handle straight metformin. In my practice, over 90 percent of patients who cannot tolerate regular metformin can tolerate metformin ER.

Vitamin B_{12} and folic acid deficiency. Metformin interferes with the enzyme that enables vitamin B_{12} to be absorbed in the terminal ileum of the small intestine. That enzyme needs calcium as a nutrient cofactor. The vast majority of patients on metformin do not become vitamin B_{12} deficient, but the risk is there; one analysis of the problem said up to 30 percent of patients on metformin can suffer from low vitamin B_{12} levels. Low vitamin B_{12} can cause peripheral neuropathy, weakness, intestinal issues, vision loss, and many other problems. Research has shown that by giving patients on metformin calcium supplementation, it pushes the enzyme in the gut that enables vitamin B_{12} absorption to work better and overcome the blocking effect of the drug. Patients on metformin need to take a multiple vitamin-mineral that contains vitamin B_{12} (methylcobalamin), folic acid (5-methyltetrahydrofolate), and calcium. Over the years I have found that putting metformin patients on a multivitamin is effective at preserving these nutrient levels and so I no longer recommend metformin patients receive a shot of vitamin B_{12} and folic acid once per month, unless, perhaps, the patient is on a proton pump inhibitor, which further inhibits vitamin B_{12} absorption, or has pernicious anemia (an autoimmune disease that prevents oral vitamin B_{12} absorption).

KEY TREATMENT NOTE

All patients who have been on metformin should be checked for vitamin B_{12} and folic acid deficiency by having their serum B_{12}, methylmalonic acid, serum folate, and homocysteine measured.

Lactic acidosis. This is a very, very rare occurrence with metformin. Ninety percent of metformin is excreted through the kidneys within twenty-four hours. If you have liver or kidney failure, then metformin may not be a safe drug for you. Also, metformin may be a problem pre- or postsurgery if the patient becomes dehydrated or develops sepsis. Otherwise, metformin is a safe medication. If a patient does have kidney disease, their estimated glomerular filtration rate and creatinine levels help a physician know how to safely dose metformin.

Metformin dosing and kidney labs:

- Elevated random microalbuminuria level does not mean you need to change metformin dosing
- Normal metformin dose: more than 60–45 mL/min/1.73 m2 eGFR
- Reduce dose in half: at 45 mL/min/1.73 m2 eGFR
- Stop metformin at or below: 30 mL/min/1.73 m2 eGFR

When serum creatinine levels rise above these numbers, metformin should be reduced or avoided:

- Men: ≥ 1.5 mg/dL
- Women: ≥ 1.4 mg/dL

Regarding a patient on metformin undergoing a radiographic dye study, since both are excreted through the kidney, the American College of Radiology states that in general a patient does not need to stop metformin. Contrast media is a potential concern in patients with significant renal damage or acute kidney injury. Their recommendations are as follows.

Category 1. Patients with no evidence of AKI and eGFR higher than or equal to 30 mL/min/1.73 m2, do not discontinue metformin before/after contrast administration and do not need to rest kidney function afterwards.

Category 2. Patients on metformin with AKI or severe kidney disease (eGFR less than 30) or having arterial catheter study with increased risk of emboli to the renal arteries, discontinue metformin before or at time of procedure, and do not restart for forty-eight hours, when kidney function has been shown to be normal.

Gadolinium. Do not stop metformin if gadolinium dose is typical at 0.1–0.3 mmol per kg of body weight.

COST: Metformin is on many $4 price lists from pharmacies. Whether brand name Glucophage works better than generic metformin is hard to know. Overall, I feel satisfied with patients getting metformin, and insurances like that, too. It's very rare for an insurance company to agree to pay for Glucophage.

DOSE:

Metformin HCL. 500 mg, 850 mg, 1,000 mg—1 tablet twice per day
Metformin HCL ER. 500 mg, 750 mg—1–2 tablets once or twice per day

It is best to titrate up metformin when prescribing it, to help prevent the gastrointestinal upset it may cause.

- Start with 500 mg once or twice per day.
- After five to seven days, can increase to 1,000 mg twice per day, if that is the final recommended dose.

- Metformin dosed at 850 mg—start with one once per day, and then increase to one twice per day, and then, if directed, one three times per day for the maximum dose.
- Maximum daily dose of metformin is 2,550 mg per day in adults, 2,000 mg per day in children (ten to sixteen years old).
- Maximum daily dose of metformin ER in adults is 2,000 mg per day. The manufacturer states it can be taken one time a day with the evening meal. However, I never do that. I always dose this twice a day, just like regular metformin, with the same titrating up of dosage.

Metformin at maximum dosage has been shown to lower A1C after three months by approximately 1 percent.

▶ **KEY TREATMENT NOTE**

I like metformin, and if I have to use an OHA, and the patient has no contraindications, I will always choose to use metformin first, as do the vast majority of physicians. Metformin can be used with any other diabetic medication, including insulin.

Sulfonylureas

DRUG NAMES: DiaBeta/Glynase/glyburide; Glucotrol/glipizide (XL); Amaryl/glimepiride

BASIC INFO: These medicines are called "secretagogues" because they work by forcing the pancreas to secrete more insulin. We have to be very careful using these medications. They should never be used with insulin or the metiglinides. Sulfonlyureas have historically been very popular medicines, and it is typical to add one as the second medicine if metformin alone is not effective enough at lowering glucose numbers. They are also very inexpensive. Sulfonlyureas have been studied in pediatric patients but are not approved for use in them. They are also not recommended in pregnant women.

SIDE EFFECTS (THESE CAN BE SIGNIFICANT):

Hypoglycemia. As these medicines cause extra insulin to be secreted, they can easily cause hypoglycemia. There is a higher risk of hypoglycemia when a sulfonlyurea is mixed with other diabetic medications. Glyburide may have a higher risk of hypoglycemic reactions than the other sulfonylureas.

Weight gain. Extra insulin secreted from the pancreas can cause insulin resistance, weight gain, and water retention. It is very common that T2DM patients who need to lose weight not only cannot lose it but often gain it on these medications.

Pancreatic burnout. These medicines can cause "pancreatic burnout" by forcing the pancreas to secrete extra insulin over time; that is, the pancreas may simply be unable to secrete any more insulin. The earlier in a patient's life this medication is prescribed, the more likely pancreatic burnout is to develop. For example, prescribing sulfonylurea to a forty-year-old puts him at higher risk for pancreatic burnout than an eighty-year-old who is introduced to it, as it does take some years for the burnout to occur. Because of pancreatic burnout risk, sulfonylureas are contraindicated in patients with LADA.

COST: Many of these are on $4 price lists.

DOSE:

DiaBeta/glyburide. 1.25, 2.5, 5 mg single/twice per day dosing. Maximum 20 mg per day.

Glynase/glyburide micronized. 1.5, 3, 4.5, 6 mg single/twice per day dosing. Maximum 12 mg per day.

Glucotrol/glipizide. 5, 10 mg per day single/twice per day dosing. Maximum 15 mg once per day. Maximum 40 mg twice per day.

Glucotrol XL/glipizide ER. 2.5, 5, ten tablets once per day. Maximum 20 mg per day.

Amaryl/glimepiride. 1, 2, 4 mg once per day. Maximum 8 mg per day.

Sulfonylureas have been shown to lower A1C after three months by approximately 1.25 percent.

▶ KEY TREATMENT NOTE

I suggest avoiding these medications as much as possible. Their interference with weight loss is real. They are the first OHA I will take the patient off if their glucose decreases significantly with my comprehensive protocol.

Metiglinides (Glinides)

DRUG NAMES: Starlix / nateglinide; Prandin / repaglinide

BASIC INFO: These medicines work by increasing insulin secretion from the pancreas but do not last as long as the sulfonylureas. They are short-acting and thus are used to raise insulin levels specifically with meals. As a result, they are rarely, if ever, prescribed, because patients would prefer to take a sulfonylurea one or two times a day rather than a metiglinide with each meal. They should never be taken with sulfonylureas or with insulins. Metiglinides are not approved for pediatric patient dosing and are not recommended in pregnancy.

SIDE EFFECTS:

Hypoglycemia. As with sulfonylureas, forcing the pancreas to secrete more insulin causes a risk of low blood sugar, but the risk is less than with the long-lasting, stronger sulfonylureas.
Pancreatic burnout. Same as with sulfonylureas.
Weight gain. Same as with sulfonylureas.

COST: Around $80–150 / month out of pocket.

DOSE:

Starlix / nateglinide. 60–120 mg 30 minutes before meals.
Prandin / repaglinide. 0.5–4 mg 30 minutes before meals.

Metiglinides have been shown to lower A1C after three months by approximately 0.75 percent.

▶ **KEY TREATMENT NOTE**

It makes more sense to dose a sulfonylurea than a metiglinide if pancreatic insulin secretion is desired.

Thiazolidinediones (TZDs)

DRUG NAMES: Avandia / rosiglitazone; Actos / pioglitazone

BASIC INFO: This type of medicine works by lowering insulin resistance in body cells so that muscle and fat cells accept insulin more effectively and absorb glucose, lowering serum levels. These were the only medications actually developed that treated the actual cause of T2DM, insulin resistance. These medications were also helpful in reducing fatty livers.

Unfortunately, these medicines have a sordid history and, in general, are now rarely used by any physician. In 2007, there was a study that reported patients on Avandia (and other TZDs) were found to have an increase in weight gain, water retention, edema, congestive heart failure, and cardiovascular disease. Thousands and thousands of patients on these medications had heart attacks and died.

In 2011, the FDA restricted the use of TZDs, and combination products of TZDs with metformin or sulfonylureas were banned in the United States. TZDs have also been banned entirely from European countries.

In June 2013, the FDA voted to reduce the restrictions on Avandia and since then it can be given to patients who were already successfully treated with this medication and could not successfully control their glucose with other antidiabetic medicines, and did not want to use Actos.

The FDA recently removed all restrictions on dosing Avandia, although I haven't seen any patients back on it.

Actos was once shown to significantly increase the risk of bladder cancer. In fact, one study showed patients had an 83 percent increased risk of bladder cancer if they had ever taken Actos, especially if it was for more than two years. But, after a follow-up ten-year study by the FDA, published in 2015, it was shown that Actos is not associated with bladder cancer, but rather is linked to a 41 percent increased risk of pancreatic cancer.

I feel it's probably best if both of these medications are entirely avoided, and I believe that is the general feeling of the vast majority of medical practitioners prescribing diabetes medications. Avandia and Actos contain a black box warning (the most stringent warning the FDA demands) that they can cause or exacerbate congestive heart failure.

TZDs are not recommended for pediatric patients or pregnant women.

COST: $15/month with insurance; $200–300 a month out of pocket.

DOSE:

Avandia/rosiglitazone. 2, 4, 8, mg single/twice per day dosing. Maximum 8 mg per day.

Actos/pioglitazone. 15, 30, 45 mg once per day. Maximum 45 mg per day.

TZDs have been shown to lower A1C after three months by approximately 1 percent (pioglitazone) and approximately 1.25 percent (rosiglitazone).

▶ **KEY TREATMENT NOTE**

If you are on a TZD, you should request your physician change it to a safer medicine. If you are not on one, it's likely one will not be prescribed to you.

Alpha-Glucosidase Inhibitors

DRUG NAMES: Precose/acarbose; Glyset/miglitol

BASIC INFO: These pills are not commonly used. They block the digestion and absorption of carbohydrates. Undigested carbohydrates make lovely meals for microorganisms in your intestinal tract, creating smelly flatulence, bloating, abdominal pain, and diarrhea. Most people would rather have poorly controlled diabetes than be farting all the time! Plus, undigested carbohydrates can feed the wrong bacteria in the gut that may produce gastrointestinal dysbiosis (an unhealthy bacterial balance). Integrative physicians stress that a healthy gut and healthy gut bacteria are a vital foundation for overall good health. Plus, we now know healthy gut bacteria encourage your systemic body to have less insulin resistance and reduce the risk of autoimmune disease. We do not like drugs to mess with gut bacteria!

On the other hand, alpha-glucosidase inhibitors do not cause weight gain and water retention.

These medications are not approved for pediatric patients but can be prescribed to pregnant women.

SIDE EFFECTS: Abdominal pain, bloating, diarrhea, flatulence.

Do not take if you have a chronic intestinal illness, inflammatory bowel disease, intestinal obstruction, colonic ulceration, or liver disease.

COST: Approximately $35–60/month.

DOSE:

Precose/acarbose. 25, 50, 100 mg pills taken before meals three times per day. Maximum 300 mg per day.

Glyset/miglitol. 50–100 mg taken before meals three times per day.

These can be used with any other diabetic medication.

Alpha-glucosidase inhibitors have been shown to lower A1C after three months by approximately 0.5–0.8 percent (not very impressive with all the unpleasant gut side effects).

KEY TREATMENT NOTE

I have never prescribed these, and never will prescribe these, and have never seen a patient from another physician on them.

DPP-4 Inhibitors: Gliptins

DRUG NAMES: Januvia/sitagliptin; Onglyza/saxagliptin; Tradjenta/linagliptin; Nesina/alogliptin

BASIC INFO: These medications work by suppressing an enzyme that breaks down the incretin hormones. Incretin hormones—glucagon-like peptide 1 (GLP-1) and gastric inhibitory peptide—are secreted by the intestines and help to lower glucose levels.

These medications are prescribed when a physician is trying to extend the life and action of the leptins. The idea is that if we can stop an enzyme from breaking down GLP-1 in the body, its glucose lowering effects will last longer. It is a great idea, but in practice, I rarely see any significant clinical benefits to these medications. I doubt I am alone as, again, I do not see many patients coming in to see me on one of these medications.

They do not, however, cause weight gain, edema, or hypoglycemic reactions. And, they are conveniently dosed at one pill a day, making it easy to take them. These medications are not recommended for pediatric patients or pregnant women.

SIDE EFFECTS:

Associated with increased risk of acute and chronic pancreatitis and pancreatic cancer.

Associated with causing chronic joint pain, which tends to go away a month after stopping the medication.

These drugs are cautioned in renal disease.

- If the eGFR is higher than 50 mL/min, full dosing of a DPP-4 inhibitor is safe.
- If the eGRF is between 30 mL/min and 50 mL/min your physician might wish to lower your dose or stop.
- If your eGRF is lower than 30 mL/min, these medications ideally should be stopped.

COST: Approximately $400/month.

DOSE:

Januvia/sitagliptin. 25, 50, 100 mg pills—100 mg once per day with healthy kidneys, 50 mg once per day with moderate kidney disease, 25 mg once per day for severe kidney disease.

Onglyza/saxagliptin. 2.5, 5 mg pills—5 mg once per day with healthy kidneys; 2.5 mg once per day with moderate or severe kidney disease.

Tradjenta/linagliptin. 5 mg pill—5 mg once per day. This is the only DPP-4 medication that does not require dose adjustment.

Nesina/alogliptin. 25 mg with healthy kidneys, 12.5 mg once per day with mild kidney disease, 6.25 mg once per day with moderate kidney disease.

Gliptins have been shown to lower A1C after three months by approximately 0.75 percent.

▶ KEY TREATMENT NOTE

Although these do not seem to be problematic drugs, I have not found them clinically effective at lowering glucose. If a patient is on one of them, I do not consider it a problem, and, if necessary, I may use one with a patient, as they are overall fairly safe medications.

Sodium-Glucose Co-transporter 2 Inhibitors: Gliflozins

DRUG NAMES: Invokana/canagliflozin; Farxiga/dapagliflozin; Jardiance/empagliflozin

BASIC INFO: The sodium-glucose co-transporter 2 (SGLT-2) system in the kidney is responsible for reabsorbing back into the bloodstream up to 90

percent of the glucose that enters the kidneys. The kidneys filter 180 grams of glucose per day, all of which is reabsorbed, 90 percent by the SGLT-2 transporter. Diabetic patients can even reuptake more glucose, since they have higher glucose levels in their bloodstream. This class of drug prevents that reabsorption so a patient will lose 70–100 grams of glucose a day as the glucose passes through the kidneys into the urine. That can cause up to 200–300 kcal being lost a day. So, on this drug patients can more easily lose weight as they urinate out calories. This class of medications is not approved for use in pediatric patients or pregnancy.

SIDE EFFECTS:

Significant polyuria. Increased urination can lead to dehydration and renal impairment.

Glycosuria. Increased urine glucose.

Some weight loss and fatigue.

Genital fungal infections. Affects 10 percent of patients. Usually, after treating these infections, they do not tend to recur.

Urinary tract infections.

Thrush (fungal infection in the mouth).

Volume depletion. Low blood pressure, dizziness, fainting. Most diabetic patients are on two to four hypertension medications when they come to see an integrative physician, so it is important to alert patients that due to increased urination their blood pressure may decrease significantly, leading to a need to reduce or remove their blood pressure medications.

May raise cholesterol levels. Both HDL (good cholesterol) and LDL (bad cholesterol).

Diabetic ketoacidosis. By far, the most significant side effect recently uncovered is that SGLT-2 medications are shown to increase the risk of diabetic ketoacidosis (DKA) in both Type 2 and Type 1 patients. DKA is extremely rare in Type 2 patients—almost unheard of—and usually seen only in T1DM patients. Moreover, these drugs are not FDA approved for Type 1 patients. In Type 2 patients, DKA occurred at relatively low serum glucose levels—lower than 200 mg/dL; typically when a T1DM patient develops DKA, it is at glucose levels much higher than 250 mg/dL. The median time for DKA onset after beginning the medication was only two weeks. The risk of DKA in patients on these medications can be increased by illness, surgery, extensive exercise, heart attack, stroke, infection, trauma, reduced calorie intake, and reduced insulin dosing. However, in some patients, there was no identifiable reason the DKA occurred. DKA occurred mostly in patients who were insulin deficient, such as those who had LADA and T1DM. DKA signs and symptoms include abdominal pain, nausea, vomiting, fatigue, and dyspnea (problems breathing). If at any time you are on one of these medications and develop one or more of those, call your physician immediately. The AACE recommends in their "AACE/ACE Position Statement on SGLT-2 Inhibitors and DKA Risk" the following to reduce the risk of DKA developing in patients on these medications:

- Consider stopping the SGLT-2 inhibitor at least twenty-four hours prior to elective surgery, planned invasive procedure, or severe stressful physical activity such as running a marathon.
- Avoid stopping insulin or decreasing the dose excessively.
- For emergency surgery or any extreme stress event, the drug should be stopped immediately.
- Routine measurement of urine ketones is not recommended during use of SGLT-2 inhibitors because this measurement can be misleading. Only use measurement of blood ketones for DKA diagnosis.
- Patients taking SGLT-2 inhibitors should avoid excess alcohol intake and very low carb diets.

Kidney injury. The FDA has put out stronger warnings about canagliflozin (Invokana and Invokamet) and dapagliflozin (Farxiga and Xigduo XR) regarding the risk for acute kidney injury. Acute kidney injury has been seen

Table 5.1. SGLT-2 Inhibiter Dosing Adjustments with Renal Disease

eGFR	Invokana/canagliflozin	Farxiga/dapagliflozin	Jardiance/empagliflozin
> 60	No dose change	No dose change	No dose change
45–60	100 mg/day	NOT RECOMMENDED	10 mg/day
30–45	NOT RECOMMENDED	N/A	NOT RECOMMENDED
< 30	Contraindicated	Contraindicated	Contraindicated

in patients within one month of starting these medications; most patients improved upon drug cessation, but some needed to be hospitalized and get dialysis. It may not be a good idea to use either of these medications if you have chronic renal insufficiency, congestive heart failure, decreased blood volume, or are on a diuretic, angiotensin-converting enzyme inhibitor, angiotensin receptor blocker, or nonsteroidal anti-inflammatory drugs. Your physician should assess your kidney function before starting you on this drug and monitor it periodically while you stay on it. At any sign of renal impairment the medication should be stopped immediately and care should be initiated. Two early signs of kidney damage are decreased urination and the development of edema (swelling in the lower legs). Empagliflozin/Jardiance actually was shown in the EMPA-REG OUTCOME trial to significantly slow the progression to kidney disease in T2DM patients. It seems that just based on this concern, if your physician wishes to give you a SGLT-2 inhibitor, empagliflozin (Jardiance, Glyxambi, Synjardy) seems to be the safest one. See table 5.1 for SGLT-2 inhibitor dosing adjustments with renal disease.

Bone loss. Canagliflozin is also associated with an increased incidence of bone fractures. The fractures affected the upper limbs, and began occurring as early as three months after drug initiation, resulting from minor trauma events. However, hip and low spine bone density was also seen to decrease. The FDA is studying the other drugs in this class to see if they also may increase bone fracture risk. The reason may be due to these drugs increasing serum phosphate, which can over time adversely affect bone density.

Other contraindications to using these medications:

- Digoxin is particularly contraindicated in patients on SGLT-2 inhibitors (higher levels of digoxin will be required).
- Higher doses of SGLT-2 medications will be needed for patients taking rifampin, phenobarbital, phenytoin, or ritonavir but these are not commonly used drugs.
- If eGFR is lower than 45 mL/min/1.73 m2, the medications should not be given.
- Hyperkalemia (high serum potassium).

As we see with any class of medications, we need to think about the benefits of the drugs and carefully watch for potential problems.

COST: Approximately $400–450/month.

DOSE:

Invokana/canagliflozin. 100 mg or 300 mg once per day.
Farxiga/dapagliflozin. 5 mg or 10 mg once per day.
Jardiance/empagliflozin. 10 mg or 25 mg once per day.

Start at the lower dose and titrate up to the higher one if necessary.

SGLT-2 inhibitors have been shown to lower A1C after three months by approximately 0.9 percent.

KEY TREATMENT NOTE

It seems using empagliflozin is the best choice in this category of medications. These drugs are new, and I am willing to try them with patients when they seem like a necessary and appropriate choice, though I have not yet had the need to do so. I am aware that they may have some serious side effects, and over time, we'll learn if we truly can consider them safe and responsible drugs. Physicians will be eagerly watching for future studies on the safety of using this medication.

Oral Mixed Hypoglycemia Agents: Combination Products

In general, I like to use medications individually to dose them specifically and also to wean them down or remove them as is possible, and that seems to be a common practice among medical practitioners. The main combination medication I've seen patients prescribed is Janumet. I suggest you never use any combination medicine that contains a TZD. Table 5.2 lists various combination oral hypoglycemic agents and their dosages.

Non-insulin injectables

There are two different types of non-insulin medications that are injected into patients to help control glucose numbers.

Synthetic Glucagon-like Peptide: GLP-1

DRUG NAMES: Byetta/exenatide; Bydureon/exenatide ER; Tanzeum/albiglutide; Trulicity/dulaglutide; Victoza/liraglutide; Adlyxin/lixisenatide

BASIC INFO: These drugs are injected subcutaneously into the abdomen, thigh, or posterior upper arm. They are FDA approved for T2DM, though they are used off-label for prediabetic patients, Type 1, or LADA patients for appetite control. It concerns me to mix GLP-1s with insulin, sulfonylureas, and metiglinides, as the risks of hypoglycemia are significantly increased, but these risks can be managed successfully with good attention to glucose numbers.

These medications should not be prescribed to pediatric patients or pregnant women.

GLP-1 injectables have the following methods of action:

- Decreases glucagon, the pancreatic hormone that signals the liver to increase glucose production
- Increases insulin secretion, to help lower glucose
- Slows gastric emptying so food is digested slower, and that lowers glucose elevation after meals
- Signals appetite suppression in the brain

In general, these medications reduce appetite, aid weight loss, help decrease glucose, and are easy to use if you do not mind self-injecting a medication. They may also help preserve pancreatic beta cell functioning.

SIDE EFFECTS:

Nausea. By far the main side effect.

Headache.

Vomiting, diarrhea, constipation. If the vomiting and diarrhea are extreme, renal impairment can occur.

Dyspepsia.

Risk of acute and chronic pancreatitis and pancreatic cancer. All patients on these medications should be alerted that if they begin suffering left upper abdomen pain, indicating they may be developing pancreatitis, they should immediately stop dosing and call their physicians.

Table 5.2. Combination Oral Hypoglycemic Agents and Their Dosages

Combination Oral Hypoglycemic Agent	Components	Dosage(s)
Actoplus Met XR	Pioglitazone and metformin HCL	15 mg pioglitazone/500 or 850 mg metformin HCL: 1 tablet 1–3x/day
Avandamet	Rosiglitazone and metformin HCL	2 mg rosiglitazone/500 or 1,000 mg metformin HCL: 1 tablet 2x/day
		4 mg rosiglitazone/500 mg metformin HCL: 1 tablet 2x/day
Avandaryl	Rosiglitazone and glimepiride	4 mg rosiglitazone/1, 2, or 4 mg glimepiride: 1 tablet 1–2x/day
		8 mg rosiglitazone/2 or 4 mg glimepiride: 1 tablet 1x/day
DueTact	Pioglitazone and glimepiride	30 mg pioglitazone/2 or 4 mg glimepiride: 1 tablet 1x/day
Glucovance	Glyburide and metformin HCL	1.25 mg glyburide/250 mg metformin HCL: 1–2 tablets 1–2x/day
		2.5 mg glyburide/500 mg metformin HCL: 1–2 tablets 1–2x/day
		5.0 mg glyburide/500 mg metformin HCL: 1–2 tablets 1–2x/day
Glyxambi	Empagliflozin and linagliptin	10 or 25 mg empagliflozin/5 mg linagliptin: 1 tablet 1x/day
Invokamet	Canagliflozin and metformin HCL	50 mg canagliflozin/500 mg or 1,000 mg metformin HCL: 1 tablet 2x/day
		150 mg canagliflozin/500 mg or 1,000 mg metformin HCL: 1 tablet 2x/day
Janumet	Sitagliptin and metformin	50 mg sitagliptin /500 mg or 1,000 mg metformin HCL: 1 tablet 2x/day

Combination Oral Hypoglycemic Agent	Components	Dosage(s)
Jenadueto	Linagliptin and metformin HCL	2.5 mg linagliptin/500 mg, 850 mg, or 1,000 mg metformin HCL: 1 tablet 1–2x/day
Kazano	Alogliptin and metformin	12.5 mg alogliptin/500 mg or 1,000 mg metformin HCL: 1 tablet 2x/day
Kombiglyze XR	Saxagliptin and metformin HCL ER	2.5 mg saxagliptin/1,000 mg metformin HCL ER: 1 tablet 1–2x/day
		5.0 mg saxagliptin/500 mg or 1,000 mg metformin HCL ER: 1 tablet 1–2x/day
Metaglip	Glipizide and metformin HCL	2.5 glipizide/250 or 500 mg metformin HCL: 1 tablet 1–2x/day
		5.0 mg glipizide/500 mg metformin HCL: 1 tablet 1–2x/day
Oseni	Alogliptin and pioglitazone	12.5 mg alogliptin/15 mg, 30 mg, or 45 mg pioglitazone: 1 tablet 1x/day
		25 mg alogliptin/15 mg, 30 mg, or 45 mg pioglitazone: 1 tablet 1x/day
Prandimet	Repaglinide and metformin HCL	1 mg or 2 mg repaglinide/500 mg metformin HCL: 1 tablet 2–3x/day
Synjardy	Empagliflozin and metformin HCL	5 mg empagliflozin/500 mg or 1,000 mg metformin HCL: 1 tablet 2x/day
		12.5 mg empagliflozin/500 mg or 1,000 mg metformin HCL: 1 tablet 2x/day
Xigduo XR	Dapagliflozin and metformin HCL	5 mg dapagliflozin/500 mg or 1,000 mg metformin HCL: 1 tablet 1x/day

Risk of developing medullary thyroid cancer. Patients with thyroid nodules should not be prescribed these medications.

Hypoglycemia. If a GLP-1 is mixed with a sulfonylurea or with insulin, the person is at higher risk for developing hypoglycemia.

Administer with caution in the following situations:

- Gastroparesis—a neurological complication in diabetes whereby the stomach does not empty its contents smoothly and regularly (see chapter 14); GLP-1 injection should be avoided in this condition
- Malnourishment, irregular dietary intake, dietary intake deficiency—the state of debility
- Intense muscular exercise
- Excessive alcohol intake

Table 5.3. Dosing Information for GLP-1 Medications

Drug	**Dosing**	**Mixing Needed**	**Pre-inject Waiting**
Byetta/exenatide	2x/day	No	None
Bydureon kit/exenatide extended release	1x/week	Yes	None
Bydureon pen/exenatide extended release	1x/week	Yes	None
Tanzeum/albiglutide	1x/week	Yes	15–30 minutes
Trulicity/dulaglutide	1x/week	No	None
Victoza/liraglutide	1x/day	No	None
Adlyxin/lixisenatide	1x/day or 1x/week	No	None

- Adrenal failure
- Fever, trauma, infection, or surgery

This class of medicine should not be used in cases of serious renal failure: that is, with eGFR lower than 30 mL/min/1.73 m2.

COST: Approximately $230–$650/month.

DOSE: These drugs do not need to be refrigerated after opening as long as the injectable is kept in the temperature range of 36–77° F. They come in prefilled pen form. They are dosed before breakfast either once per day, twice per day (before breakfast and supper), or once per week. Most patients, of course, now prefer to be given a type of GLP-1 that only requires one shot per week. Each insurance company is deciding which GLP-1 to cover, so your medical practitioner should know which yours covers before giving you a prescription. See table 5.3 for detailed dosing information.

Dosing Strength	Smallest Needle Size	Needle Included	Can Use with Basal Insulin	Auto Injector
5 mcg 10 mcg	32 gauge 4 mm	No	Yes	No
2 mg	32 gauge 8 mm	Yes	No	No
2 mg	32 gauge 7 mm	Yes	No	No
30 mg 50 mg	29 gauge 5 mm	No	Yes	No
0.75 mg 1.5 mg	Built into device: 29 gauge 5 mm	Yes, part of device	No	Yes
0.6, 1.2, 1.8 mg	32 gauge 4 mm	No	Yes	No
Day: 10 then 20 mcg Week: 20 mcg	32 gauge 4 mm	No	Yes	No

The patient is always started on a lower dose for a month and then titrated up if a stronger dose seems helpful and manageable.

GLP-1 medications have been shown to lower A1C by approximately 0.9 percent when using a daily dose and by approximately 1.6 percent when using a weekly dose.

KEY TREATMENT NOTE

I like these drugs overall. It's pretty easy for patients to inject once a week to aid lowering their glucose. These drugs are fine if used carefully and with good attention to how a patient tolerates them. A GLP-1 is a good addition to metformin.

Synthetic Amylin

DRUG NAME: Symlin/pramlintide acetate

BASIC INFO: Symlin is a subcutaneous synthetic injection of amylin, the other hormone that is made in the beta cells of the pancreas, with the idea that if the beta cell has failed and cannot produce insulin, then it likely might not produce this hormone, either. So, injecting some amylin might also be beneficial to diabetic patients. It was designed to use with Type 1 or Type 2 patients on insulin for meals. It comes in prefilled pens.

Amylin has the following actions in the body:

- Signals satiety, so people eat fewer calories and can lose weight.
- Slows gastric emptying, so food is digested slower, leading to lower glucose levels after eating.
- Suppresses glucagon, so the liver is not signaled to produce glucose.

That is, it does what GLP-1 does without raising insulin secretion.

This all sounds good and logical, but this product is not currently used by physicians because it also does the following:

- Increases the risk of severe hypoglycemia.
- Causes nausea and vomiting.
- Is confusing when dosed with insulin. Patients cannot mix the medications, so they have to inject both insulin and aymlin at a

meal, and it is hard to figure out how much of both are necessary to lower the glucose effectively without causing a significant hypoglycemic reaction.
- Having to inject insulin and amylin separately means patients inject in two different areas at every meal. This is a hard sell for most patients.
- Adding it into a patient's protocol has not been shown to change A1C in any significant way.

Aymlin is contraindicated to use in the following situations:

- A1C is higher than 9 percent.
- Patient does not do excellent monitoring of their daily glucose levels.
- Patient has a history of hypoglycemic reactions.
- Patient has poor insulin compliance.
- Patient has hypoglycemic unawareness.
- Patient has gastroparesis.
- Patient is a child.
- Patient is on a drug that promotes gastrointestinal motility.

COST: $850 per 2 pens.

DOSE: This product comes in prefilled pens—one for T1DM and one for T2DM. A patient should reduce their mealtime insulin by 50 percent while beginning amylin. The patient starts with the lower dose and then titrates up the amylin dosage every three days as needed or as doctor directed.

T1DM. 15 mcg, 30 mcg, 45 mcg, and 60 mcg pens
T2DM. 60 mcg and 120 mcg pens

Amylin has been shown to lower A1C by 0.4 percent.

This is a perfect example of a great idea simply not playing out well clinically. I do not know any patient who has been prescribed amylin for the last decade.

KEY TREATMENT NOTE

There is no need to consider amylin.

Summary of Oral and Injectable Hypoglycemic Medications

The most effective oral hypoglycemic agents are metformin, sulfonylureas (with all the problems associated with them), and SGLT-2 inhibitors (which, being new, we have to watch for more information on significantly negative side effects). None of them actually treat the disease driving T2DM, insulin resistance, except perhaps metformin, which may have a slight benefit in that regard. The other OHAs are simply not commonly prescribed. The GLP-1 injectables are good medications, though patients need to be screened for thyroid nodules beforehand. This is why relying solely on medications for T2DM is a problematic prospect for treatment and generally fails in reaching the goal of reversal.

Cholesterol-Lowering Medications: Statin Drugs

Other prescription medications are part and parcel of being diagnosed with diabetes in conventional care. They are regularly given to diabetic patients due to studies supporting their preventive or therapeutic effects. While I agree that it is imperative to reduce lipid panels to normal, keep the kidneys healthy, and lower blood pressure, I know that prescription medicines are not usually necessary to achieve those clinical goals. I've seen numerous patients have success without using medicines, and for the patient who comes to me on those drugs, usually we can remove them while responsibly ensuring the patient's diabetes is still well controlled and her health is being safeguarded. The key is working with an integrative physician and being aware of the specific contexts and circumstances of your disease. Also, remember to be tested for more than just your cholesterol and triglycerides, and to have more extensive lipids analyses done, as discussed previously.

Cholesterol is a substance made by the liver and absorbed from animal foods. Cholesterol is needed to activate vitamin D_3 from sunlight exposure; it is the core of all our hormones; it is needed for neurotransmitter function in the brain; and it is anti-inflammatory.

One in four Americans over forty-five years old is on a statin drug. Statin drugs are supposed to be added to any patient's regimen if they are diagnosed with T2DM. In fact, when I do not have a patient on a statin drug, the pharmacy that is receiving his prescriptions for glucose meter strips or other tools or medications I am prescribing may fax me a form reminding me to prescribe him a statin drug. The protocol is ingrained in the conventional system.

KEY TREATMENT NOTE

If you are on a statin drug, you must also be taking CoQ10 as a supplement! A good CoQ10 supplement is "crystal free." If you are on a regular CoQ10, you would want to take 100–400 mg per day. A crystal-free form of CoQ10 can easily be taken at only 50–100 mg per day.

Designed to lower cholesterol, statins block the HMG-CoA reductase enzyme pathway in the liver (and adrenals). This pathway makes three separate substances: cholesterol, CoQ10, and dolichols.

CoQ10 is used therapeutically to treat congestive heart failure, arrhythmias, and other diseases of the heart. It is also anticarcinogenic and is a great antioxidant. Since diabetic patients usually die of cardiovascular disease, it does seem odd that using a drug that prevents the production of one of the most important agents for keeping a heart healthy is promoted so adamantly, without at least the strong suggestion to add CoQ10 back in.

Most supplemental CoQ10 is produced as a large crystalline molecule that is hard to absorb through the gut; only around 1–2 percent can be absorbed. Some companies make a much smaller crystal-free molecule that is much easier to absorb, resulting in up to 8–15 percent absorption, so lower doses are fine. There are two forms of CoQ10 currently being sold: ubiquinone and ubiquinol. The cheaper ubiquinone is what I recommend in a crystal-free form.

The lack of dolichols is not usually mentioned when discussing statins. Little known, dolichols are substances in our cells that regulate the production of protein/sugar combinations called "glycoproteins." Dr. Duane Graveline, MD, MPH, has created a presentation about a lack of dolichols being associated with deficiency of neuropeptides, which can be associated with aggression, hostility, depression, and suicidal ideation—problems associated at times with the use of statins.

Conventional care medicine sets the following cholesterol goals for patients with diabetes. See table 5.4 for additional guidelines.

Table 5.4. ADA 2016 Guidelines for Statins

Patient Description	Therapy for Lipid Management
Individuals with diabetes and atherosclerotic cardiovascular disease (ASCVD)	High-intensity statin therapy and lifestyle therapy
Age < 40 with diabetes and ASCVD risk factors	Moderate- or high-intensity statin therapy and lifestyle therapy
Age 40–75 with diabetes without ASCVD risk factors	Moderate-intensity statin therapy and lifestyle therapy
Age 40–75 with diabetes and ASCVD risk factors	High-intensity statin therapy and lifestyle therapy
Age > 75 with diabetes without ASCVD risk factors	Moderate-intensity statin therapy and lifestyle therapy
Age > 75 with diabetes and ASCVD risk factors	Moderate- or high-intensity statin therapy and lifestyle therapy

Note: The intensity of statin therapy may require adjustment based on an individual's response.

LDL. Lower than 100 mg/dL and lower than 70 mg/dL if the patient with diabetes has risk factors for cardiovascular disease.

Total cholesterol. Lower than 200 mg/dL and lower than 170 mg/dL if the patient with diabetes has risk factors for cardiovascular disease.

One's risk of cardiovascular disease can be determined by using the risk calculator at www.cvriskcalculator.com. This calculator also interprets, based on your percentage risk, whether you should or should not take an aspirin or a statin, and if so, at what doses. However, note that the ADA recommends that every patient with diabetes should be on a statin drug, at least at moderate dosing, even if the patient does not have any cardiovascular disease risk. The ADA also recommends mixing statins with other lipid management medications in some populations.

The American Heart Association (AHA) has their own guidelines for statin use, dividing users into four groups. Group 1 includes patients who have had a cardiovascular disease (CVD) event or who have CVD and take statin drugs for secondary prevention. Group 2 are those whose low density lipoprotein cholesterol (LDL-C) is higher than 190 mg/dL. These patients are considered very high risk, and intensive statin therapy is recommended in high doses. Group 3 are diabetic patients, who are also considered very high risk. The AHA recommends that patients in this group who are between the ages of forty and seventy-five be prescribed a moderate or high-intensity statin regimen. Group 4 includes everyone else aged forty to seventy-five based on their estimated ten-year risk for a CVD event. If their risk is equal or greater to 7.5 percent, the AHA recommends they use a statin.

Studies on statins show they are most effective in patients who have advanced coronary disease, positive inflammatory labs, elevated calcium scores in their arteries, and are middle-aged men (and also women who have very severe coronary artery disease).

There is much controversy about how important it is to have low cholesterol. Books like *Overdosed America*, by Dr. John Abramson, and *The Great Cholesterol Myth*, by Dr. Stephen Sinatra and Dr. Jonny Bowden, bring this topic into a glaring light. In cases where my diabetic patient has already had a heart attack or stroke, or smokes and refuses to stop, or refuses to follow my comprehensive protocol (which is very uncommon) and maintains very elevated cholesterol with low HDL levels and elevated inflammation levels, studies do support using statin drugs to lower cholesterol to prevent a second event. I support the use of statins in those situations.

However, in Dr. Abramson's work we learn that there are no studies showing, for example, that women or men over age sixty-five who have not had a cardiovascular event previously will have any decrease in morbidity or mortality on statins. In these cases I recommend removing a female patient's statin if she is over sixty-five and has not already had a heart attack or stroke. But, of course, if this is your situation, please check with your physician first.

To further the case for doubting the need for statins, half of all people who have a heart attack also have normal cholesterol levels. In addition, there are many serious complications for patients on statin drugs, including:

- Severe memory loss, referred to as "transient global amnesia," though this goes away upon stopping the drug.
- Muscle weakness, fatigue, pain, aching. This can be so bad that it prevents patients from being able to exercise. Stopping statins and giving CoQ10, acetyl-l-carnitine, and R-alpha-lipoic acid can usually eradicate those muscle symptoms.

- Rhabdomyopathy, a condition where the muscles break down and cause kidney failure. This is not a common side effect.

However, I think there is more compelling evidence for being wary of using statins. Statin drugs given to prediabetic patients caused a 9 percent increased risk of developing diabetes. The level of risk was shown to be dose dependent; the higher the statin doses, the more risk of becoming a diabetic. Statins simply cause hyperglycemia.

In a study in March 2009 by the *Journal of Investigative Medicine*, statins were shown to raise glucose levels by 7 mg/dL in nondiabetic patients. In diabetic patients, statins can raise glucose levels by 39 mg/dL. That is enough to raise one's A1C by 1.5 percent! This rise can easily turn a prediabetic A1C of 5.7 percent to a diabetic A1C of 7.2 percent. In the JUPITER study of patients taking rosuvastatin/Crestor, 270 became diabetic patients compared to only 216 cases of diabetes in the placebo-treated patients. An analysis by the Women's Health Initiative showed a 48 percent increased risk of diabetes in women on statins. Another study with long-term data reported a 363 percent increased risk of diabetes after being on statins for fifteen to twenty years. And another showed a 46 percent greater risk of T2DM onset in patients with metabolic syndrome when they were on statin therapy for almost six years. It seems the longer one is on a statin, the worse the risk of raising glucose levels and causing diabetes. As a result, the FDA changed the label for the entire class of statins to warn medical practitioners that statin therapy can raise glucose and A1C levels.

The question therefore is whether the effect of lowering cardiovascular disease occurrence offsets the increased risk of becoming a diabetic patient or of having worse glucose control. Since the main cause of death of diabetic patients is cardiovascular disease, it does seem questionable to use a medication to prevent heart disease in people with prediabetes while that same medication promotes the development of diabetes, in which their risk of dying from cardiovascular disease significantly increases. And it seems questionable to give it to diabetic patients who are trying to lower cardiovascular disease risk when the result is a rise in glucose levels, the cause of blood vessel damage in these same patients.

In a study published in *Clinical Lipidology* in 2013, statin drugs were shown to cause proteinuria, the loss of protein through the urine, the first sign of kidney failure. Fifteen percent of those on statin medications experienced proteinuria, while only 6.9 percent of those not on statins lost protein. Although we do not understand the long-term effect on the statin-induced microalbuminuria, it is a concern to me that it happens at all.

On the other hand, a 2014 study in *Lancet Diabetes and Endocrinology* showed that diabetic patients who were on statins developed less retinopathy and nephropathy than patients not on statins, which may be due to the anti-inflammatory aspect of the drug. However, since none of my patients have ever developed either of those complications, without using statins, I am confident in my comprehensive integrative protocol without using statins.

I know that by following my diabetic protocol there is usually a substantial improvement in the lab values even in the first three to six months. Lipids can come down significantly by changing diets, reducing insulin use, using appropriate supplements, exercising, sleeping well and managing stress, and ensuring other hormones are well controlled. I've seen a patient's triglycerides lowered from 688 mg/dL to 88 mg/dL and total cholesterol from 344 mg/dL to 192 mg/dL after three months on my protocol, with no statin drugs. Those levels are not uncommon among patients on an effective integrative protocol.

The Great Cholesterol Myth coauthor Dr. Stephen Sinatra, an integrative-minded cardiologist whose son became a naturopathic physician, has written repeatedly that high sugar, not high cholesterol, causes cardiovascular disease. He advised not to prescribe statins to healthy diabetic patients with no cardiovascular disease history, but to use statins with middle-aged men, between fifty and seventy years old, who have had a heart attack or stroke, or who have coronary artery disease. He also pointed out that statins are anti-inflammatory and can help make the blood thinner, but instead of using them for that purpose, he recommends the following supplements, in addition to a healthy diet: fish oils, digestive enzymes, bromelain, garlic, and nattokinase. I find these to be great naturopathic recommendations. Supplements will be discussed later in this book, including specifics on how to use alternatives to statins in situations where it is safe and responsible to do so.

COST: \$10–\$230/month.

DOSE:

Lipitor/atorvastatin. 10, 20, 40, 80 mg
Zocor/simvastatin. 5, 10, 20, 40, 80 mg
Pravachol/pravastatin. 10, 20, 40, 80 mg
Crestor/rosuvastatin. 5, 10, 20 mg
Mevacor/lovastatin. 10, 20, 40, 80 mg

▶ **KEY TREATMENT NOTE**

You may get a recommendation to be on a statin drug if your cholesterol is outside the ranges I listed above and you are a diabetic patient. First, get a more comprehensive cardiovascular lab panel done at a specialty lab, as discussed in chapter 4, and learn more about your cardiovascular risk. Unless you are a middle-aged male and have already had a heart attack or stroke, there are alternatives to starting a statin drug. Find a good integrative diabetic physician to help guide you to safe and effective treatment. If you are on a statin drug, you should take crystal-free CoQ10 to make up for the lack of formation of that antioxidant.

— CHAPTER SIX —

The Eighth Essential: Medicine (The Insulins)

Insulin: both a blessing and a burden.

Invented in 1922 by two enterprising Canadians, Frederick Banting and Charles Best, insulin was intially exceedingly difficult to use; patients had to reuse and sharpen their needles, as well as boil them for sterility before injecting. Today, patients are able to choose between different types and forms of insulin and accessories that are much simpler to use and have success with. I encourage medical practitioners reading this book to connect with the representatives of the makers of glucose meters, pumps, pens, continuous glucose monitor systems, and even syringes. Having an office full of samples for patients is helpful when you are discussing the varied ways of using insulin.

Although insulin injections were used historically only for people with T1DM—who by the nature of their disease generally do not make enough insulin to sustain life and usually require multiple daily injections to stay alive—now, due to the epidemic of T2DM and poorly controlled T2DM, it's typical, though sad and unnecessary, that T2DM patients often progress to the point of requiring insulin use as well.

According to conventional medicine, insulin levels are high only in the prediabetic state (such as in metabolic syndrome / insulin resistance) and once T2DM develops, the pancreas in T2DM patients no longer makes enough insulin; that is, patients are not producing enough to overcome their insulin resistance, and that is why their glucose numbers are elevated. Yet, when I measure insulin or c-peptide levels in T2DM patients, they are often making normal amounts of insulin, or sometimes too much—proof of insulin resistance, even when they have been prescribed insulin. Sometimes, though, long-term poorly controlled T2DM can show very low insulin production.

In general, the problem is usually that the patient is overweight or obese, eating a high-carbohydrate diet that his or her pancreas cannot keep up with. When the diet is changed, oftentimes with resultant weight loss, the pancreas of a T2DM patient often makes plenty of insulin on its own.

To be blunt, no person with T2DM should ever wind up on insulin if they follow the protocol established by an integrative physician. In my opinion, conventional care management, however, is not designed to control diabetes, given its lack of focus on diet and the other Eight Essentials. A T2DM patient requiring insulin over time illustrates previous medical treatment failure or lack of compliance if a valid diabetic protocol was given but not followed.

Nevertheless, when needed, insulin is a very helpful medication, and we are lucky it was invented.

We need to initiate insulin in diabetic patients when:

- T1DM has been diagnosed (although many pediatric patients can reduce and even remove insulin through an undefined honeymoon period).
- The patient has LADA. Over time, many LADA patients may not be able to control glucose levels and keep their A1Cs down without the addition of insulin.
- Gestational diabetes is not well controlled with diet, exercise, and oral hypoglycemic agents.
- A patient has MODY, although this is very uncommon.
- A T2DM patient has progressed to either having damaged beta cells that no longer produce appropriate amounts of insulin, or is so insulin resistant that even multiple OHAs cannot control their glucose levels. If the T2DM patient is on two or three OHA medicines and has an A1C that is higher than 6.5 percent, even on a good diet and lifestyle insulin may indeed be required.
- Complications are developing in a T2DM patient.

Diabetic ID

The need for a diabetic ID if the patient is injecting any type or amount of insulin is one of the more sensitive things I discuss with patients. A diabetic ID is a necessity for the safety of the patient, so that if something goes wrong, all emergency responders will immediately know that a diabetic reaction must be considered.

There are many different types of diabetic IDs. I've even had one patient tattoo "Diabetes Type 1" on her wrist. There are shoelace IDs, bracelets, or necklaces made of basic metal, silver, gold, or platinum. Many people now prefer wearing a plastic wristband with "diabetes" on it. Psychologically, it can be tough for some patients to wear an ID, and I understand that. It's as if they are defined by their condition instead of their unique personality, and they are lost to their disease. That is a valid feeling, and a patient should be able to discuss this topic with their physician without feeling judged. Nonetheless, as a physician, the safety of my patient is always the top concern, and having an ID just makes good sense. In a positive physician/patient team, this can be processed in a way that ensures the patient is still seen as an individual and allows the physician to feel the patient is protected.

- T2DM has been newly diagnosed. There are newer studies wherein patients diagnosed with T2DM are prescribed insulin right away to "rest" their pancreas, if their hyperglycemia is particularly high. As I mention later in the chapter, while studies are showing this is efficacious, very few physicians and patients are willing to engage in this protocol. Since I've seen patients' postprandial blood sugars drop from 400 mg/dL to 150 mg/dL in just a couple of weeks *without* the use of insulin, I do not initiate insulin immediately with T2DM patients.

The use of insulin is understandably a big concern both for patients and physicians. For many patients with diabetes, avoiding the use of insulin is their entire focus; I feel it should instead be keeping their glucose under the most excellent control possible. However, the use of insulin is a very emotional phenomenon, and many patients who should be on insulin are not, because their physicians do not want to deal with it and because the patients are adamantly against it themselves.

Barriers to Using Insulin

One observational study showed that diabetic patients spent an average of four years in suboptimal glucose control, their A1Cs above 8 percent, before starting insulin therapy. Why is this? When everything is not working, and the patient's A1C is showing the patient is out of control and their glucose levels are causing damage to their body, why does it take so long for insulin to be initiated? It is no doubt due to the multiple barriers that both physicians and patients must overcome about starting insulin.

What are those barriers? For health care professionals, they can include:

Pessimistic attitude. Many physicians do not believe patients will do well on insulin; they believe that insulin will not stop the development of complications; and they think that insulin is not a good methodology for treating diabetes.

Too much to know. There are many different types of insulin, different insulin protocols, and different situations to feel mastery in, such as travel, illness, and so on. Many physicians simply do not have good knowledge bases for all the nuances in order to ensure their patients are using the least amount of insulin in the most precise ways, avoiding both hyperglycemic and hypoglycemic reactions.

Lack of confidence using insulin. Though this may surprise patients, many physicians are not good at, and in fact, may be terrible at, prescribing insulin and managing patients on it. Many physicians do not feel comfortable either having patients on insulin or having to deal with all the complexities that come with it.

Time-consuming. Believe it or not, there are physicians who refuse to see patients on insulin because managing insulin for diabetic patients can be time-consuming. I do not find it to be excessively time-consuming because my patients are well trained, and with the entirety of their protocol their diabetes is typically very well controlled.

Cost to patients. For patients paying out of pocket or who have bad insurance policies, using insulin can be very expensive.

For patients, there are also several notable barriers:

Fear of gaining weight. Gaining weight on insulin is a real risk for patients, particularly if they are dosed too high in order to control their glucose and are not on a low-carbohydrate diet. Patients can avoid gaining weight if they are guided to the right diet, if their insulin dosing as a whole is kept as low as is possible, and if they are being treated comprehensively with the other Eight Essentials.

Worries about insulin resistance. This is a very sensible worry, as again, injecting massive amounts of insulin (and some patients are on massive amounts of insulin!) does indeed lead to insulin resistance, weight gain, and the inability to lose weight.

Fear of needles. This is now easy to curtail. Insulin dosing needles are extremely small and thin. I have patients inject themselves with an empty insulin syringe in my office, and they realize they cannot even feel it. Teaching proper injection technique is very helpful, too.

Psychology. Some patients feel like a failure for having to use insulin, especially when everything they've done with diet, exercise, and previous medications has not controlled the disease. This is why it is important that physicians working with patients with diabetes set the tone that no treatment is a sign of failure. The focus has to be on controlling glucose; however that happens is a winning situation. Another psychological aspect is typified by a T2DM patient with a family history who believes "insulin killed Aunt Mary." That is, after Aunt Mary went on insulin, her leg was amputated, and then she had a heart attack and died. The patient may honestly believe it was the insulin that killed her. This is a fairly common association for many patients with a family history of T2DM, but of course, the reality of such a situation is that the patient's diabetes was poorly controlled, she was put on insulin, and still her diabetes was poorly controlled, and she wound up developing severe complications that led to her morbidity and mortality. A well-trained physician can assure patients that their control will be very different than "Aunt Mary's."

Too much to learn. Patients on insulin have to live their lives wondering about how much insulin is in them, how much needs to be in them, matching the entirety of their lives—food, rest, exercise, travel, and stresses—to figuring out how much insulin they need to inject. Working with insulin is complicated for patients, and it can be frustrating when they work hard to get everything matched and their glucose numbers are still not ideal.

Fear of hypoglycemia. This is a very understandable fear. In general, I can confidently state that the majority of diabetic patients feel more comfortable being high than having a hypoglycemic episode. But, I have found that excellent training on using insulin, particularly in an integrative fashion, can truly allay that fear in a patient. Matching an appropriate diet, lifestyle, and supplements with appropriately managed insulin significantly reduces risks of hypoglycemia, in both adults and children.

Cost. If a patient is paying out of pocket, insulin can be enormously expensive. I refer patients to www.canadianinsulin.com for significant savings on insulin products if they are paying out of pocket.

Fear of allergy to insulin. This does happen now and then. I've had patients who were allergic to basal insulin and also allergic to Humalog insulin. However, this is very uncommon and switching to another brand will often suffice.

Patients need calm and compassionate counseling when starting to use insulin, but they also need to understand that they must commit to the program and ensure excellent communication with their physician. Patients on insulin have the responsibility to get a diabetes ID, as well as a glucagon kit and glucose tabs/gels to treat hypoglycemia; test glucose levels regularly; alert their physician when they're sick, are vomiting, have diarrhea, or cannot eat; and keep diet diaries and glucose graphs prior to office visits.

A physician must give the patient on insulin methods to contact the physician twenty-four hours a day, seven days a week. I give patients on insulin my personal email address and cell phone number, so they can always reach me in case a crisis occurs after normal office hours, although since most patients are very well controlled on my program, I have only received a call once or twice a year.

Insulin Use

To best use insulin, you must be on a low-carbohydrate diet. If you eat too many carbohydrates, it will be nearly impossible to have stable, low glucose numbers without having hyperglycemia or hypoglycemia as a regular occurrence.

Using insulin requires being calm, patient, and attentive. It can take weeks, and sometimes months, until a full protocol is figured out. There is no need to rush—getting good control without hypoglycemia is the key. Physicians and patients need to know that there is always some "winging it" when using insulin, and educated guessing is common. When done with a confident physician who is in close contact with patients and has created a comprehensive protocol for a patient, educated guessing in a step-by-step process is effective and safe. It is important to change only one variable at a time with insulin and always to keep good glucose levels.

Finally, when analyzing glucose numbers, especially for patients on insulin, it is vital to look for trends. As a general rule, do not focus on individual glucose numbers, but look for daily or weekly trends. For example, if I see that every afternoon at 3 p.m. a patient's glucose levels are high, or their fasting glucose is usually high, or that the patient has hypoglycemia after exercise in the morning, I can easily use these trends to adjust insulin doses. But one odd elevated glucose level standing alone on a glucose graph that shows excellent numbers otherwise probably means some indiscretion occurred, or it may be some mysterious outlier. I wouldn't prescribe a change in insulin dosing in that case.

General Insulin Information

Insulin in the United States and Canada is U-100 insulin. That means that there are 100 units of insulin per 1 cc. Thus, a 10 cc bottle, the typical vial of insulin sold in North America, contains 1,000 units of insulin. Not all countries in the world are standardized to U-100, so when you are traveling overseas, ensure you have extra insulin, although I will discuss in chapter 13 how to adjust to using U-40 or another type of insulin if you must when you are overseas.

When insulin is unopened, refrigerate it; the range for maintaining potency is between 36° F and 84° F (Apidra, one of the rapid-acting insulins, should not be stored above 77° F). Once insulin is opened and in use, however, do not refrigerate it. It is not only unnecessary, but injecting cold insulin can sting. It is best to inject insulin at room temperature.

Most insulins last twenty-eight to thirty days, so they shouldn't be used for more than one month. Not all patients are aware of this; I've had numerous patients presenting to me with numbers in the 300s when their numbers should be lower, and the reason was that they were using three-month-old insulin, which simply wasn't active anymore. If you only use 10 units of insulin a day, 300 units a month, you are going to have a lot of insulin left in the bottle at the end of the month, but nonetheless, you need to throw it all away and get a new bottle, or it will stop working.

Insulin pens have essentially the same limitations related to temperature and length of time as vials of insulin do, though the Levemir pen can be used for forty-two days. Mixed insulin pens, however, are only good for ten to fourteen days.

There are three main categories of insulins, all of which can cause hypoglycemia and need to be finely controlled.

Basal/background. This type of insulin is used to control the liver's production of glucose between meals and during sleep.

Bolus/meal/correction. This type of insulin is used to cover food eaten at meals. Some bolus insulin can also be used to make corrections, which is when insulin is used to lower an elevated glucose number, either at a meal or between meals.

Mixed. This type of insulin contains both a basal and a bolus insulin. It is nonstandard now. If you are on a mixed insulin product, tell your physician you want to get off that product and use a better insulin protocol that is more updated and more effective. No one should be prescribed mixed insulin vials or mixed insulin pens if

Medicines and Insulin

As a quick review, here is a list of all the diabetic medicines safe to use with insulin.

- Metformin
- DPP-4 inhibitors
- SGLT-2 inhibitors
- Symlin
- Hypertensive medications
- Statins

Diabetic medicines that are usually stopped with insulin are as follows.

- GLP-1 injections (although this is not totally avoided by those on insulin)
- Sulfonylureas
- Meglitinides

they want excellent control. Luckily, it's very rare to see a patient who is prescribed a mixed insulin dosage, and I change the protocol immediately when I do.

Insulin can be used in several different ways. Multiple daily injections (MDI) is when patients use insulin vials and syringes *or* disposable pens *or* pens with cartridges and inject one or many times throughout the day either basal alone or both basal and bolus insulin. The other method of insulin dosing is using a continuous subcutaneous insulin infusion, also known as a pump. This is only used for patients who need both basal and bolus insulin, usually T1DM patients, but an increasing number of T2DM patients are unfortunately progressing to that scenario as well. With a pump, only one type of insulin is used.

Either of these ways is valid, and I prefer allowing patients who need insulin to choose which one they wish to use and are most comfortable with. Some studies show that patients on pumps have better control than those doing MDI, and I have to agree that pumps are a better way to control basal insulin levels, as we'll discuss later. However, no matter the insulin-dosing method, a patient's diabetes can be out of control on any or all of them, or a patient's diabetes can be in control on any or all of them.

The Different Insulins

The different insulins available for use are made by the three main companies: Lilly (Humalog); NovoNordisk (NovoLog, Levemir); and Sanofi (Apidra, Lantus). All of the insulins are discussed below; the specifics of how to dose them will be covered in depth after this introductory section.

All insulins are expensive if paid for out of pocket. I've listed estimated prices for the insulins in each category as found via internet searches. The insulin companies have programs, such as the Lilly Cares Patient Assistance Program, Novo Nordisk's Diabetes Patient Assistance Program, and Sanofi's Patient Connection, to help individuals pay for or even receive free insulin.

Another option is that most of my patients ordering insulin out of pocket buy it for much less at www.canadianinsulin.com.

Rapid Insulin

NAMES: NovoLog/aspart, Humalog/lispro, Apidra/glulisine

ACTIONS:

Onset: 15–20 minutes
Peak action: between 30 minutes and 2.5 hours
Duration: 3–4 hours

Rapid-acting, or rapid, insulin is a clear, analog insulin. "Analog" means that it has been genetically altered to create an insulin nearly identical to human insulin except for an amino acid change in the insulin molecule. It acts quicker in the human body, and has a quicker peak time and a shorter duration of action than regular insulin.

It is used in four main ways:

1. For bolus injections with meals
2. As a correction insulin dose (to lower high numbers)
3. In pumps
4. To treat diabetic ketoacidosis

Rapid-acting insulins take effect within fifteen to twenty minutes after injection and last for three to four hours. Thus, they should be injected fifteen to twenty minutes before a meal. In the last few years, I've seen more and more diabetic patients getting into the really bad habit of injecting their rapid insulin right at the beginning of a meal, not before. To have the insulin meet the glucose breakdown from food smoothly, it is necessary to inject fifteen to twenty minutes before the meal.

The only patients who should inject their rapid insulin after meals are young pediatric patients, as we are never sure how much food a young child will eat. So, parents will see how much of the meal the child eats, and then inject a dose to cover that meal afterward. There will be a slight lack of control, but it's the safest way to go. By around ten years old, children are usually eating what is on their plate, and when this happens, starting the injection before the meal is recommended. However, parents have to ensure their children will eat their plate of food on which the insulin dosing is based, no matter what their age, before injecting fifteen to twenty minutes before the meal, to prevent hypoglycemia (which will occur if the insulin injected is for more food than the child actually eats).

Rapid insulin is also used to make corrections—that is, if a patient's blood glucose gets too high, rapid insulin is dosed to lower the glucose to the correction goal number. Ideally, there should be few corrections to make, as the diet and insulin dosing should merge well. A correction dose should ideally be done upon waking and before meals, added to the insulin designed to cover the meal. Injecting insulin in between meals to correct puts a patient at a higher risk of having hypoglycemia, and only patients experienced in injecting insulin should do it. Of course, the most important thing to learn about going high and needing a correction is what caused the glucose elevation in the first place and how can that be avoided in the future.

Typical corrections should be injected subcutaneously with the meal bolus, but at times, such as if the patient is ill or the numbers are very high, one can inject a correction dose directly into the muscle. Doing so will markedly enhance the speed of the insulin reaction in the body, as it will enter into the blood much quicker than if injected into the subcutaneous tissue. But, injecting subcutaneously works best the vast majority of times.

Under good comprehensive care, the correction goal (that is, the glucose level we wish to achieve after the correction is injected) is generally a range from 80 to 100 (depending on age).

For some reason, most patients are prescribed a rapid pen that only allows a full-unit dosing change; for example, a patient can only inject 2, 3, or 4 units at a time. When a patient is on a low-carb diet, injecting by full units can cause poor control, leading to hypoglycemia or, if underinjected to avoid lows, leading to hyperglycemia.

I want my patients on rapid insulin, whether pediatric or adult, to only use rapid pens that allow half-unit dosing. That way a patient can inject 1 or 1.5 units, for example, and better match their insulin needs to the meal eaten. Half units can make a big difference on a low-carb diet! These half-unit pens usually have to be ordered by the pharmacy, because the full-unit pens are by far the most commonly prescribed, and pharmacies do not keep the half-unit pens in stock.

RAPID PENS I DO NOT USE WITH PATIENTS BECAUSE THEY ARE SET FOR ONLY FULL-UNIT DOSING:

NovoLog FlexPen. Prefilled, disposable pens: five per box
Humalog KwikPen. Prefilled, disposable pens: five per box
Apidra SoloSTAR. Prefilled, disposable pens: five per box

RAPID PENS I USE WITH MY PATIENTS BECAUSE THEY ARE SET FOR HALF-UNIT DOSING:

NovoPen Echo. One refillable pen and five cartridges per box
HumaPen Luxura HD. One refillable pen and five cartridges per box

Rapid insulin is one-third stronger than regular insulin, so they cannot be substituted equally. If a person injects 6 units of regular, he would only inject 4 units of rapid. But please note: although I discuss regular insulin next, almost no one uses regular anymore, and it's likely it will be taken off the market in the near future.

Last, the cost difference of prefilled and refillable pens is also a concern, if a patient has to pay out of pocket. One box of five prefilled rapid pens costs around $510 and one box of five cartridges costs around $310.

Humalog U-200 KwikPen

Humalog is now made in a form that is twice as strong as typical Humalog. It contains 200 units per ml, instead of the 100 units per ml that is in typical

Inhaled Insulin

I am not sure why pharmaceutical companies continue to bother with inhaled insulin, since the methodology has not, I feel, developed into anything worth recommending.

The only inhaled insulin product is called Afrezza. It is a rapid-acting insulin used for meals. The use of Afrezza has been shown to reduce A1Cs only 0.4 percent, which is unimpressive. Also, our lungs are designed to breathe in pure air, not pancreatic hormones. Side effects of inhaling insulin include throat pain, cough, hypoglycemia, and acute bronchospasm. I highly disagree with breathing in insulin.

Afrezza is a poor choice to use for meals for another reason, as well. It comes in cartridges that are either 4 units of insulin (blue colored) or 8 units of insulin (green colored). That means that a patient has the capacity to only dose 4, 8, 12, and so on units for a meal, which is not helpful. Patients need many different sizes of insulin doses per meal, not only 4-unit doses, and not being able to specifically dose the exact units needed sets patients up for all kinds of problems, ending up with their glucose levels either too low or too high after meals. Due to the odd cartridge setup, a patient will have to keep changing the blue and green cartridge doses and use one to three of the cartridges per bolus dosing at each meal.

The last nail in the coffin is that Afrezza has been shown to only last two hours after meals, which is not long enough to cover all the food that a patient has eaten. Afrezza is now being marketed to T1DM patients, using one cartridge for smaller meals and two cartridges for larger meals or if a correction is needed. I teach how to precisely dose insulin later in the chapter, and so I do not agree with using doses in Afrezza's 4-unit increments.

Afrezza is contraindicated in patients in ketoacidosis, smokers, and patients who already suffer from a lung condition, like asthma or chronic obstructive pulmonary disease (chronic bronchitis or emphysema). In general, I would say avoid Afrezza. Afrezza seems to be an option only for a person who has to use insulin at higher doses at meals and refuses to use any insulin injection. I've never met that type of patient!

Humalog. Thus, it comes in a pen that contains 600 units of insulin, instead of the 300 units a standard Humalog pen contains.

For patients who are injecting a lot of rapid-acting insulin at meals, Humalog U-200 can cut their insulin in half, which may help them lose weight. For example, if a patient injects 16 units at a meal three times a day, he is injecting 48 units a day, and goes through a pen—filled with only 300 units—every seven days, or four pens a month. Injecting Humalog U-200 can lower that to 8 units a meal, so that a pen lasts for fourteen days, or only two pens a month. It is bioequivalent to U-100 Humalog in all other ways.

Patients inject the same amount of U-200 insulin as they did U-100, so there is no confusing conversion factor. The pen simply injects half the insulin the dose indicates, but the insulin is twice as strong. This insulin comes in Humalog U-200 KwikPens: prefilled, disposable—two pens per box. A box with two pens may cost up to around $500 out of pocket.

Regular Insulin

NAMES: Novolin R, Humulin R

ACTIONS:

Onset: 30–45 minutes
Peak action: 2–3 hours
Duration: 5–6 hours

Regular insulin is also known as short-acting insulin. It is only used for bolus dosing before meals. It is a clear insulin.

As regular is not an analog insulin, it takes between thirty and forty-five minutes to "kick in," because the body first has to disassociate the insulin from the zinc molecule it is attached to. Patients often do not want to have to inject their insulin dose for their meal that far ahead of time. However, it does last significantly longer in the body, up to six hours, so that it can cover a meal better than a rapid insulin. Regular insulin is steadier in its effect than rapid-acting insulin, too.

In addition to patients not wanting to inject that far ahead of their meal, another problem with regular insulin is that it is not a good correction insulin, so patients using it for meals will still have to have some rapid insulin available in case a correction dose is needed before a meal. That would mean, ideally, that the patient would inject a rapid insulin for their correction dose, and then inject another shot of regular for their meal. Insulins are not supposed to be mixed if they do not come that way already. However, a patient can pull up a rapid and then a regular insulin into the same syringe, in that order, if they need to correct at their meal. The quicker insulin should always be pulled up first if you are using two insulins with one syringe. Still, patients are hardly interested in having to carry around two insulins, one for a meal and one for corrections, when a rapid-acting on its own is designed to cover both.

Humulin R and Novolin R insulins only come in a 10 cc vial. Regular insulin is a little less expensive than rapid insulin, around $200 for a 10 cc vial out of pocket.

Humulin R U-500

Humulin R U-500 is a very concentrated insulin prescribed to patients who need to take excessively high units of insulin for their meals, injecting over 200 units a day. Using U-500 allows a patient to inject a lot fewer units to get high unit dosing. Remember, U-100 means that each 1 ml contains 100 units of insulin, and U-100 insulin vials come in 10 cc doses equaling 1,000 total units per bottle. So with U-500, each 1 ml is 500 units of insulin, and each vial is 20 cc; equaling 10,000 units per bottle. U-500 insulin contains, therefore, as many units of insulin as 10 vials of U-100 insulin.

A patient can use a U-100 syringe with this insulin. Dosing entails dividing the U-500 by 5 to get the U-500 injection dosing using a U-100 syringe, or by 500 to get the U-500 dose in a volumetric syringe. It is pretty complicated, and it is easy to make a dosing error. Thank goodness a Humulin U-500 cartridge KwikPen was recently created, which contains 1,500 ml of U-500; each click is the equivalent of 5 insulin units. This insulin cannot be transferred from the pen to a syringe, as that would significantly increase the risk of a severe hypoglycemic episode.

Switching from U-100 to U-500 insulin starts with either giving the same U-500 dose as was the patient's U-100 dose (if the patient's A1C is greater than 8 percent and mean glucose in the last week was greater than or equal to 183 mg/dL) or giving 80 percent of the U-100 dose (if the patient's A1C was lower than or equal to 8 percent or mean glucose in the last week was lower than183 mg/dL). U-500 is given either twice a day, with 60 percent of the total daily dose before breakfast and 40 percent of the total daily dose before supper or three times a day, with 40 percent of total daily dose before breakfast and 30 percent of the total daily dose before lunch and supper.

U-500 is very rarely needed in a typical diabetes protocol, and it can be very confusing to use. I've never had a patient require U-500. I imagine that people using that much insulin are obese, eating a very high-carbohydrate diet, and in need of instruction on improving their lifestyle, too. The Humulin U-500 KwikPen is prefilled, disposable, and has 600 units per pen, with two pens included per box. Out-of-pocket costs can be between $600 and $1,500.

Intermediate Insulin

NAMES: Neutral protamine Hagedorn (NPH)
Protamine molecule: Humulin N, Novolin N, NPH Purified
Zinc molecule: Novolin L (lente), Humulin L (lente)

ACTIONS:
Onset: 2–4 hours
Peak action: 4–10 hours
Duration: 8–16 hours

NPH is a cloudy insulin that needs to be rolled between one's hands around twenty times before use to ensure the molecules are all mixed equally in the fluid. NPH is a basal insulin; that is, it is used to keep glucose levels down between meals and during sleep. It is much less popular now, as this type of insulin has the highest incidence of causing hypoglycemia. Also, the long-acting insulins are now the standard basal insulins. NPH is not used for meal or correction dosing. In mixed insulins, NPH is typically (though not always) the insulin used with a rapid or regular insulin. NPH costs about the same as other insulin 10 cc vials, around $200 out of pocket, though a box of pens is around $570.

NPH lasts between eight and fifteen hours, so patients need to inject it two or three times a day. When patients are on NPH insulin and their physicians wish to change them to a long-acting basal, the following protocol is used:

- If NPH is given once a day, we'd switch by dosing an equal dose of long-acting insulin.
- If dosing two or more NPH shots a day, the long-acting basal would be 80 percent of that NPH total daily dose. So, for example, if the NPH dose is 15 units total a day in two shots, we'd start with 12 units of long-acting insulin.
- The formula to switch from long-acting insulin to NPH is to convert equal units to units.

Due to the risk of hypoglycemia, it is important with NPH to titrate up doses as required every three to five days. NPH is not used to treat diabetic ketoacidosis.

NPH insulin comes in the following forms.

Humulin N or Novolin N U-100. 10 cc vials
Humulin N KwikPen. 100 units / mL, 3 mL per pen, box of five pens

Long-Acting Insulin

NAMES: Lantus / glargine (U-100); Lantus—generic Basaglar (U-100); Toujeo / glargine (U-300); Levemir / detemir (U-100); Tresiba / degludec (U-200)

ACTIONS:

Onset: 1–4 hours
Peak action: None
Duration (Lantus / Basaglar / Levemir): 11–24 hours, depending on dose and age. In a younger patient the insulin can last 24 hours. In adults higher doses of insulin may promote 24-hour duration. Levemir states that two doses are typical for their product, while Lantus says one dose can last all day. In many adults, though, even from adolescence, two shots of either insulin are often required, morning and evening.
Duration (Toujeo / Tresiba): Up to 36 hours, but most patients inject these daily.

Long-acting insulin is a basal analog clear insulin. These insulins are "peakless"; they are at their height of action five hours after injection and stay stable in activity. They are generally injected one or two times a day.

Lantus (Glargine U-100)

Lantus advertises itself as lasting twenty-four hours and only needing one shot a day, but the study behind this claim required injecting huge amounts of insulin. Levemir states a patient should require one or two shots a day. In general, for pediatric T1DM patients, one shot a day may be effective, as the insulin's effects are so strong in their little bodies. Once puberty kicks in, though, and in all adults, it's typical that two doses are needed in a twenty-four-hour period, an evening shot and a morning shot. In T1DM patients, more is usually needed at night and less in the morning, but T2DM patients may need equal doses of insulin evening and morning. A physician who has expertise in using insulin will help create the perfect dosing pattern for patients.

Some patients have injected this type of insulin three times a day—at bedtime, in the morning, and then in the afternoon—the way we used to dose intermediate NPH insulins. I have not done that with patients myself, and if a patient is that uncontrolled with basal insulin, I feel using a pump is a better idea and is less likely to cause hypoglycemia, or I choose to move to one of the stronger basal insulins.

This is the insulin we start with if insulin is required for new T2DM patients, with initial dosing at bedtime. In pediatric T1DM patients it's very common to inject once a day in the morning, so the child would not be asleep if any significant hypoglycemic episode were to occur, and the parents would be aware of the incident. When the child is in her teens, the basal can be moved to nighttime to be more effective against the dawn phenomenon.

Long-acting insulins cannot be used to treat diabetic ketoacidosis. They should be slowly titrated up, waiting three to five days before increasing a dosage; absolutely do not keep increasing the dose each night. It takes several days for basal insulin to have its full effect in the body. Each time the long-acting insulin evening dose is increased, a patient's blood glucose should be checked around 3 a.m., for a couple of nights, to ensure no hypoglycemia is occurring.

Long-acting insulin cannot be mixed with any other insulin.

Lantus is slightly acidic in nature, with a lower pH than Levemir, and that can be irritating and cause burning in some patients. In such cases, it's easy to change to Levemir; if the patient's insurance prefers Lantus, a pre-authorization is required, but in my experience it is nearly always approved.

Lantus was associated with causing cancer some years back, but that association was not proved; researchers agree that it does not increase the risk of cancer. In general, poorly controlled diabetes as a whole increases the risk of cancer, due to elevated glucose and increased inflammation, but it is safe to use Lantus as a basal insulin.

U-100 long-acting insulins come in the following forms.

Lantus U-100. 10 cc vial
Lantus SoloSTAR pen. Prefilled, disposable, 1 unit dosing—five pens per box
Levemir U-100. 10 cc vial
Levemir FlexPen. Prefilled, disposable, 1 unit dosing—five pens per box

One of my largest frustrations right now is that in the United States we cannot get the JuniorSTAR Pen, which is available in Europe and Canada. This is a half-unit pen one can use with Lantus cartridges, thus allowing the patient to inject half-unit basal doses. For pediatric patients using Lantus, and even adults, this would be a valuable option to have.

As for out-of-pocket costs, they are expensive. Basal insulin per vial is around $275. Basal pens, 3 per box, cost around $400. Getting the generic Basaglar Kwikpen is around $375 per box.

Toujeo (Glargine U-300) and Tresiba (Degludec U-200)

Toujeo insulin is a stronger form of Lantus, equal to U-300; that is, there are 300 units per cc. It is designed to be injected at the same time every day, once a day. It is not recommended for patients under eighteen years old, while regular Lantus or Levemir are safe for pediatric patients. This insulin should be considered if a patient is on a very high unit dose of Lantus or Levemir.

Toujeo comes in a pen, and the pen is set up so that the patient will continue to inject the same Lantus or Levemir dose they were injecting previously; each unit dose of the Toujeo pen actually doses only one-third as much insulin as a Lantus or Levemir pen, but because it is three times stronger it winds up having the same insulin effect. Toujeo is supposed to last up to thirty-six hours, but it is usually injected daily by patients. It is mainly designed for very insulin resistant T2DM patients. These pens are designed so that patients use less insulin and require fewer pens.

To switch from Toujeo to long-acting U-100, inject 80 percent of the Toujeo dose. Patients may need to titrate up or down from that starting dose to get an effective dose.

To switch from long-acting insulin to Toujeo, inject the same long-acting dose. However, in general, we are seeing that an equivalent dose of a stronger insulin does not always work for patients, and sometimes patients may need to titrate up the dose of Toujeo to establish good control. Still, a patient would be injecting a lot fewer units of insulin at a given time, and that might help with weight loss.

Tresiba is a long-acting insulin of Levemir, with the strength of U-200, and comes in a FlexTouch pen. It advertises that it can be used for up to eight weeks if kept at appropriate temperatures. Like Toujeo, there is no conversion and a patient can inject the same dose of Tresiba they were injecting of Lantus or Levemir.

Neither of these stronger basal insulins should be used with diabetic patients younger than eighteen or with pregnant women. They also cannot be used to treat diabetic ketoacidosis or be mixed with other insulins. Great care should be taken in dosing, as a mistaken overdose could have serious, potentially fatal consequences due to extreme hypoglycemia.

These high-unit dose insulins are available in the following forms.

Toujeo SoloSTAR pen. Prefilled, disposable, 1-unit dosing: three or five pens per box

Tresiba FlexTouch pen. Prefilled, disposable, 1-unit dosing: three pens per box

I have had some good feedback from patients who were using U-100 insulin and switched to Toujeo. Patients feel they have good stability of dosing even at just once a day. I think these stronger insulins are worth looking into and using with appropriate patients.

Toujeo pens are also, unfortunately, another expensive out of pocket, around $410, and Tresiba (degludec) may be even more at around $630.

Mixed Insulins

Mixed insulins are not ever recommended, and are not generally used very much. For physicians who are not that comfortable dosing insulin, mixed insulins may still be prescribed, but it is an inferior form of dosing.

Here is the latest list of mixed insulins. Remember that if they have NPH in them, they need to be rolled between the hands twenty times:

- Humulin 50/50 (NPH + regular)
- Humulin 70/30 (NPH + regular)
- Humalog 75/25 (lispro + protamine lispro)
- Humalog 50/50 (protamine lispro + lispro)
- Novolin 70/30 (NPH + lispro)
- Novolin 70/30 (aspart + protamine aspart)
- Novolin 50/50 (aspart + protamine aspart)

I am not listing the out-of-pocket costs for mixed insulins because I never use them, and I strongly suggest they be avoided.

Diabetic Accessories

When you are using insulin, there are many accessories that come with it.

Syringes

In general, syringe needles come in 6 mm, 8 mm, and 12.7 mm lengths. Moreover, they come in 28, 30, and 31 gauges; the larger the gauge number, the thinner the needle. They can hold 30 ml (30 units), 50 ml (50 units) or 100 ml (100 units), respectively.

There are a lot of different companies making syringes, but I prefer patients to stay with the BD brand. The most common syringe I prescribe is the 30 cc (0.3 ml) half unit 6 mm 31 G. This means the syringe can inject a maximum of 30 units at a time. It is very, very rare that any of my patients inject more than 30 units at one time, and the only patients doing that came to me taking even higher doses and were weaned down little by little. If your pharmacy does not carry this, the NDC order number is 08290-3249-10, and it can usually be ordered for next day delivery. This syringe with half-unit markings also comes with an 8 mm–sized needle, but none of my patients need that long a needle. Stick with a 6 mm–sized needle. While the largest insulin needle length available is 12.7 mm, there is no reason anyone has to use a needle that long, ever!

KEY TREATMENT NOTE

A number of times pharmacies have not given my patients the exact syringe I wrote on my prescription pad. I always ask patients to check the syringes they get at the pharmacy and make sure they are exactly what I requested.

The syringe I recommend has half-unit markings, so patients can dose using 3.5 units instead of just 3 or 4 units. For patients following a low-carbohydrate protocol, having half-unit markings on the syringe is vital to help them use the specific low amount of insulin needed per meal dose.

What do you do with a used syringe? There are several ways to be responsible when disposing of the syringes you use for your injections. What you absolutely cannot ever do is throw out a used syringe in a traditional garbage container; doing so puts any person dealing with the garbage at serious risk of being punctured by your needle. Never flush syringes down a toilet, either! If you are away from home or traveling, or even at home, one of the best ways to dispose of your used syringes is to use the BD Safe-Clip. This is an amazing tool that I always keep in my office to show to patients who use syringes. The BD Safe-Clip can be bought online for around $5. It is a small plastic container into which you can insert the syringe needle and then the Safe-Clip clips off the needle, leaving the needleless syringe safe to throw out with any type of trash. A Safe-Clip mechanism can hold up to 1,500 needles, which can last nearly a year for patients on basal/bolus insulin and even longer for those just injecting basal doses. It will cut needles that are 5 mm to 12.7 mm in length.

If you do not use a BD Safe-Clip, most city laws allow patients to put syringes in a thick, heavy container through which the needle cannot poke, such as a bleach bottle or coffee container. When the container is full, close it, place duct tape around the lid, and then throw it out. Patients can also order the same sharps containers that physicians use in their offices for use at home, but there is a charge for it. BD has a mail-in sharps container program, but it's likely that local companies in your town do, too. Using syringes is still a common method for many patients, and disposing of needles in these ways helps patients be good, legal citizens, protective of others in society.

Temperature Stability Kits

Most people in the United States live in an area of the country where it either gets cold in the winter or very hot in the summer or both. Insulin is quite sensitive to temperature changes, and if it is frozen (temperature below 34° F) or heated (temperature above 85° F), it can lose its utility. I practice in Tempe, Arizona, and it is not uncommon for at least one patient to call every summer wondering why their glucose numbers are very high when they are stringently following their protocol; we deduce that their insulin became too hot. A quick change to a new pen or a new vial, and the patient's glucose numbers come down.

There are reusable kits that maintain glucose at a good temperature, never too hot or too cold, and can be used in Tempe in the summer and Minneapolis in the winter, as they maintain a room temperature range all the time, between 64.4° and 78.8° F. These are helpful if you are outside a lot with your insulin exposed to extreme temperatures. One brand is the FRIO Insulin Cooling Case, which is listed as an FDA-approved medical device and works as an evaporative cooler. The gel should be re-immersed in cool water for five to fifteen minutes every forty-five hours. These come in all sizes and fit whatever you need—vials, pens, or pumps. There are also other insulin cooling kit companies you can find through an online search.

Insulin Pens

Diabetic patients who need to inject insulin usually prefer insulin pens over a vial and syringe. Pens are convenient and easy to use. There are two types: One is a prefilled disposable pen, filled with 300 units of insulin, which comes five to a box; patients use the pen and then dispose of it each month or when the insulin is used up. The other is a pen you keep, which is reusable month to month but is filled with a cartridge that is inserted for use and then removed and replaced. Each cartridge also holds 300 units and also comes five to a box.

Pens require needles that are prescribed separately. Generally, insulin pen needles come in lengths of 4 mm, 5 mm, 8mm, and 12.7 mm and in widths of 29 gauge, 31 gauge, and 32 gauge. I believe the only length to use with any diabetic patient is a 4 mm needle; studies have shown that this length works well for all diabetic patients no matter their body size or shape. If you are using a longer needle than 4 mm, ask your physician for a new prescription for the smallest 4 mm size. Pen needles fit all brands of pens. The 4 mm 32 gauge is the thinnest pen needle available.

Pens come with rules that must be followed: Keep the cap on when it is not in use. Put the needle on directly before the injection and then remove immediately after the injection is over. Do not leave the needle on the pen.

It is best to keep the pen at a steady temperature or wait a little if it has gone through a cold-to-warm or warm-to-cold change. Going from warm to cold may cause insulin shrinkage that can create air bubbles. Going from cold to warm can cause insulin expansion that may cause insulin to lose a little potency. There are temperature stability kits for pens.

Pen needles at 4 mm are too small to fit into the BD Safe-Clip. It's best to collect those during the day and then put them in a thick container, to be thrown out when full. For those traveling and using pen needles, carrying an appropriate container in which to collect your used needles for proper discarding is a thoughtful, responsible gesture.

Insulin Pumps

NAMES OF PUMPS CURRENTLY SOLD: Medtronic MiniMed 670G, MiniMed 630G*, MiniMed 530G*; Omnipod; Animus OneTouch Ping, Animus Vibe*; Tandem t:slim X2, t:slim G4, t:flex; Accu-Chek Aviva Combo. The asterisk (*) denotes pumps that come combined with continuous glucose monitors, which are discussed in the next section.

An estimated 350,000 patients in the United States have an insulin pump; of these around 30,000 have T2DM. A pump is a small unit about the size of a pack of cards. It is worn outside the body and injects insulin into the body via an infusion set, which consists of a catheter attached to a cannula or needle.

For patients on basal/bolus insulin, switching from multiple daily injections (MDI, with either syringes or pens) to a pump is a serious consideration. If a person is injecting two basal doses and three rapid injections for meals, five injections a day, the pump can replace all of those to inject insulin twenty-four hours a day as directed. Basal insulin is preprogrammed into the pump, and bolus dosing is dosed per meal. Pumps tend to hold between 180 and 315 units of insulin in their reservoirs, but the insulin is refillable when it gets low; patients use the same vials for syringe injections to refill the pumps. Only rapid insulin is used in pumps, and pumps are used only when a patient requires both basal and bolus dosing.

Only one of the available pumps is a "closed loop" system—the new Medtronic MiniMed 670G. This pump is designed to measure your glucose and then automatically dose insulin as required. It will be exciting to see how well the pump functions!

Overall, a physician shouldn't mind either way if their patient wants to use MDI or a pump. The biggest benefit of a pump for patients is establishing basal control. Instead of dosing 1 to 3 units of basal insulin a day, a patient's basal can be specifically dosed via smaller increments with a pump. For example, here is what a typical diabetic patient's basal pump setting might look like (do not set your pump to these numbers; this is strictly an example):

Midnight to 3 a.m. 0.65 units per hour
3 a.m. to 6 a.m. 0.85 units per hour
6 a.m. to 9 a.m. 0.95 units per hour
9 a.m. to noon. 0.75 units per hour
Noon to 10 p.m. 0.55 units per hour
10 p.m. to midnight. 0.60 units per hour

Thus, throughout the day, intricate dosing protocols can be established, instead of injecting basal insulin one to two times a day and hoping it evenly covers the background glucose effectively.

To broadly generalize, most patients utilize between four and eight pump settings throughout the day and night for basal dosing. Dose settings tend to change with dietary changes, new daily schedules, exercise, new sleep schedules, growth spurts, hormonal fluctuations (e.g., before menstruation), or when the glucose is not well controlled.

The bolus dose for meals is independent of the basal settings. Pumps come with a "pump wizard," or a capacity to figure out, supposedly, how much insulin is still in a patient's system, to help her eat between meals and inject a proper intermeal insulin dose. But pumps only count carbohydrate intake, not protein intake, and both need to be covered. As a result, I do not like "pump wizard" aids and ask patients not to use them as a tool. Instead I have patients figure out how much insulin they need to inject for their meals based on the math I teach them (or the phone app I created), including carbohydrate and protein foods in their calculations, as well as any correction doses. This math is described later in this chapter.

If a patient's glucose is too low, one can lower or stop the insulin delivery from the pump. If a patient's glucose is too high, one can inject a correction dose via the pump, or manually. It is exceedingly helpful for my diabetic athletes to use a pump because of the flexibility of basal pump dosing, which includes even disconnecting the pump when a patient is engaged in long, intensive exercise, such as running a marathon.

Talking with pump distributors and your physician should help you determine which one is best for you. Pump representatives have trial models that patients can try for free to see if the particular pump works for the individual patient. Most insurances cover the cost of pumps and continued supplies if the patient is on basal/bolus dosing; any pump representative can investigate if your insurance will cover their pump.

When a patient gets a pump, he is assigned a pump trainer who teaches him how to use the pump and shows him all the settings it features. The pump trainer establishes basic basal rates, but after that the patient's medical practitioner takes over regulating those doses.

The pump consists of a pump, pump batteries, the refillable insulin cartridge, and the infusion set. There are many infusion sets, which consist of a length of tubing and a type of catheter needle. The pump trainer will know which one to start with. They can be covered with Skin-Tac-H, Tegaderm, or Skin-Prep to enhance skin adherence and prevent sweat from loosening the connection. To help remove the adherence aids, Detachol or Uni-Solve can be beneficial.

Pumps contain alarms for battery changing, tubing blockage, and other technological problems. Some are waterproof. Pumps can be disconnected for showering, swimming, and other activities where the pump might be damaged or it might be awkward (such as during sexual intimacy). Of course, patients should not remove their pumps for long, as they will not receive basal insulin protection during the disconnection.

Patients can carry a pump in many different ways. They can wear them like pagers on their belts, or put them in their pockets—there are clothes with special pump pockets. I've even had female patients wear them in their bras. Some pumps have decorative covers. There are a number of websites that can help kids and adult personalize their pumps.

Most pumps are attached to tubing, and the patient uses the pump itself to set up dosing and monitor insulin use. The Omnipod pump, however, does not require any tubing. It is an oval, white pump that is directly applied to the skin; the insulin cannula enters the skin, and the insulin is directly inserted into the body. Because it is an independent unit, it can be administered in areas unique to a pump, like on the upper outer arm, or the back hip area. The Omnipod is controlled by a personal diabetes manager (PDM), which is held in the patient's hand. I have numerous patients, both children and adults, who enjoy using an Omnipod. They are changed every three days, so patients need ten per month. Omnipods do stop working at times; however, the manufacturer will send a new one overnight.

There is also a disposable pump called V-Go; this pump holds 20, 30, or 40 units of rapid insulin for twenty-four hours. There are only three set basal rates available for use: 0.83 units per hour; 1.25 units per hour; or 1.67 units per hour, and then the bolus doses are dosed independently as a 2-unit dose. V-Go is recommended only for T2DM patients. It is waterproof. I do not recommend using this pump, however, as the basal rates are very high and are not specific to what any individual might need throughout the entire day and night.

There are both pros and cons to using a pump.

PROS

- No daily multiple injections are needed—pump needle changes occur every three to seven days.
- They can provide precise basal dosing throughout the day and night, broken down into individual doses needed per patient individually at different times.
- Some come with a continuous glucose monitor system to aid in glucose control.
- They can accurately inject very low doses of insulin.

- They give more freedom for regulating insulin during exercise.
- They can be removed for water/bathing.
- They record insulin usage that can be viewed for dosing analysis.
- Bolus dosing is easy.
- Insulin usage is simplified—pumps use only one type of insulin.
- Pumps may help reduce hypoglycemic events.
- They send glucose level information to cell phones.
- Patients can have more freedom—they can sleep late and still be getting basal doses instead of missing their morning dose if they did MDI.
- Pumps are okay for both children and adults (though the new Medtronic MiniMed 670G will not be available for children under seven years old).

CONS

- Some patients do not like the idea that a needle is always inserted into their body, or that they have to deal with the tubing, which can get stuck on things at times (like doorknobs!).
- There is increased risk of infection, but this is not common with good hygiene.
- There is scarring at catheter sites.
- Technology can be faulty—pumps can have problems with alarms, catheters, tubing, and insulin reservoirs. The FDA has stated that more pump failures occur than are known—including over or under dosing insulin, sparks, battery failures, and so forth. However, pump companies are very good at customer service and also replacing broken pumps. Nonetheless, patients using pumps should have insulin and syringes or pens as backups in case their pump breaks, in order to continue dosing insulin until a new pump is received.
- Pumps are expensive out of pocket.

SO, WHO SHOULD GET A PUMP?

- Patients who are fully dependent on basal/bolus insulin
- Patients who have problems with hypoglycemia and hyperglycemia (especially nocturnal or postprandial hypoglycemia)

- Patients who travel or have unpredictable schedules
- Patients who exercise frequently or intensely
- Teenagers with pubertal growth
- Patients motivated to have very tight control of their insulin
- Patients with a needle phobia
- Patients with a stubborn dawn phenomenon problem
- Patients with gastroparesis

Continuous Glucose Monitor Systems (CGMSs)

MODELS CURRENTLY AVAILABLE: Medtronic Guardian Real-Time (though this is no longer manufactured by itself, as Medtronic is turning to their new "closed loop" pump); Abbott FreeStyle Libre; Dexcom G5 Mobile; GlySens ICGM System, with an insert that lasts up to a year (currently undergoing studies)

A CGMS is a machine that records a patient's glucose level every one to fifteen minutes, up to around 288 glucose readings in twenty-four hours. It requires a sensor to be inserted under the skin and worn continuously for up to a week (although many patients leave them in for up to two weeks). Its sensor is separate from the pump sensor, and one needs a separate monitor as well, except in pumps that come with a CGMS contained within them, as those pumps incorporate a monitor for both insulin dosing and CGMS recordings.

One needs to calibrate a CGMS daily with between two and four glucose checks, except with the Abbott Libre, and it is typical also to record when one has eaten, exercised, and taken medications. The CGMS can be downloaded to a computer and that data can produce extraordinarily helpful graphs and charts showing glucose highs, lows, and trends. Having this visualized clearly helps enable the patient and physician to pinpoint insulin adjustments throughout the day and night. The Abbott Libre is a unique system that doesn't require multiple calibrations during the day. With this CGMS, a diabetic patient goes to a physician's office and has the water resistant sensor placed on the back of their arm. It lasts for fourteen days, after which the patient returns to the physician's office and the sensor data is scanned and downloaded.

The information we can learn from a CGMS includes the following:

- A twenty-four-hour chart of glucose levels—including during sleep
- Average glucose in a day, week, or month
- Percentage of glucose levels that were high or low
- Percentage of glucose levels in target ranges and when they occurred
- How exercise, meditation, and other influences affect glucose levels

I find CGMS charts to be exceedingly helpful. I mostly prefer the five-day graph that plots daily lines of glucose levels throughout each twenty-four-hour period; this is the most helpful medical tool for me to view trends in glucose control, as it helps me understand where to raise or lower glucose basal rates and how a patient's diet and lifestyle are affecting his or her glucose levels.

The CGMS is expensive, however, and before they agree to cover it, most insurances require proof that the patient has been following good dietary protocol yet is having consistent glucose highs/lows and their A1C is not under good control. The best way to get a CGMS (and the best way to get a pump) is by having your physician contact the CGMS company representative; representatives are usually very helpful—meeting with the patient and organizing all the paperwork and insurance billing.

CGMSs still struggle with accuracy, and it can frustrate patients when their accuracy is not dependable. For example, the Abbott Libre website states that this CGMS may inaccurately indicate hypoglycemia. A study on the Libre showed that 40 percent of the time when the machine reported the patient was at or below 60 mg/dL, they were actually in the range of 81–160 mg/dL. I've had patients stop using other CGMS devices because they were so consistently inaccurate; using them was more frustrating than helpful. They can also fail to work at all, and their alarms can be faulty—not going off when they should, or going off too frequently. They also represent another insertion and monitor unit to carry around and work with each day.

However, a CGMS can certainly help a physician better adjust the patient's insulin, learn when diet is not working, prevent hypoglycemia and hyperglycemia events, and overall attain better control and lower A1Cs. There are also many alarms incorporated into the CGMS machine. Predictive alarms can be set to alert the patient when their glucose levels are notably rising or falling. If a patient does not want their glucose levels to fall below 70 mg/dL, they can set an alarm to ring when their glucose is falling to 85 mg/dL (for example, so that they can disconnect their pump, or correct with glucose/food). If a patient does not want their glucose to go above 150 mg/dL, they can set an alarm to ring when it is at 140 mg/dL (for example, so they can perhaps give a correction dose before their glucose goes too high). These are the four typical predictive alarms in CGMSs:

KEY TREATMENT NOTE

I enjoy having patients use a CGMS. They are extremely helpful for enabling accurate insulin dosing. Trends of glucose numbers are much more important than individual random numbers.

Very high. Glucose seems to be rising significantly (add enough insulin or exercise to offset 50 mg/dL rise).
Mild high. Glucose seems to be rising mildly (add enough insulin or exercise to offset 25 mg/dL rise).
Mild low. Glucose seems to be lowering mildly (reduce insulin dosing to offset 25 mg/dL decrease in glucose; be prepared to treat the low).
Very low. Glucose seems to be lowering significantly (reduce insulin dosing to offset 50 mg/dL decrease in glucose; be prepared to treat the low).

Parents who were using Dexcom's CGMS who wanted to connect the CGMS to cell phones, computers, tablets, and other devices, so they could check on their child's glucose readings at will created a website for that purpose, but Dexcom also created Dexcom Share, a type of receiver that allows wireless communication between the Dexcom receiver and various users when the receiver is in its cradle. There is also a patient-created way to connect available on iCloud called Nightscout. Medtronic has Carelink software, where CGMS information can be accessed by computer hookups.

How to Inject Insulin

It is always good when opening up a new bottle of insulin to write the date on the label, so you know when to throw it out (a month later). There are also little elastic bands of various colors you can wrap around the top of the vial if you need help immediately knowing which vial is basal and which is bolus—for example, blue means basal and red means bolus. However, you should check the label twice before drawing the insulin to ensure you are using the right insulin. Injecting the wrong insulin is a mistake I've had numerous patients make, who then call me at night to help them work through the error safely.

There are several steps to injecting insulin in the best, least painful way.

THE FOLLOWING IS A GOOD GUIDE FOR SYRINGE AND VIAL INJECTIONS:

1. Double check your vial to make sure it is the correct insulin to inject.
2. Fill your syringe with air to the level of insulin you need to inject and inject that into the insulin vial. Then pull back the insulin so that the amount you need is leveled off at the bottom of the black plunger.
3. If there are bubbles in the syringe, they will not harm you if injected into your body, but they are taking up valuable insulin space. If you draw slowly, it is uncommon to have bubbles enter the syringe; if some do, just push the insulin back into the vial and redraw. You can also draw more insulin into your syringe and then tap the syringe a little to get the bubbles to collect in the needle area. Then you can squeeze out the bubbles with the extra insulin you do not need.
4. These are subcutaneous injections that enter the fat directly under the skin. No matter how lean or overweight a person is, the skin is pretty much always the same depth, so using small needles is okay for everyone.
5. You can inject into the stomach (avoiding the belly button by a full two-inch radius), the upper outer buttocks, the upper thigh, and the upper outer arm.
6. You usually do not pinch the skin if using a 5 mm needle or smaller and inject straight into your skin at a 90-degree angle.
7. If you are using a longer needle, say 6–8 mm, then pinch the skin and inject at a 90-degree angle.
8. If you are using a longer needle, which is very uncommon, and you have very little fat, inject at a 45-degree angle.

9. Inject a maximum of between 7 and 10 units in one area. This is based on a key tip from the personal history of Dr. Richard Bernstein, a highly regarded, well-respected T1DM patient and diabetologist, and an endocrinologist who focuses on diabetic patients. The University of Minnesota conducted a study showing that for very large injections of insulin, between 29 and 39 percent of it could be inactivated by the immune system. So, if you injected 40 units in one area, up to 16 units could not work! Why? Because when large amounts of a foreign protein enter the body, the immune system will attempt to attack and destroy it. Thus, if a person injects a huge amount of insulin in one spot, the immune system will attack and destroy some of it, and that amount will not be active. Dr. Bernstein did his own experiments and discovered that if he injected more than 7 units of insulin in any one area, his glucose lowering was less effective. So he teaches that injecting 7 units is the maximum in any one area. I use that as guidance, but if someone is injecting 16 units, to inject 7, 7, 2 is a lot, so I expand it to between 7 and 10 units of insulin in each area for the convenience of patients, and that still tends to work very well.
10. Leave the syringe in for five seconds to ensure all the insulin is injected.
11. Do not rub the injection site after the injection.
12. Inject insulin at room temperature.
13. Do a quick jab in a straight line—just poke it into the skin. Going slowly makes it hurt more. You can practice poking into an orange to get the movement smooth and quick.
14. Do not reuse needles; needles are destroyed with the first injection, and this is visible under electron microscopy. Reusing a needle makes it more jagged and will hurt more. Also, a little insulin remains in the syringe and polymerizes; if you pull more insulin into the used syringe, the new insulin can also polymerize, which will inactivate some of it. If you must, must, must reuse a syringe after your injection, then pull some saline solution into it, and squirt it out, to try to clean out any remaining insulin.
15. Use magnifiers if you have trouble seeing the syringe or switch to a pen. There are magnifiers that fit over the syringe so you can clearly

What Raises Insulin Needs

There are several reasons insulin needs can be raised both temporarily and in an extended fashion in both Type 1 and Type 2 diabetes. Reviewing the chapter on what causes T2DM to develop will be helpful in understanding these. However, there are a few specific key areas.

DIET

A diet high in carbohydrates is always going to require a lot more insulin than a diet low in carbohydrates. You can often cut your insulin dosage in half, and have significantly better glucose control, by simply changing to a low-carb diet. Overeating is another reason you will require more insulin.

HORMONES

Growth and puberty are key times when children and adolescents will require more insulin. The sex hormones naturally create insulin resistance in adolescents, and diabetic patients will require more insulin during those years. Also, growth spurts will hormonally drive more insulin requirements, which can come and go with each spurt.

Many women note that they require more insulin before menstruation—this is because the increase in estrogen secretion that occurs before menses each month causes slight insulin resistance. Women will also need more insulin during pregnancy.

see the amount of insulin you are extracting from the vial. But most patients prefer using pens.

THE FOLLOWING ARE STEPS FOR INJECTING USING A PEN:

1. When you are ready to shoot a pen, remove the pen cap.
2. Check the insulin to see that it is still clear and pure.

DECREASED PANCREATIC FUNCTIONING

Decreased functioning of the pancreas will cause a need for more insulin. Patients with poorly controlled diabetes, for example, start off needing just basal insulin, but over time, as their glucose remains too high, more damage occurs to the pancreas, requiring them to add in bolus insulin, too. For T1DM patients, when decreased pancreatic function is caught very early and they are put on a very specific diet (as discussed in chapters 7 and 8), they can often have a very long honeymoon period. Over time, the pancreas will no longer be able to cover the diet, and insulin will be necessary. Certainly by puberty, it's nearly certain the diabetic child will require insulin.

INCREASED INSULIN RESISTANCE

Insulin resistance in T1DM or T2DM patients is likely to increase the need for insulin. Excess abdominal weight is one reason for insulin resistance. Injecting too much insulin is another. Some diseases, such as Cushing's or hepatitis C, can cause insulin resistance as part of how they present in a patient, and this can cause the patient to require more insulin. Some medications, such as glucocorticoid steroids, can also cause insulin resistance.

MISCELLANEOUS

Fevers usually cause an increased need for insulin. If you are on insulin and develop a fever, you must contact your physician right away. If insulin is losing its potency by spoiling due to age or temperature fluctuations, patients may mistakenly believe they require more insulin.

3. Attach the needle and remove the two caps that come with the needle.
4. A pen needs to be "primed" or have an "air shot"; two terms for the same activity. You need to click your pen to 2 units and then press the button for an injection before each and every injection to ensure you see a tiny drop of insulin form on the needle. That proves that

What *Lowers* Insulin Needs

There are a few things that might lower one's need for insulin, including a low-carb diet; weight loss (in a T2DM patient); supplementation of nutrients, nutraceuticals, and botanicals that promote better insulin sensitivity; regular exercise; controlling sleep apnea; stress management; environmental detoxification; and a healthy microbiome. All of these will be discussed in upcoming chapters.

the pen is working and ready to go, the needle is correctly attached, and there are no air bubbles. If you do not see a drop, make sure there is insulin in the syringe, and try again. If it is not working, you may need a new pen.

5. After you inject, leave the needle on your skin for 6–10 seconds to allow all the insulin to enter the body, until the dose window shows "0." If you withdraw the needle too soon and see any insulin dripping from the needle, that is a problem! The insulin did not get fully into your body.
6. When the injection is done, remove the needle via the outer cover sheaf and discard it appropriately, as discussed above. Do not reuse pen needles. Replace the pen cover.

It is not necessary to alcohol swab an area before an injection (though it is before checking your glucose with a glucose meter), but you can if you wish. However, injecting into wet alcohol can be more painful, so most people do not bother swabbing before they inject. You will not cause an infection if you do not swab. If you get a little blood on your clothes, immediately dabbing it with hydrogen peroxide will help clean it off. Carry some hydrogen peroxide in a small container—an empty vitamin container works well.

Is there ever a time you should inject insulin into muscle? Injecting into a muscle gets the insulin into the bloodstream much quicker than injecting it into the fat, so we tend not to want to do that as the insulin will be used quicker, with a stronger effect, but will not last very long. However, yes, there is a time to inject into the muscle. You can inject into a muscle for a correction dose when your glucose is very high and you wish to bring it down to normal as soon as possible. Injecting into muscle will significantly shorten the time to lower your glucose level. Injecting into the upper arm deltoid muscle is a good site to use.

For a correction shot injected into muscle, in a time of high-glucose crisis, it is helpful to have at least a 6 mm needle; however, most corrections are not injected into muscle, because they are not typically made in a time of crisis. Most patients correct into the same subcutaneous areas they do for their main injections. Corrections are often done at meals; when corrections are done inbetween meals, or when patients snack and inject for food inbetween meals, it's called "stacking," and there is a higher risk of developing hypoglycemia as a result. Experienced diabetic patients who are comfortable with insulin can inject a correction inbetween meals, but for new diabetic patients injecting insulin, it's best to inject with a meal.

It is very important to rotate injection sites. Avoid injecting near the belly button, or near scars or moles. Do not inject into your inner thigh or inner buttocks in order to avoid hitting large arteries, veins, and nerves. If you inject into the same areas all the time, you are putting your body at risk of scarring, localized lipohypertrophy (fat overgrowth), lipoatrophy (fat atrophy), lipodystrophy (fat scarring), bruising, infection (this is very rare), and allergic reaction (also very rare, but it has happened, and a patient who has an allergic reaction needs to change their brand of insulin). If the fat in an injection site undergoes any changes, that area can no longer be used for injections. If the patient bruises frequently, I like to prescribe blueberry capsules and/or citrus bioflavonoids, as the proanthocyanidins in berries and the citrus bioflavinoids enhance the strength of the blood vessel walls and can help reduce the bruising.

Using Insulin: How to Dose Insulin Safely and Efficiently

Every person with diabetes needs to work with a competent, caring medical practitioner when insulin is involved, to ensure glucose levels are well

The Dawn Phenomenon

The rise of glucose levels early in the morning, known as the "dawn phenomenon," is well known to all diabetic patients. Insulin has a very short life span in our bodies, only 4–7 minutes long. In a person who does not have diabetes, the liver clears 60 percent of insulin from the portal venous system (the blood vessels from the abdomen), and the kidneys clear around 30 percent to 40 percent. However, for those injecting insulin, the percentages are reversed.

So, why are early morning fasting glucose numbers usually higher than the bedtime glucose numbers, and at times the hardest to get under control even with insulin?

There are several reasons why the dawn phenomenon occurs.

Liver insulin resistance. During the night, in abdominally overweight or obese T2DM patients, the fat cells "dump" free fatty acids into the portal venous system and take everything absorbed into it directly to the liver, to be screened before it enters the systemic body. Excessive free fatty acids rushing to the liver during the night cause the liver to become insulin resistant. (This is also another reason the liver can develop nonalcoholic fatty liver, discussed further in chapter 14). The liver does not have glucose receptors on its cells, but it does have insulin receptors. When the liver senses insulin, it realizes that the person has just eaten, and starts uptaking glucose and storing it. When the liver does not sense insulin, it realizes it is inbetween meals and secretes glucose by breaking it down from starch (glycogenolysis) and amino acids (gluconeogenesis). So when the liver problematically develops insulin resistance from the free fatty acids during the night, it cannot perceive if insulin is in the serum. As a result, it will act as if it is not in the serum, even if it is there, and secrete glucose throughout the night, leading to elevated morning glucose levels. This is one reason metformin is so helpful for many patients, as it works by slowing down glucose secretion by the liver.

Elevated levels of cortisol. Elevated levels of cortisol are secreted by the adrenals in the morning. This is a normal physiological process. When we eat dinner and then do not eat more before we go to bed, we may fast for ten to twelve hours before we wake in the morning. To give us energy to get us up and active even before breakfast, our body produces cortisol, which is a hormone that signals the liver to produce glucose from the same biochemical processes mentioned above.

Growth hormone secretion. Growth hormone is secreted in between meals and during our sleep. The surge of growth hormone is associated with elevated morning glucose. Growth hormone has been shown to induce a state of insulin resistance in people.

The Somogyi effect. This is a controversial effect whereby it is understood that when a patient has a hypoglycemic reaction in the middle of the night, the body puts out enough counterregulatory hormones, such as cortisol and epinephrine, and stress hormones from the adrenals to signal the liver to produce glucose. The liver may make too much glucose, causing higher glucose in the morning. Some physicians do not believe this effect occurs, but I have heard from patients now and then who believe they have experienced it. Of course, the key to this is ensuring your patient's diabetes is well controlled enough to not have serious lows during sleep in the first place!

While it is frustrating for patients and physicians at times, overcoming the dawn phenomenon is certainly possible without needing massive amounts of insulin.

covered, without having high or low numbers. Having worked with diabetic patients for twenty-five years, I can certainly help patients understand how to use insulin in safer, more effective ways, whether for basal, bolus, or correction dosing during normal times, or during exercise, sickness, traveling, and other situations.

There is always some educated and experience-based "guesstimation" when working with establishing insulin protocols. That is why it is best to go slowly and take time to ensure proper dosing is formulated without any hypoglycemic reactions occurring during the process.

I recommend patients use a different type of insulin dosing regimen than conventional care has established, and I will discuss my protocol in more detail later in this chapter.

When beginning or maintaining an insulin regimen, the goals are simple:

- Optimal glycemic control—good A1C (in the 5s)
- No or minimal hypoglycemic or hyperglycemic events
- No weight gain
- Minimal impact on lifestyle

In addition, when starting a patient on insulin, I consider the following patient traits:

- What is her typical day like? Does it follow a consistent pattern day to day or does it vary significantly?
- Is it consistent in terms of timing of meals and types of foods eaten?
- Is it consistent in terms of time and intensity of exercise?
- Is it consistent in terms of time and length of sleep?
- What is her age and vitality—does she require help for living her life?
- Is she entering puberty?
- Does she have good cognitive abilities?
- Does she have any limitations in dexterity or vision?

Insulin is a strong medication and can cause serious, even life-threatening, hypoglycemia if the patient cannot inject correctly as prescribed and treat any low-glucose event that occurs.

Dosing Insulin

In this section I will discuss the best ways to inject insulins for a variety of patients and situations.

T2DM Patient Starting Basal Insulin

Insulin loss due to pancreatic damage varies greatly among T2DM patients. If the diabetes has worsened, usually years after diagnosis, insulin may be required.

T2DM patients need to begin basal insulin when:

- Their fasting glucose is too high.
- Their comprehensive protocol treatment has not been successful in controlling their glucose numbers.
- They are on maximum oral hypoglycemic agents and non-insulin injectables, and glucose is not well regulated.
- They have low c-peptide/insulin.
- They have elevated A1C.
- Complications are developing or they are at risk of developing due to elevated glucose and A1C.
- They have acute onset of severe T2DM with high glucose numbers and high A1C.

It is always best to start at a lower starting dose of basal insulin and then titrate up. Avoiding a hypoglycemic reaction is best to earn a patient's trust and faith.

The typical way of starting basal insulin in patients with T2DM is to start with one shot of basal at bedtime, using either a syringe and vial or a pen. There are two dosing methodologies:

- Start with 10 units—a typical starting dose.
- Body weight starting dose—0.15–0.2 units per kilogram of body weight. For example, if you weigh 200 pounds (approximately 91 kg): 91 × 0.15 = 13.65. So, 13 units would be your starting dose.

Unless your patient weighs less than 150 pounds, injecting 10 units will always be less than when calculating based on body weight. If your patient

KEY TREATMENT NOTE

A patient should wake up around five hours after starting an evening (or morning) basal injection, even just 1 unit, to check his glucose level. For most people who go to bed around 10 or 11 p.m., waking around 3 a.m. is suggested. This is vital to catch any hypoglycemic event occurring as soon as possible. If there is no hypoglycemic reaction after two to three days, this check can be stopped, but it needs to start again with any new increase in basal insulin dosing.

weighs 150 pounds and has T2DM, then use the body weight formula. However, since most T2DM patients (who are not mistakenly LADA) are overweight, starting with 10 units is a typical methodology.

Once the starting dose is decided, and the patient knows the proper way to inject, she must wait three to five days to see how low her fasting glucose levels go before raising her evening basal insulin dose. I usually wait four days. It takes basal insulin a few days to get settled in the body and start having a consistent effect on fasting glucose; patients can notice day by day that their fasting glucose is lowering. The target fasting glucose is lower than 100 mg/dL. Ideally it's lower than 90 mg/dL, but starting out at lower than 110 mg/dL is acceptable to prevent lows in a patient just getting used to using insulin.

After three to five days, the titrating formula for increasing the evening injection if the fasting/waking glucose is still not ideal is as follows:

- If glucose is higher than 180 mg/dL, increase by 4–8 units.
- If glucose is higher than 140 mg/dL, increase by 2–6 units.
- If glucose is 120–140 mg/dL, increase by 2–4 units.
- If glucose is 110–120 mg/dL, increase by 1–2 units.

I usually increase by the lowest amount, to be safe, so if it says 2–6 units, I'll usually recommend my patient go up just 2 units. It is better to be cautious and not cause a low glucose event than be aggressive and have the patient develop hypoglycemia.

When I begin working with patients on insulin, I give them my personal cell phone number and email account, so they feel comfortable that they can contact me after hours as needed, particularly for a hypoglycemic episode, which rarely happens. During office hours patients contact me there. When they are starting insulin, I want patients to be able to contact me twenty-four hours a day, seven days a week, for the first couple of weeks until we get their dosage on target. After that, it is rare that a patient calls me, even parents of pediatric patients. Taking the time in the office to educate patients effectively means they leave the office very capable of initiating discussed regimens. Within one to three weeks it is typical to have their evening dose safely determined.

KEY TREATMENT NOTE

Regarding basal dosing, when a patient presents to my office on a certain basal dose, the day they start a low-carbohydrate diet I reduce that basal dose by half. A low-carb diet will significantly reduce the need for basal insulin! If cutting the dose in half is too much, we might have to titrate the dose back up a little to find the correct dosing, but it will prevent any hypoglycemic reaction to the low-carb diet.

T1DM or LADA Patient Starting Evening Basal Insulin

With these usually lean patients, who have no excess abdominal fat to initiate hepatic insulin resistance, it is best to start with very low doses of insulin, such as a half or single unit, and titrate up slowly as necessary. If after three to five days fasting blood glucose is still very high, then it is sensible to add another unit, but do so as per the directions of your physician, and always check glucose levels five hours after any increased dosing.

When to Add a Long-Acting Morning Dose?

There are good signs that indicate when it's necessary to add a long-acting morning basal dose to a T2DM or T1DM patient's insulin regimen: The patient's fasting blood glucose is lower than 100, showing that the evening basal dose is correct; the patient's postprandial glucose levels are well controlled at lower than 120 mg/dL (ideally at lower than 110 mg/dL), yet glucose numbers still begin rising in the afternoon and remain high into the evening.

When this situation occurs, it is a clear indication that the evening dose of basal insulin is wearing off and a morning dose of basal insulin is necessary. How much should you start with in the morning? In general, it is very typical that patients need to use more basal insulin in the evening than in the morning due to all the conditions causing the dawn phenomenon. For adults with T2DM who are overweight or obese, in general (but adapting to each patient's individual specifics) I'd start with around 4 units in the morning. With lean T1DM patients, children with T1DM, or LADA patients, I'd start with half to a single unit in the morning. Insulin can be carefully titrated up to the required dose. You should follow the insulin dosing directions of your physician, who knows you best.

In pediatric patients injecting their main dose first thing in the morning, waking elevated glucose would be the clue that their morning dose is wearing off during their sleep at night and an evening dose is required.

Checking to See If Basal Doses Are Accurate

If you are on basal insulin alone, it is easy to determine if your dosing is correct: Both your fasting glucose numbers and your glucose numbers for the rest of the day should fall well within a definable goal. However, when you are on both basal and bolus insulin, or mealtime and/or correction dosing, it can be harder to figure out if the basal dose is correct, as you are dealing with other insulin injections at least three times a day.

Remember that basal insulin concerns the glucose made by your liver and kidneys inbetween meals and during sleep. If food is not impacting your glucose, it will all come from liver and kidney production, and we can specifically pinpoint basal management of that. If your glucose numbers remain good through that time, your basal is the correct dose.

When you want to see if your basal doses are controlling your glucose numbers, here are ways to do that:

Evening basal dosing check. Eat a low-fat dinner, so your body processes it more quickly, and inject for it if you inject for meals. Do not inject any correction at bedtime, even if the glucose is a little high (however, if the glucose is higher than 150 mg/dL, correct that with rapid insulin, injecting your basal, though this will mean you cannot then do the basal analysis that night). If you did not need to correct, then inject your basal dose and fast to breakfast, recording glucose every other hour (losing one good night's sleep). Some people say just check twice—once during the middle of the night and then the fasting glucose—but if possible, getting more readings is very helpful and more precise. Analyzing those numbers will inform you if you stayed in the desired glucose range on that dose of basal.

Morning basal dosing check. Do not eat breakfast, and if your glucose is inbetween 80 and 150 mg/dL, begin the test. Do not inject your meal or correction dose. Fast from morning to a late lunch (around 2 p.m.), and record your glucose levels every hour. You can stop the test at lunch if you wish and then do an afternoon basal insulin test. However, if you are a real trooper, you can fast until supper and get the whole day in one shot. If glucose rises at any time above a desired number, either evening basal needs to be higher or a morning basal dose may be required.

Afternoon basal dosing check. Eat breakfast and inject (if you do), and then do not eat lunch. If your glucose is between 80 and 150 mg/dL, then begin the test and record glucose every hour until 10 or 11 p.m., when you inject your evening basal. If glucose rises above the desired number in the afternoon or evening, either evening basal needs to be higher or a morning basal dose may be required.

The easiest way to check basal efficiency is to use a CGMS to record your glucose levels throughout the day, if you have one. You can do the basal test in the same way, but if you are using a CGMS, you do not have to test your glucose each hour, you just need to calibrate the meter two to four times a day as you've been trained to do (unless using an Abbott Libre, which does not require calibration). You can then print out the CGMS daily graph showing where your glucose was during your testing period.

It is good on those testing days to not do extreme exercise or any other very stressful activity. Do not conduct the test during sickness or before menses, as many women's glucose levels rise in those days due to the output of estrogen. Also, do not drink alcohol on the day of the test, as that lowers glucose by interfering with the hepatic production of glucose.

If you have low glucose during the test (lower than 70 mg/dL), stop and treat it. If you have high glucose during the test (higher than 150 mg/dL), stop and correct.

For people using a pump, if their glucose rises more than 40 mg/dL during a four-hour span, they should increase their basal insulin during that time span by around 0.05–0.1 units per hour, as per the directions of their physician. If the glucose falls more than 40 mg/dL, leading to hypoglycemia, the pump should be adjusted lower by the same 0.05–1.0 units per hour, again after discussing an insulin change with your physician.

Basal Dosing for Pumps

For patients using pumps, a diet diary and glucose graph or a CGMS report are helpful tools for monitoring any trends due to the pumps' segmented basal dosing. Since most patients on pumps have divided their twenty-four-hour basal dosing into four to eight segmental delineations, a good physician has the skill to adjust the appropriate basal times, raise or lower the insulin dose, or even change the established basal times, and see if different timing would be more beneficial.

For example, let's say a patient has the following basal guidelines:

Midnight–2 a.m. 0.75 units/hour
2 a.m.–6 a.m. 0.80 units/hour
6 a.m.–9 a.m. 0.85 units/hour
9 a.m.–2 p.m. 0.80 units/hour
2 p.m.–midnight. 0.75 units/hour

Based on a CGMS report that shows the patient's glucose levels were too high early in the morning, and then rose again later in the afternoon from 3 to 6 p.m. I would suggest the patient adjust their basal levels in these ways:

Midnight–2 a.m. Maintain 0.75 units/hour
2 a.m.–6 a.m. **Increase** to 0.85 units/hour
6 a.m.–9 a.m. Maintain 0.85 units/hour
9 a.m.–3 p.m. Maintain 0.80 units/hour but change to **3 p.m.**
3 p.m.–6 p.m. **Increase** to 0.80 units/hour (I would add a new basal time segment here)
6 p.m.–midnight. Maintain 0.75 units/hour

We would try that for approximately one week and see what happens. The idea is that by lowering the initial high dose of insulin starting at midnight, we might be successful in getting consistently ideal glucose levels. If necessary, we can also raise the 6 a.m.–9 a.m. insulin, too. However, a good dosing of insulin is a step-by-step process, and it is not wise to be too aggressive. Having patients maintain diet diaries and glucose graphs, and use their CGMS if they have one, is vital during this insulin evaluation time.

We do the same type of evaluation if a patient is having lows to figure out what basal segments need to be lowered.

Bolus Insulin Dosing for All Diabetics

Since we start with basal dosing in T2DM, bolus is always added after. However, bolus dosing is usually added concurrently when starting a new T1DM on insulin.

Who tends to require both basal and bolus insulin dosing?

- Most T1DM patients, over time
- Many LADA patients, either soon after diagnosis or over time
- Many T2DM patients, although ideally this should never happen

The main clue that a patient requires meal dosing is that the patient's postprandial glucose tends to rise even if their fasting glucose is fine due to basal insulin.

The medical standard now for basal/bolus insulin is using long-acting insulin (basal) with rapid insulin (bolus). Although regular insulin is a better insulin for meals, most patients do not wish to use it, for the reasons described earlier in this chapter. Insulin that is a mixture of NPH and rapid or regular is significantly more difficult to work with, and patients will simply not have as good control as when injecting long-acting and rapid insulins separately, or using a pump.

The standard methodology for basal/bolus insulin is to inject basal insulin at night or both night and morning (as needed), and then to inject bolus insulin before each meal, three times a day, for a total of four or five separate shots a day.

To accurately dose bolus insulin in order to superbly control glucose levels, one must eat a low-carbohydrate diet. Why? Because FDA food guidance and regulatory information allows nutrient labels on foods to have a 20 percent variance. Dr. Richard Bernstein calls this "the low of small numbers." Let me explain. Suppose you are going to eat a plate of pasta for dinner, and the food label says that if you eat this much pasta, you will be eating 100 grams of carbohydrates. However, since the FDA allows food manufacturers to have a positive 20 percent error in defining the actual amounts of carbohydrates in each portion of the food eaten, that means you might be eating 100 grams of carbs, or you might be eating up to 120 grams of carbs. In general, each gram of carbs raises the glucose of a person who weighs 140 pounds by 5 mg/dL, so that means you might have to cover a rise of between 500 and 600 mg/dL of glucose (more or less depending on your weight). How can you cover that amount accurately? That is a spread of 100 mg/dL! If you cover for 500 mg/dL, and it rises 600 mg/dL, you will be high after the meal. If you cover for 600 mg/dL, and it rises only 500 mg/dL, you will be low after the meal. For children, 1 gram of carbs raises their glucose significantly more than 5 mg/dL; the spread gets much wider.

If, however, you eat some steamed vegetables and salmon, a meal that only contains 12 grams of carbs, and that is off 20 percent in accuracy, it means you might have eaten between 12 and 14.4 grams of carbs, which translates to a between 60 and 72 mg/dL rise in glucose, a much narrower range of only 12 mg/dL, which affords a much lower risk of having either a high or low after dosing for insulin.

A low-carb diet is the best for any diabetic patient, but it is really important for diabetic patients who need to inject insulin at meals. If a patient is told to "eat what you want and cover it with insulin," as so many T1DM pediatric patients are directed, they are almost guaranteed to have highs and lows all the time. A patient cannot closely cover a high-carb meal with insulin, and so will wind up high, and then correct, and go low, and then eat too much and go high again, over and over each day. Or, a patient will overinject for his meal, and have a low, and then eat too much and go high, correct and . . . well, you get the picture! I really do not believe there is any "brittle" diabetic patient who cannot attain easy, smooth diabetes control upon going low carb and being taught proper usage of insulin.

Conventional Dosing of Insulin

There are three foundational problems with conventional insulin dosing for food. The first is that a high-carb diet is allowed, at least for pediatric T1DM patients. The second is that protein intake is not included in the insulin dosing. Protein breaks down in our bodies into amino acids, and amino acids can be transformed into glucose, and thus protein also needs to be covered by insulin. The third is that conventional dosing does not base insulin on a person's individual weight, and one's weight can indeed help specify exactly how much insulin is needed, particularly with meal-bolus dosing.

Conventional insulin dosing is based on the total daily dose (TDD) metric, which includes the total amount of insulin injected as basal, bolus, and correction insulin. The average amount of insulin needed to cover all those doses is the TDD. So, if you injected 22 units of Levemir in the evening and 18 units of Levemir in the morning; and you injected Novolog at 7, 6, and 8 units respectively at breakfast, lunch, and supper; and you had to inject a 2-unit correction dose before supper; and you added up all those units, your TDD would be 60 units and insulin.

In general, the typical TDD breaks down to basal insulin covering 45–65 percent and bolus insulin covering 35–55 percent of daily insulin. If one is getting too many lows, it is suggested to lower the TDD by 5–10 percent. If one is getting too many highs, it is suggested to raise the TDD 5–10 percent.

The starting basal rate can be determined by dividing the TDD in half. That is the usual starting dose. So, with a TDD of 60, one would be directed to have around 30 units as basal dosing.

The key to bolus dosing in conventional methodologies is the insulin/carbohydrate ratio; that is, how many grams of carbs are covered by one unit of bolus insulin. Dividing 500 by one's TDD equals the amount of carbohydrate grams covered by one unit of insulin. So, if you are injecting a total of 60 units of insulin a day, 500 divided by 60 equals about 8, so you would be told to inject one unit of insulin for every 8 grams of carbohydrates you ate. Every diabetic patient who has seen a conventional physician will have been given their insulin/carborhydrate ratio, even though it is a very inaccurate way of covering meal glucose elevation.

In conventional methodologies, medical practitioners use a correction factor to figure out how much insulin to inject to make a correction. There are many different rules used, with many different starting numbers, but the "1800 Rule" seems to be the most common. In this rule, we take 1,800 divided by TDD, and find out how much glucose is lowered per unit of insulin. If you are injecting 60 units a day, then your correction factor is 1,800 divided by 60, meaning 1 unit of insulin lowers you 30 mg/dL. Different practitioners use a variety of rules: 1600, 1700, 2000, and 2200. The 1500 Rule has been suggested if patients are using regular insulin for corrections, but that is not the best insulin to use for corrections; rapid insulin is better.

Once the correction factor is established, the correction dose can be determined in this way:

Actual blood sugar
- target glucose
÷ correction factor
= How much insulin is needed to get to your target glucose range

For example, let's say the patient comes to the meal with a glucose of 200 mg/dL, and their goal for after the meal is 100 mg. Having done the math with the TDD, which is 60 units a day, this patient has a correction factor of 30 mg/dL. So the correction dose should be 200 minus 100 divided by 30, which equals 3.3 units. That correction dose would be added to the meal insulin designed to cover the food about to be eaten.

Here is the total math for an example patient. A pediatric patient has a insulin/carbohydrate ratio of 1/15; correction factor is 30; glucose target after meals is 120. This patient comes to a meal with a glucose level of 180

Table 6.1. Conventional Correction Dose Amounts

Units/24 Hours (TDD)	Rapid Insulin	Short-Acting Insulin
20	90 mg/dL	75 mg/dL
30	60 mg/dL	50 mg/dL
40	45 mg/dL	38 mg/dL
50	36 mg/dL	30 mg/dL
60	30 mg/dL	25 mg/dL
70	26 mg/dL	21 mg/dL
80	23 mg/dL	19 mg/dL
90	20 mg/dL	17 mg/dL

mg/dL and is eating 50 grams of carbohydrates at the meal. How much does he inject for his meal and correction? Fifty carbs divided by 15 equals 3.3 units, while the correction dose (180 minus 120 divided by 30) equals 2 units. So, the total insulin dose would be 5.3 units.

I dose insulin a little differently, as you will see in the next section.

Nota Bene: I have an Android phone app called the CarbProtein Insulin Calculator, which makes it very simple to use the upcoming math in your daily life. You can purchase lifetime use of the app for $1.99 (it's more expensive to have an app made than you think, so I charge this nominal lifetime user fee) at the Google Play Store. I strongly suggest that those with Android phones use my app, if allowed by your physician, in order to help to determine how much insulin to inject at meals. Parents can use it for their children. Unfortunately, Apple, unfairly from my point of view, rejected allowing me to put my app on their iPhones.

Ideal Insulin Dosing Methodology

This information is adapted from Dr. Richard Bernstein's book, *Dr. Bernstein's Diabetes Solution*, as well as information I learned years ago when he was my mentor.

The benefit of this different, better methodology is that it is based on the patient's weight and includes protein intake at meals, so it is more inclusive of what the insulin has to cover.

The system is based on a 140-pound man using regular insulin for meals, because Dr. Bernstein believes that regular is the best insulin for meals and he weighs 140 pounds. He figured this out to help match his food with his insulin intake. Since his protocol is based on his weight and regular insulin, and many people neither weigh 140 pounds nor use regular insulin for meals, we need to do a little math to transform it to your weight, and for rapid insulin.

If you weigh 140 pounds, 1 unit of regular insulin lowers your glucose around 40 mg/dL. If you weigh 140 pounds, 1 unit of rapid insulin lowers your glucose around 60 mg/dL. If you do not weigh 140 pounds, here are the calculations for determining how much insulin lowers your glucose:

140 ÷ (your weight) × 40 = (about) how much 1 unit of regular lowers your glucose number.
140 ÷ (your weight) × 60 = (about) how much 1 unit of rapid lowers your glucose number.

For example, if you weigh 200 pounds:

140 ÷ 200 × 40 = 28 mg/dL (how much 1 unit of regular lowers your glucose)
140 ÷ 200 × 60 = 42 mg/dL (how much 1 unit of rapid lowers your glucose)

These numbers are good unless a person gains or loses 20 pounds or more. Then they have to be recalculated.

Then we divide the regular number for a 140 pound person (40) by your regular number for your weight. In this case:

40 ÷ 28 = 1.4

I call the result (in this case, 1.4) "my regular weight number" (MRWN). People who weight more than 140 pounds will need more regular insulin to have it work (their MRWN will always be more than 1) and people who weigh less than 140 pounds will have to use less regular insulin (their MRWN will always be less than 1). This number is important for the final calculation.

The final equation proceeds as follows—and again, it was Dr. Bernstein's brilliance that figured this out:

Number of grams of carbohydrates ÷ 8 = units of regular insulin to inject before a meal for a person who is 140 pounds.
Number of ounces* of protein ÷ 1.5 = units of regular insulin to inject before a meal for a person who is 140 pounds.
Adding up those carbs and protein units equals total regular units (TRU) needed to inject if you weigh 140 pounds.

Now we need to turn that number to the amount of rapid insulin you'll need at your weight.

---

* Ounces, not grams; the ratio for protein is 6 grams = 1 ounce of protein (see chapter 7, on diet).

For regular dosing based on your weight: Multiply TRU by your MRWN to get the units of regular you need to inject based on your weight.
Since rapid insulin is stronger than regular insulin by one-third, multiply your regular dose by 0.66 to get your rapid dose, if that insulin is used at that meal.
In summary, carb + protein insulin units × MRWN (× 0.66) = your rapid insulin for a given meal.

I know, unless you are an engineer who loves this stuff, you are probably very confused right now. Let's use again the example of a patient who weighs 200 pounds, and therefore has an MRWN of 1.4. If he eats 12 grams of carbs and 5 ounces of protein at a meal, he calculates (or my Android cell phone app calculates automatically) how much rapid insulin he needs to inject as follows:

12 grams of carbs ÷ 8 = 1.5 units of regular insulin for a person weighing 140 pounds.
5 ounces of protein ÷ 1.5 = 3.3 units of regular insulin for a person weighing 140 pounds.

Total regular dose: 4.8 units for a person weighing 140 pounds.

4.8 units × 1.4 (the patient's MRWN) = 6.72 units of regular, the amount of regular insulin he would inject for his meal (he needs more because his weight makes him more insulin resistant).
6.72 units × .66 = 4.4 units of rapid insulin for that meal.

If he is using a pump, he can self-direct the pump to inject 4.4 units exactly. If he is using a vial and syringe with half-unit markings or a pen dosed in half units, he would round up to 4.5 units. Rounding up or down is based on how close the dose is to the higher or lower half-unit marking. The guidelines in table 6.2 can be used with any denomination of insulin units; 2 units is just an example.

Table 6.2. Guidelines for Rounding Insulin Dose Up or Down, If Using Syringe or Pen

Meal Insulin Result	Dose
2–2.25 units	2 units
2.25–2.5 units	2.5 units
2.5–2.75 units	2.5 units
2.75–3 units	3 units

Although calculating ideal dosage seems complicated, once a patient learns the math it is a pretty quick process, and the calculator on your cell phone will help with the math. The phone app makes it even simpler. And, having a physician who is a whiz at this is always helpful! The handout I go over with patients has many examples of how the math works, so I can ensure patients have some skill figuring this all out by the end of the office visit.

Also, people tend to eat the same meals over and over; we are culinary creatures of habit. Once a particular favorite low-carb meal insulin dose is figured out, it can automatically be injected from then on.

The combination of this dosing methodology and a low-carb diet means that within a week patients (and pediatric patients' parents) are very excited because they are becoming truly successful at glucose control, with no more highs and lows all day long, have better energy, and now have hope that they will successfully manage their diabetes.

CORRECTION DOSING

A correction dose lowers a glucose number to the goal glucose level. If a person comes to a meal with their glucose at 180, and covers their meal with insulin perfectly well, they will wind up at 180 after their meal. The correction dose brings the glucose down to that goal level.

Correction dosing is simple in this format; the correction dose equals the amount by which 1 unit of rapid insulin lowers a patient's glucose according to their weight. So for the 200-pound patient, we've already calculated this as 42 mg/dL (140 ÷ 200 × 60 = 42 mg/dL). For a patient who weighs 100 pounds, 1 unit of rapid insulin will lower her 140 ÷ 100 × 60 = 84 mg/dL.

Though imperfect, this calculation is very close to the actual correction dose, and works unless the patient's glucose number is greater than 170 mg/dL; the higher the glucose, the more insulin resistance develops (even in T1DM patients), and more insulin will be needed to correct than if the glucose is less than 170 mg/dL. Thus, if a 100-pound patient comes to lunch with glucose at 160 and has a correction goal after meals of 100, she would want to lower her glucose by 60 mg/dL, which would equal 0.71 units (60 mg/dL ÷ 84 mg/dL = 0.71) of rapid insulin to correct that. If she has a pump, we can add that exact dose. If she is using a syringe or pen, she can inject either 0.5 units or 1 full unit and see how her body responds. A few guesstimations of that type and the dose will be clarified.

Let's go through one last patient example, all the way through:

Sara is a nine-year-old T1DM patient. She weighs 70 pounds. She comes to a meal at 180 mg/dL, with a correction goal of 100 mg/dL, and she will eat 8 grams of carbohydrates and 3 ounces of protein for dinner. She is using syringe and vial for rapid insulin with meals.

Her math:
$140 \div 70 \times 40 = 1$ unit of regular would lower her around 80 mg/dL
$140 \div 70 \times 60 = 1$ unit of rapid would lower her around 120 mg/dL
$40 \div 80 = 0.5$ (MRWN to change her regular insulin from 140 pounds to her weight)

Her meal:
8 grams of carbs $\div 8 = 1$ unit of regular insulin
3 ounces of protein $\div 1.5 = 2$ units of regular insulin
3 units $\times 0.5 \times .66 = .99$ rapid units for her meal

Rounding up, she would inject 1 unit of rapid for her meal. Remember, that one unit is just to cover her food. As a result, without a correction dose, she would start her meal at 180 mg/dL, and if her meal were perfectly covered, she would wind up at 180 mg/dL.

For her correction dose, she needs to lower from 180 mg/dL to 100 mg/dL. Since 1 unit of rapid based on her weight lowers her 120 mg/dL, the math is $80 \div 120 = 0.67$ units. Rounding down, she would inject 0.5 units for her rapid correction dose. (She may need a little more insulin as a glucose level of 180 mg/dL can cause insulin resistance.)

This becomes an easy process with practice, and of course, we all eat many repetitive meals, so the mealtime insulin for various common meals could either be remembered or could be written on a piece of paper or in a computer or cell phone file.

On Changing Patients from the Standard to the Ideal Dosing Methodology

Although engineers love learning these calculations, many patients' eyes glaze over going through the math, and having the phone app makes things much quicker and simpler for patients. However, with enough practice, patients do

KEY TREATMENT NOTE

Working with a physician who is confident with dosing insulin, takes the time to educate patients, and has innovative methodologies is a great way to get your glucose under fantastic control.

understand the math, and I have worksheets for them to use with me watching to ensure they are doing everything accurately.

And, this new way ultimately does make sense to patients. They know their old way is not working well, and their glucose numbers are not well controlled. What seems to be most interesting to them is that they were never told that proteins can raise their glucose numbers. Once patients fully comprehend the math, everything goes very smoothly.

— CHAPTER SEVEN —

The First Essential: Diet

Entire books have been written that promote one specific type of diet for diabetes. I would like to discuss the best diets for diabetes, giving the details and both pros and cons, so you can then choose which one is best for you. The goal for every patient is to commit to an achievable, sustainable dietary regimen.

As the one-line definition of diabetes is "a condition whereby patients have lost the ability to metabolize dietary carbohydrates," it only makes sense to have low carbohydrates as the foundational basis of any diet. A person with diabetes either does not make insulin or makes it but it doesn't work well in the body. Since insulin is designed to clear glucose out of the bloodstream, if insulin secretion or sensitivity is a problem, removing sources of glucose from the diet will logically and rationally be of great help.

Carbohydrates turn directly into blood glucose. In the liver and kidneys, amino acids, which are breakdown products of protein, can also be turned into sugar, though at a lower percentage than carbohydrates. Nonetheless, we do have to monitor the intake of proteins. Fats do not need any insulin to be properly metabolized, because they do not turn into carbohydrates. As a result, based on common sense and science, diabetic patients of all types ideally should eat a low-carbohydrate diet, sensibly eat protein, and indulge in healthy fats.

There are innumerable studies showing that a low-carb diet is more effective than a low-fat diet for weight loss, fat loss, decreased cardiovascular risk factors, lower glucose, lower triglycerides, and lower A1Cs. I will not discuss those studies in depth; they are well established in medicine. Perhaps the

The Pros and Cons of Low-Carb Diets

There are several pros and cons to low-carb diets. On the "pro" side, a diet containing fewer carbs helps reduce one's appetite as well as one's blood glucose, promotes weight loss, and reduces insulin resistance. There are many nutritionally complete ways to implement low-carb diets.

On the "con" side, low-carb diets may also be lower in fiber, which may have a negative impact on the health of colon cells and may cause constipation, so care should be taken to make sure fiber intake is adequate. As with other restrictive diets, low-carb diets can make mealtimes with friends and family more complicated, as well as require creative thinking to come up with new ways and habits to keep the diet fresh and enjoyable. Low-carb diets are strict, and need to be committed to by diabetic patients. Lastly, because they don't allow many processed foods, low-carb diets often require more work in the kitchen.

KEY TREATMENT NOTE

In my practice, both the diet diary and glucose graph forms are required before any diet discussion is initiated with a patient.

best article to read proving the efficacy of a low-carb diet as the foundational treatment of diabetes is "Dietary Carbohydrate Restriction as the First Approach in Diabetes Management: Critical Review and Evidence Base," put together by twenty-six researchers and physicians, including Richard Feinman, PhD (founder of the Nutrition and Metabolism Society), Dr. Richard Bernstein, Dr. Jay Wortman, MD, and their colleagues. This published article presents major evidence for a low-carbohydrate diet as the leading diet for treating diabetes, noting that a low-carb diet reliably reduces blood pressure, and can reduce or eliminate the need for medication. There are also no side effects accompanying changing one's diet, as opposed to the many potential side effects of being on more and more medications.

Dr. Feinman is also the author of *The World Turned Upside Down: The Second Low-Carbohydrate Revolution*, which is full of further research on using low-carb diets for people with diabetes.

Important Dietary Terms

Before we get to the individual specifics of the different diets promoted to treat diabetes in the next chapter, it's important first to establish some basic knowledge that will be applicable to most of the diabetic diets we will be discussing, including ingredients, carbohydrates, protein, fats, vegetables, fruits, genetically modified organisms, and fermented foods.

Ingredients

I encourage you to read the labels of everything you consider purchasing. Do not be fooled by the unhelpful advertising gimmicks companies put on their prepared foods, such as use of the words *natural* or *lite*. A food label contains the nutritional facts, showing you the amounts of total carbohydrates, fiber, fat, and protein, below which is the ingredient list. Ensuring the ingredients are healthy ones, even if the food is low in carbs, is important. I need patients to eat food that has both the right carbohydrate and protein levels and is healthy to eat!

Foods that contain preservatives, flavorings, colorings, and any unpronounceable words should generally be avoided, although some additives are not harmful, such as sunflower lecithin (a fat emulsifier) and natural colorings that come from plants. When I promote a whole-foods, low-carb diet, I want food to contain the fewest added ingredients with the greatest health benefits. It's best to have a medical practitioner who is a specialist in nutrition working with you, so you can bring products and labels to him or her to see if the ingredients are acceptable.

Glycemic Index

The glycemic index is a laboratory numerical rating of foods describing how quickly and completely foods break down into glucose in our bodies within two hours. The higher the number, the more quickly and intensely glucose

KEY TREATMENT NOTE

I suggest patients avoid glycemic index categorization of foods as the methodology of figuring out how they should eat.

is produced by that food. The lower the number, the slower the transformation of that food into glucose. The glycemic load is a more accurate rating that measures the potential of foods with the same amount of carbohydrates to turn to glucose.

There are problems with both the glycemic index and load, however, and I do not use either in choosing which foods my patients can or cannot eat. Problems with the glycemic index include the fact that foods can have a different glycemic effect based on whether they are mixed together versus eaten separately; the ripeness of the food (for example, a very ripe and a barely ripe banana have different glycemic ratings; if the food is raw or cooked; the fact that an individual's variable digestion affects how food is broken down and processed; the fact that individuals have their own glucose response to foods, which can affect the number; and the fact that laboratory numbers can never accurately represent what happens in each unique human body.

Since many foods that should not be eaten by patients with diabetes may seem "low" on the glycemic index, using the index is not part of a methodology I use with patients, and I feel it is more confusing than helpful.

Organic Foods

Certainly, as much as possible, buying organic foods is vital. When a food is organic, it means that no chemical pesticides, herbicides, antibiotics, hormones, fertilizers, or other dangerous and disease-causing substances have been directly put on the food. Organic food is not irradiated; it is GMO-free. Organic food may not be 100 percent free of all pesticides or herbicides, because those chemicals sprayed on other fields enter the atmosphere and can travel across countries and oceans and, through rainfall, land on organic farms even on different continents. However, organic food does have a lot less of those chemicals on it than conventional, directly sprayed food does.

Organic foods have more nutrients, vitamins, minerals, and antioxidants than conventionally grown nonorganic foods. They are obviously the best choice to make, as far as your pocketbook can allow. Organic foods can be more expensive to buy; if organic foods are available where you live and are affordable, then choose to buy them. As mentioned earlier in the section on diabetic etiological risk factors and later when we discuss environmental detoxification (chapter 9), an enormous amount of environmental chemicals, including the pesticides and herbicides sprayed on food, are associated with causing both insulin resistance in body cells and autoimmune diseases. Thus, the cleaner your foods are, the less likely it is that you will develop T2DM or an autoimmune disease like T1DM or LADA.

The Environmental Working Group produces its Dirty Dozen and Clean Fifteen lists each year, noting which foods have the most chemical contamination and should be eaten organically, and which foods are safe enough to be purchased conventionally, in case you live on a budget like so many of us do. In the must-buy-organic list are usually most of the healthy greens, such as kale, collards, and spinach, as well as celery, blueberries, strawberries, bell peppers, cucumbers, and cherry tomatoes. The Clean Fifteen list includes foods with thick skins, such as avocados, onions, cauliflower, eggplant, asparagus, and cabbage.

Genetically Modified Organisms (GMOs) or Genetically Engineered (GE) Foods

A GMO is the result of a laboratory process where genes from one species are inserted into another to attain a particular trait or characteristic. This is a very new science, and the transfer of interspecies genes can disrupt the finely controlled organization of DNA in the receiving organism. GMOs are developed mainly to allow commercial crops to withstand massive amounts of herbicides or insecticides. Most nations in the world, including the entire European Union, Australia, and Japan, do not believe GMOs are safe and either restrict or simply do not allow them to enter their countries or be sold there.

At the time of this writing, there are eight GMO foods in America: soy (94 percent of crops), canola (90 percent of crops), corn (88 percent of crops), cotton, alfalfa, sugar beets (95 percent of crops), Hawaiian papaya, and zucchini/yellow summer squash. Common ingredients made from GMO crops include aspartame, hydrolyzed vegetable protein, maltodextrins, monosodium glutamate, sucrose, textured vegetable protein (TVP), and xanthan gum. A genetically modified salmon was FDA approved for consumption a couple of years ago.

GMOs themselves are poorly regulated by the US government and can be harmful to both animals and humans. I believe science has proven that GMOs are also incredibly unsafe to eat. Not only that, genetic engineers themselves have stated that GMO crops are neither safe nor necessary. There are many published false and misleading studies that tell untruths about the safety of GMO foods, so you need to be vigilant in checking sources. GMO soy and corn seem to be significantly increasing allergic responses in humans to those foods. GMOs fed to animals have caused higher death rates, organ damage, infertility, and infant mortality, and have contributed to the toxic and allergic properties of genetically modified foods.

But, more importantly, there is now science showing that GMOs are indirectly associated with causing both T1DM and T2DM via the increased use of Roundup herbicides on GMO crops. GMO crops are often designed to allow a crop to survive massive doses of glyphosate herbicide, most notably Roundup Ready. The excess Roundup herbicides on crops is a toxic burden to humans and our environment and is associated with an increased rate of obesity, diabetes, autism, and other medical conditions. Even if you cannot purchase organic foods all the time, at least avoid eating GMO foods. Look for the food label to say "GMO-free" and avoid foods that simply list any of the eight GMO foods above, unless they specify that they are organic.

Carbohydrates

Motivation is the key for any physician hoping to entice a diabetic patient into eating well. If you're reading this book, you are probably willing to consider learning about the value of eating a low-carbohydrate diet, which is the key to controlling your diabetes.

Eating large amounts of carbs over time can impair one's capacity to metabolize them, especially once diabetes sets in. Diabetic patients need to be strict in eliminating refined sugar and high glycemic white flours, potatoes, and so forth, from their diets—even small amounts of these foods can pose big problems for regulating glucose.

The human body requires very little glucose to run well and with good energy. How much blood sugar in the human body equates to waking up and having a nice, healthy fasting glucose number of 80 mg/dL? The surprising answer is only 4 grams of sugar, or about four-fifths of a teaspoon. It may sound far-fetched, but that small amount of glucose will energize your entire body and all your cells.

How much sugar equates to 99 mg/dL, the highest fasting blood sugar you can have and not be diagnosed as prediabetic? The answer is 4.95 grams, or just about one full teaspoon of sugar.

How much blood sugar is in your body when it reaches the fasting level of diabetes, 126 mg/dL? The answer is 6.25 grams of sugar, one and one-quarter teaspoons, or the amount you probably stirred into your coffee this morning.

So, the difference between being nondiabetic and diabetic is a little more than one quarter of a teaspoon of sugar!

Imagine what happens when you drink a soda pop with *ten* teaspoons of sugar in it, if the whole body prefers only to have four-fifths of a teaspoon in it at any given time. Add this type of excess sugar and carbs into your body for years, and your body will gradually lose control of its ability to maintain good glucose levels, develop insulin resistance, and likely develop diabetes.

Small indiscretions cause huge glucose changes in your extremely tightly regulated, glucose-controlled blood. Three Oreo cookies, for example, contain 14 grams (or two and three-quarters teaspoons) of sugar. Washed down with a Starbuck's Caramel Macchiato drink (32 g of sugar), this snack is guaranteed to raise your glucose very high, and over time, ruin your body's capacity to process it. There is a clear lesson: If you are a patient with diabetes, cheating with one cookie here, or a piece of chocolate there, will affect your blood sugar! Other foods that do not necessarily contain refined sugar, but are very high in carbohydrates (a bowl of oatmeal, for example) will break down into glucose that will overwhelm your system, too.

Working with a physician who understands, respects, and can help guide you through a low-carb diet to prevent or treat your diabetes is necessary and can be a positive, helpful, informative, and effective way to get your glucose under excellent control.

A low-carb diet is the only way for people with diabetes who are on insulin to eat in order to know exactly how much insulin they need to inject accurately to cover their meals, as I discussed in chapter 6, in the section on insulin bolus dosing. A low-carb diet is also best for patients *not* on insulin to ensure glucose control, reduction of lipids, reduction of insulin resistance, reduction of weight loss, and reduction of blood pressure.

So, what exactly are carbohydrates? Carbohydrates are biological molecules consisting of carbon, hydrogen, and oxygen atoms, but we also use the term as shorthand for foods that contain a lot of starches or sugars. A low-carb diet means restricting carbohydrates to less than 45 grams per day, and even down to 20 grams per day. If you eat 1,500 calories a day, and only eat 30 grams of carbohydrates, and each carbohydrate burns 4 calories per gram, your daily carbohydrate caloric intake would be around 120 calories or 8 percent of your calories. For a diet of 2,000 calories, it's about 5 percent of calories a day. Twenty grams of carbs, or 80 calories, would mean your carbohydrate intake is only about 5 percent of a 1,500 calorie diet, and only about 4 percent of a 2,000 calorie diet: all very low amounts of carbs each day.

Carbohydrates are listed on nutrition labels as total carbohydrates, fiber, and sugar. A diabetic patient reading a nutrition label only needs to take into account total carbohydrates minus fiber, as fiber is not absorbed into the body and so does not raise glucose levels. The result equals how many carbs will be absorbed by your intestine and affect your glucose level.

We do not focus on the sugar content of the label, because it is not helpful to us. If a label says each serving of food contains "19 grams of total carbohydrates, 1 gram of fiber, 4 grams of sugar," and a patient does not understand how to interpret that label, he might feel it is safe to eat on a low-carb diet because the sugar content is fairly low. In reality, what that label says is: Of the 19 grams of total carbohydrates, we can subtract 1 gram because it is fiber, for a total carbohydrate content of 18 grams. Of those 18 grams, only 4 are "sugars," but the rest of the 14 grams will also raise the glucose. So, looking at total carbohydrate grams minus fiber is the only math I want patients to do—it represents all the carbs, starches, and sugars combined. *That* is the total carbohydrate intake of the serving of food, and what will affect their glucose.

Focusing on eating 30 grams of carbs a day would mean you would strive to eat along these lines:

Breakfast. Approximately 6 grams
Lunch. Approximately 12 grams
Supper. Approximately 12 grams

On this diet, we want to eat fewer carbs in the morning due to the natural glucose elevation that occurs via the dawn phenomenon. Your physician can help you figure out your specific carb intake. Morning intake of fewer than 10 grams is best.

If you agree to eat an impressively low 20 grams of carbs a day:

Breakfast. Approximately 4 grams
Lunch. Approximately 8 grams
Supper. Sppproximately 8 grams

The higher the carb intake—up to 45 grams a day as the limit ideally—the more one should eat at lunch. As mentioned, higher carbs in the morning can be a problem, and having a lot of carbs for supper can also increase your fasting glucose the next morning. With lunch, a patient can still be up and active, and more effectively burn off the glucose produced by the carbs.

The good news about pulling back on your intake of carbohydrates is that these are what drive your insulin resistance and interfere with good appetite control. Even though this diet sounds difficult, within a week, diabetic patients immediately see their appetite decreasing and smaller amounts of food filling them up. They usually come back after a week or two for a follow-up appointment saying "This isn't that bad," "I feel full," or "I'm fine with the diet."

Low-carb intake is the key, so the low intake is not flexible. Now let's discuss which carbs you should and should not eat.

KEY TREATMENT NOTE

Most people do not innately know how many carbs or proteins are in a food. Using a digital scale is an easy way to help figure out just how much carbs, protein, and fat you are eating. You can purchase an inexpensive one from any department store or online.

Grains

Grains are complex carbohydrates, and those carbs will raise your glucose levels substantially. Diabetic patients should avoid anything made from a grain, including wheat, oats, rice, quinoa (a high-carbohydrate seed), millet, barley, spelt, kamut, corn, rye, amaranth, and teff. You need to avoid all the manifestations of how grains are prepared: bread, oatmeal, noodles/pasta, muffins, rice, tortillas, pizza crust, hamburger and hot dog buns, crackers, and so on.

What can be eaten as replacements for grains? Many things! Shirataki noodles are noodles made from konjac/yam root or soy. They are sold in bags of water and are 100 percent fiber. They are stretchy and shiny like rice noodles. You can add them to a stir fry or salad in lieu of grain-based noodles. Miracle Rice is the same type of food but is made into rice instead of noodles.

Some people eat grain (such as flax) crackers that are very low in carbohydrates, a serving of which contains 11 grams of total carbs but all of it from fiber, so it will not raise glucose levels. Flax crackers can also easily be made at home.

Instead of grains, I recommend patients use nut flours, coconut flours, cauliflower, and other vegetables to make alternative "grain" products like muffins, breads, pancakes, waffles, pizza crust, granola—everything a person with diabetes wants to eat, but should not in their basic grain form.

Whole grains contain fiber (and so do beans, which diabetic patients should also mostly avoid). Fiber is eaten by beneficial bacteria and transformed into short-chain fatty acids (SCFAs). SCFAs are the food for the colon cells. Colon cells starved of SCFA can atrophy and die in days. Also, since the majority of our microbiome, our healthy gut bacteria, is in the colon, it is vitally important to ensure there is fiber in the diet to maintain a healthy colon. Fiber also reduces appetite, enhances satiety, lowers postmeal glucose levels, and helps increase beneficial bacteria in the intestine. This is why I always suggest that patients on a grain-free diet add a daily fiber powder into their diet. Any type of fiber is acceptable, from ground flax seeds, chia seeds, psyllium, and pectin, to guar gum, rice or oat bran, and inulin; whatever you like to mix with water or put in your smoothie or food.

Some patients of mine have wondered about resistant starch. Resistant starch means the starch is resistant to digestion and passes through the gut more slowly before being broken down. As a result, it produces a slow, steady glucose elevation over a number of hours. Thus, resistant starch has historically been used in diabetes as a food given at bedtime to pediatric patients with a serious risk of going dangerously low during their sleep. Resistant starch exists naturally in some foods, but has also been purposefully added to some processed products; it is usually uncooked corn or potato starch. There are a couple of products on the market that contain resistant starch, such as Extend Bars, but I do not like any of the other ingredients in those products and so I do not recommend them. There are other basic resistant starch products in plain powder form: Bob's Red Mill resistant potato starch, Anthony's Goods organic potato starch, and Honeyville Hi-Maize resistant starch.

Some patients think adding resistance starch to their meals will lower their postprandial glucose rise, but in reality, the addition is not very effective. Overall, I do not use or recommend resistant starch for patients. I don't mind if a patient wants to try it, but I will not recommend it. I much prefer the use of a basic fiber powder.

Fats

Fats, such as animal fats and those found in oils, are excellent for patients with diabetes, as they are not and do not contain carbs, and do not break down into sugar. They can be used for calorie intake, satiation of appetite, and increasing the flavor and mouth feel of foods, all without any risk of raising glucose levels.

The fat to avoid is called "trans fat," or "trans fatty acids," which is found in partially hydrogenated oils, including vegetable shortening, margarine, and vegetable fat. Trans fats are associated with raising cholesterol, causing inflammation and interfering with cell walls, increasing the risk for depression, and heart disease. They are deficient in all the beneficial nutrients and antioxidants (such as vitamin E) that are naturally found in other oils, are usually made with GMOs, and are full of hexane, which is used to process the oil, and also preservatives and other chemicals that are added to the refining process.

Since the FDA required food companies to divulge on their labels if this oil is included in their ingredients, many companies have removed trans fats from their foods. Now the FDA has told food companies it will be illegal to use partially hydrogenated oils in any food by June 2018. While this is wonderful news, unfortunately many companies removing trans fats are instead using fully hydrogenated oils as interesterified oils. Interesterified oils were shown to raise glucose levels by up to 20 percent, so they're not good oils for patients with diabetes. Fully hydrogenated fats are closer to being plastic than food, and should not be eaten, and there is no doubt interesterified oils were involved in their manufacturing. You must read all ingredient labels, and if you see either "interesterified oils" (uncommon) or "fully hydrogenated oils" (more common), please do not eat that food. These oils are mostly found in fried foods, dessert-type foods, margarine, and foods like peanut butter, "butter" flavored popcorn, and so forth.

Saturated fat is another main type of fat we eat; it comes from animal foods such as beef, pork, lamb, poultry, cheese, and cream, as well as nuts, and oils like butter, palm oil, palm kernel oil, and coconut oil. Unlike trans fats, there is nothing wrong with including saturated fats in one's diet. Yes, research has shown that elevated plasma saturated fat can increase a patient's insulin resistance, potentially raising glucose levels. However, it seems that eating a high-carb diet, particularly high in refined sugars, is the main impetus for elevated plasma saturated fat. Saturated fats, though, can increase inflammation pathways in the body. So, although saturated fats are not believed any longer to be a risk for cardiovascular disease, we still should ensure we are eating them in balance with other beneficial dietary oils, such as omega-3 oils.

Omega-3 oil is the super oil of a diet and for a person. Foods that contain omega-3 oil include green leafy vegetables, walnuts, organic grass-fed and grass-finished meats, omega-3 eggs, dairy made from animals that were fully pasture-raised, oily fish, flax and chia seeds, and soybeans. Omega-3 oils reduce insulin resistance, inflammation, depression, anxiety, pain and stiffness, autoimmunity, lipids, and cardiovascular disease risk.

Medium-chain triglyceride (MCT) oils have carbon chains that are six to ten carbon molecules long. Saturated fats and polyunsaturated fats, as described above, have much longer carbon chains. Thus, MCT oils are easy to absorb and break down to use as energy. They are not stored in fat tissue, as the other fats are, but are broken down by the liver into ketone bodies, which nourish the body and brain cells. Coconut oil contains some MCTs, but not much. These oils are usually dosed in supplements. MCT oils may have some benefits with weight management, sustained energy for sports, and helping with cognition. With diabetic patients, the ketone bodies MCT oils produce are energy that does not require insulin. MCT oils may help T1DM patients with hypoglycemic unawareness. If I use MCT oils with patients, I recommend a very pure product from www.KetoMCT.com. Watch your dosing with MCT oils, as too much may cause diarrhea. Your integrative physician can guide you about these and help you find an appropriate dose.

Oils should be kept in your refrigerator to prevent rancidity, as light, heat, and air induce oil degradation. If the oil gets hard in the fridge, like olive, coconut, and avocado oils do, they can be kept in a dark cabinet. Keeping oils out on the kitchen counter all the time can make them go rancid quicker.

Healthy oils to keep in your kitchen include:

OILS WITH OMEGA-3

Walnut. Can be used raw and up to medium-high heat
Organic unrefined flax oil. Only use raw
Organic unrefined hemp oil. Only use raw

OTHER HEALTHY OILS

Organic butter/goat butter. If not allergic to dairy
Ghee
Organic extra-virgin olive oil. Raw or medium-high heat
Organic unrefined coconut oil. Medium heat
Sesame oil. High heat, as in a wok
Avocado oil. High heat, as in a wok
Peanut oil. High heat, even for frying food
Red palm oil (highest oil source of vitamins A and E and carotenoids). Medium heat
Earth Balance or Smart Balance

Margarine should be avoided.

Making use of oils to enrich flavors, enhance flavors, and control appetite is a very valuable dietary methodology for diabetic patients. Ignore the ADA suggestion that your diet should be low in fat. That is simply wrong. Using fats to increase calories when carb intake is limited is a fantastic way to make the diet healthy and tasty and to provide good energy all day long.

Fruit

Most fruits are way too high in carbohydrates to be eaten by those with diabetes; an apple has 20 grams, for example, and a banana up to 34 grams. Berries have the lowest amount, but even a half cup of blueberries still has around 8–10 grams of carbs. In general, patients with diabetes should avoid fruits except for avocados, cucumbers, and a small amount of tomatoes. I suggest that if a patient eats berries, they eat them at lunch, as in the morning the dawn phenomenon increases glucose, and foods at supper can easily carry over to raising waking glucose. At lunch, people can still be active during the day and are not at an innately high-glucose time of the day. Table 7.1 shows the amount of carbohydrates in a quarter cup of various fruits.

Table 7.1. Net Carbohydrates in a Quarter Cup of Fruit

Fruit	Carbohydrates, in grams
Avocado	0.5
Blueberries	4.1
Cherries	4.2
Coconut	1.3
Olives	3.0 (for every 1 oz, pitted)
Raspberries	1.5
Strawberries	1.8

Vegetables

All vegetables contain some carbohydrates, but most have little effect on glucose levels and many can be eaten and enjoyed by individuals with diabetes. I recommend eating at least three and up to nine cups a day—though nine cups is probably too high a goal for most people. Vegetables can be purchased either fresh or frozen, but I do not recommend canned or boiled vegetables, and no iceberg lettuce. I do not want patients to *always* cook their vegetables using a microwave but I do not mind if one is used briefly now and then to warm up leftovers, or to cook something quickly.

The best ways to eat vegetables are raw, stir-fried, steamed, roasted, baked, or grilled. If you steam them, it's good to drink the water that's left over, as it contains most of the potassium and several B vitamins that get leached from the veggies when they are cooked.

It's important to eat lots of leafy greens. These vegetables contain omega-3 oils, magnesium, potassium, calcium, and other nutrients that can reduce insulin resistance, increase antioxidants, decrease inflammation, and increase nutrient intake. There are many different leafy greens, including red lettuce, green lettuce, romaine lettuce, butter leaf lettuces, spinach, kale, cabbage, collard greens, beet greens, mustard greens, bok choy, chard, radicchio, arugula, and others. In general, the darker the greens, the higher the amount of nutrients. Cruciferous vegetables—broccoli, cauliflower, Brussels sprouts, radish, and cabbage—are also especially healthy. These help the liver work better, and since insulin resistance begins in the liver, and many overweight T2DM patients also have fatty livers, supporting liver function via food is a good idea. Though not a cruciferous vegetable, artichokes help the liver produce and secrete bile, which aids in fat digestion.

Cauliflower is an amazing vegetable, both by itself and turned into the equivalent of mashed potatoes, Tater Tots, bagels, rolls, breads, casseroles, pizza crust, nachos, fritters, and so forth. A cauliflower bagel! Who knew? Creative cooks have invented amazing foods with cauliflower.

Onions and garlic are great; they help the immune system, keep the gut healthier, provide sulfur to help with liver detoxification, and lower glucose levels. The orange, red, yellow, and purple vegetables are full of carotenoids and antioxidants, and since diabetic damage is oxidative damage, eating foods high in antioxidants can help prevent diabetic damage. Some colorful, diabetic-safe vegetables high in carotenoids and antioxidants include bell peppers, yellow zucchini, squash, eggplant, purple cabbage, and tomatoes. The suggestion is to eat a rainbow of different vegetable colors each week.

The variety of vegetables makes making salads interesting and fun. Try adding pickles, olives, sunflower seeds, nuts, grated cheese, turkey, chicken, salmon, and so forth for even more variety. There is a study that showed that it's important to use oil dressing on a salad to ensure one absorbs all the fat-soluble nutrients such as carotenoids and vitamin E, since these nutrients require fat for absorption. Make sure the dressing is low in carbs and consists of mostly oil and vinegar, but do not use balsamic vinegar, as it is not fully fermented (which is why it is so sweet) and can raise your glucose. Any other fully tart vinegar is okay, however, including rice, apple cider, or white vinegar. If you make your own oil and vinegar dressing, try using flax oil or walnut oil to increase omega-3 intake, or olive oil for the other cardioprotective antioxidants it contains.

It's easy to increase your daily vegetable intake via a leafy green smoothie in the morning, and then a salad or a stir fry, and cauliflower pizza crust or bagels. There is a whole world of fascinating use of vegetables in diabetic diets.

Vegetables to avoid include white potatoes, yams, sweet potatoes, tomato paste, and corn. These will significantly raise glucose levels. Tomatoes, carrots, and onions can be eaten, but not too many at one time. Table 7.2 lists typical amounts of carbs in 1-cup servings of vegetables.

Table 7.2. Net Carbohydrates in a Cup of Vegetables

Vegetable	Carbohydrates, in grams
Acorn squash	30
Artichoke	4 (in a large artichoke)
Asparagus	7
Broccoli	8
Brussels sprouts	14
Cabbage (green)	4
Cauliflower	5
Celery	4
Cucumbers	5
Eggplant	7
Lettuce or salad greens	1 to 2
Mushrooms (white button)	3
Pepper (red bell)	10
Spinach	1
Tomatoes	8 (actually a fruit but used as a vegetable)
Zucchini	5

Fermented Foods

I recommend patients eat fermented foods, as they are invaluable for healing the gut lining and enhancing our intestinal microbiome, the beneficial bacteria that make us healthier overall. A healthier gut reduces autoimmunity and systemic insulin resistance, enables easier weight loss, and helps our bodies and minds in many ways. Societies all over the world include fermented foods in their diets, as do many Western countries. Fermented foods are frequently made from vegetables or proteins, and include sauerkraut, kimchi, dill pickles, black garlic, yogurt, miso soup, and fermented fish.

I recommend the book *Fermented Vegetables* by Kirsten and Christopher Shockey. It teaches how to make all sorts of fermented vegetables in your home.

Proteins

Proteins are polymer chains made of amino acids linked together by peptide bonds. Proteins are listed on food labels in two different ways: ounces and grams. Animal products are listed in protein ounces, but the FDA requires that food companies use grams on their food labels. It's important to remember that 1 ounce of protein = 6 grams of protein. Although 1 ounce of protein weighs 28 grams, only 6 grams are actual protein; the rest is water, fat, and so forth. So, if a patient is told they can have 3 ounces of protein for breakfast, that equals 18 grams of protein.

How much protein should you eat per meal? We tend to determine ideal protein intake by body weight, to some extent. There are established levels of protein intake for all ages and both sexes. Adults are generally instructed to eat 0.8 grams of protein per kilogram of body weight. We figure out kilograms by taking our own weight and dividing it by 2.2. So, a typical 150 pound adult, based on typical protein standards, requires 54 grams of protein per day (150 divided by 2.2 multiplied by 0.8 = 54). Divide that by 6, and we wind up with 9 ounces.

However, since on a low-carb diet we remove so many calories by reducing the carb intake, I add in a little more protein for calories and satiation and multiply by 1—instead of 0.8—kg of body weight (multiplying by 1 is obviously not going to change the amount of protein, but helps to clarify the example). Thus, the formula is: your weight divided by 2.2 (no need to really multiply by 1.0). That would mean the same man would wind up with the suggestion to eat 64 grams of protein a day, or 10.5 ounces.

What about if a person is overweight and needs to lose weight? How much protein should she eat?

Let's say, for example, that a patient's present (but not ideal) weight is 200 pounds.

$200 \div 2.2 \times 1 = 91$ grams of protein, or 15 ounces ($91 \div 6 = 15$), a day.

Fifteen ounces is a lot of protein to eat in one day! I do not recommend the vast majority of patients eat that much protein. So the next step is to take one's *ideal* weight, and split the difference. For this example, we'll say the patient's ideal weight is 140 pounds.

140 ÷ 2.2 = 64 grams of protein, or 10.5 ounces a day.

So I would recommend a middle zone for this patient, around 13 ounces a day. Most patients are okay if they eat between 9 and 13 ounces of protein a day. Accordingly, this patient may wish to eat 3 ounces, or 18 grams, of protein at breakfast, 4 ounces, or 24 grams, at lunch, and 6 ounces, or 36 grams, at supper.

If the starting protein intake according to this formula is not enough and a patient is still hungry after meals, it's acceptable to increase daily protein (or fat) servings, but not carbohydrate servings. Your physician will walk you through setting up and organizing your daily protein intake with your input. Remember that protein is necessary for determining insulin dosages, so we need to have a clear idea of how much protein is eaten at meals.

Now let's talk about the quality of proteins and which proteins work on a low-carb diet.

AGRI-INDUSTRY MEAT VERSUS ORGANIC GRASS-FED OR GRASS-FINISHED MEAT

Eating meat can be controversial for a variety of reasons, including its health merits. We receive many conflicting messages, many of them partially or wholly mistaken, about the healthfulness of eating meat.

Living in Montana for thirteen years, I saw a lot of cattle. Montana is home to about 1 million people and 2.5 million cattle. Everywhere you drive it seems cattle are grazing on wild grass. As a result of eating their natural food, half the fat in those cattle is made of the same essential fatty acids we find in salmon. In fact, historically, eating animals—including cattle, pigs, deer, elk, and rabbits—was a main way humans ingested omega-3 essential fatty oils, which are vital for us to stay healthy and heal from most conditions.

When cattle are taken from the range and put in a feedlot, they are fed estrogens and GMO corn to gain weight. Because corn is not a natural food for cattle, it causes terrible stomach conditions, including ulcers. It also affects their stool bacteria, which results in now common beef recalls after hemolytic E. coli infections killed innocent people eating the bacteria-laden meat. Cattle are fed antibiotics, too. *The Journal of American Science* published a study detailing how, after ninety days in the feedlot, cattle wind up losing nearly all their omega-3 fat, which is replaced by saturated fat. The meat also contains more calories and fewer nutrients.

"Agri-industry" beef and pork can be both decidedly unhealthy and pro-inflammatory. With agri-industry poultry, according to federal law, conventional manufacturers are not allowed to feed the chickens hormones (so when a company advertises it doesn't do so, it's not because they are so progressive, it's because it's against the law), but they can give them GMO corn and soybeans that have arsenic in them, a dangerous heavy metal. The natural food for chickens is insects, worms, green plants, and seeds, not corn and soy. Agri-industry feed can contain estrogens, too, which in turn can elevate levels of estrogen in poultry. Agri-industry chickens are also often fed antibiotics and might be contaminated with staphylococcus bacteria. In fact, in America, we give antibiotics to animals more than we give them to humans, and we give a lot of antibiotics to humans!

Agri-industry meat can pose serious health problems for people—it has more unhealthy fats and fewer nutrients; has more calories; is filled with hormones, antibiotics, and GMOs; and has very little or no omega-3 oils left in it. Even organic vegetarian diet–fed meat that is not exposed to hormones or antibiotics, though cleaner, may still be low in or devoid of omega-3 oils.

I always encourage my patients to spend their money on high-quality animal products. I recommend patients buy organic meat that is both grass-fed *and* grass-finished; this means the animal's diet for their entire life was grass, without any grains added. Cows that are solely grass-fed, and not grass-finished, can start their lives eating grass on the ranch, only later to be shipped off to a feedlot for the last three months or so to "marble," fattening up on grains. I knew ranchers in Montana who raised grass-fed beef who did this. So look for "grass-finished," which means the animal was not fattened up on grains, and "organic," which means that the animal did not receive chemicals, estrogens, or antibiotics.

Organic grass-fed and grass-finished forms of poultry, beef, pork, and lamb are often sold at local health food stores and farmers markets, from butchers who only sell that quality of meat, directly from ranchers raising healthy animal products, or online. Check out www.eatwild.com to find ranchers in your state raising organic, grass-fed, and grass-finished meat and poultry.

Although I do not think most diabetic patients should snack, but instead should eat three meals a day, many T1DM pediatric patients do need snacks. Nicks-sticks.com sells organic, grass-fed, grass-finished turkey and beef jerkies that contain only organic spices—no MSG, no sugar, and no soy sauce. They are a great source of quick protein with no grams of carbs included. I have these in the waiting room of my clinic and patients go through boxes of them very quickly!

NONMEAT PROTEINS

While protein is most often associated with meat and poultry, it's also found in a number of other foods.

Beans, peas, and lentils. In general, I suggest that diabetic patients avoid eating these foods, because they raise glucose levels. Some patients can eat a little bit of hummus without a rise in glucose, perhaps due to the oil and garlic included. However, in general, avoid these foods.

Soybeans. Soy is the only bean that patients with diabetes can regularly eat, but only if the label states that it is organic and GMO-free. The best, lowest carb soy foods to eat are tofu, unsweetened soy milk, unsweetened plain soy yogurt, edamame, and soy nut butter. There are low-carb miso soups, but ensure you read the label and choose the lowest carb option. Tempeh, a fermented type of soy, is too high in carbs for excessive safe eating, though a little seems okay: Half a cup is only 8 grams of carbs and 16 grams of protein. I request patients avoid soy protein isolate, a very highly processed food created using acids, which is included in foods such as soy protein powder or soy fake meat products such as soy bologna.

Many Americans feel soybeans are dangerous to eat and cause all sorts of hormonal imbalances. In reality, soy phytoestrogens are 1⁄100th the strength of human estrogens. Women in Asian countries eating soy regularly have fewer incidences of breast cancer than women in America. Environmental xenoestrogens found in many toxic chemicals are infinitely more dangerous than eating organic, GMO-free tofu a couple of times a week.

Table 7.3. Net Carbohydrates in Soy-Based Foods

Soy Food and Serving Size	Carbohydrates, in grams
Edamame—1 cup	8
Soy nut butter—2 tbsp	7
Tempeh—½ cup	8
Tofu—½ cup	2.3
Unsweetened plain yogurt—1 cup	5
Unsweetened soy milk—1 cup	1

Soy is considered a "goitregen," as are several other foods. A goitregen can interfere with thyroid processing if eaten excessively over time. That means one should not live off of soy, as some vegans mistakenly do, and if it is eaten more than a few times a week, one should also eat some seaweed products containing iodine, which can stimulate the thyroid to work better. We do not want to take excessive iodine, though! The RDA is 150 micrograms (mcg), and we should ingest that much a day (or up to 300 mcg during pregnancy). High-dose iodine pills are, I feel, dangerous and need to be avoided.

Nonetheless, soy is a nice addition to the diet, being plant-based, and if eaten in a healthy way, soy is safe and will not excessively raise glucose levels as other beans can do. See table 7.3 for the carb levels of different soy-based foods.

Nuts, nut butter, nut flours. Nuts are used very frequently and very successfully with patients with diabetes. All nuts but cashews and chestnuts can be eaten—those two nuts have too many carbs for them to be acceptable to eat. Pistachios are relatively high in carbs, too, but I do allow patients to eat a few of them, and they seem to be okay with glucose numbers.

Go for variety, as different nuts contain different nutrients: peanuts (actually a legume diabetic patients can eat, peanuts contain a great antioxidant, resveratrol), almonds (calcium/magnesium), walnuts (omega-3 oils), sunflower seeds (zinc), pumpkin seeds (zinc), Brazil nuts (selenium, an antioxidant), macadamia nuts (calcium, potassium), filberts/hazelnuts (vitamin E), and pine nuts. The key to most low-carb diabetic diets is to use nut flours to make bread, muffins, tortillas, crackers, pancakes, and other pseudograins that easily satisfy appetites. Although most recipes call for almond flour, I recommend substituting other nut flours for both dietary and flavor variety. I have seen kids become allergic to almonds, a common food allergy, if they are fed almonds and almond flour products all the time. Other nut flours are also good to use: pecan, macadamia, and hazelnut flours, for example. You can buy many different types of nut flours at www.nuts.com. Although coconut is a fruit and not a nut, its flour also has a very low effect on glucose. Using coconut flour to bake with is very popular with patients.

Nut butters can be equally low in carbs.

Nut flours can also be acceptable on a low-carb diet, especially when used in recipes with fats, nuts, coconut flakes, and flax seeds. Tables 7.4–7.6 show carb levels for various nuts and nut products.

Table 7.4. Net Carbohydrates in an Ounce of Nuts

Nuts	Carbohydrates, in grams
Almonds	2.7
Brazil nuts	1.3
Chia seeds	1.7
Coconut	2.0
Flax seeds	0.5
Hazelnuts	2.0
Macadamia nuts	1.6
Peanuts	2.1
Pecans	1.2
Pine nuts	2.7
Pumpkin seeds	4.0
Sesame seeds	3.3
Sunflower seeds	3.2
Walnuts	1.9

Table 7.5. Net Carbohydrates in 2 Tablespoons of Unsweetened Nut Butters

Unsweetened Nut Butter	Carbohydrates, in grams
Almond nut butter	2
Macadamia nut butter	1
Peanut butter	4
Sunflower seed	3
Tahini	2

Table 7.6. Net Carbohydrates in a Quarter Cup of Nut Flours

Nut Flour	Carbohydrates, in grams
Almond	3
Coconut	3
Flax	0
Hazelnut	2
Macadamia	1
Pecan	2
Soy	2

Fish. Fish is a wonderful addition to the diet. Ensuring one eats healthy fish is vitally important. You want to focus on fish that are high in omega-3 oils while avoiding those that are high in methylmercury. Methylmercury comes from industrial smoke stacks, and then, through rainfall, enters bodies of water. It then travels up the food chain where it bioaccumulates in the bigger fish that people tend to eat. Methylmercury is toxic to the brain, kidneys, liver, heart, and nervous system, and can cause numerous medical conditions. Intake of mercury is affected by a patient's weight and whether or not she is pregnant. A pregnant woman should seriously curtail her fish intake, only eat very pure fish, and totally avoid any fish noted to have any significant mercury in it for the safety of herself and her developing baby.

Fish that are high in omega-3 and low in mercury include wild salmon, rainbow trout, sardines, mussels, herring, anchovies, and Atlantic mackerel. I recommend patients get canned salmon and make salmon salad instead of tuna salad. Fish and other seafood low in mercury, but also low in omega-3, and therefore not recommended, include shrimp, catfish, tilapia, clams, and scallops. Tilapia are often farm-raised and may not be of high quality. Catfish is a "bottom feeder" and also should not be eaten regularly. Fish and seafood that should be avoided due to noticeably high mercury levels include tuna, halibut, lobster, mahi-mahi, sea bass, king mackerel, marlin, tilefish, shark, swordfish, orange roughy, and bluefin or bigeye tuna (sushi tuna).

Dairy. Dairy is okay for diabetic patients to eat, but should ideally be organic, or at least should not contain rBGH (recombinant bovine growth hormone). Many people have sensitivities to dairy products, which can give them nasal congestion, gastroesophageal reflex disease (GERD), asthma, and other conditions. Some people have lactose intolerance and get digestive upset eating dairy. Some people do not wish to eat dairy because they are concerned about its quality and how it may be affecting their immune system. If a patient cannot or chooses not to eat dairy, I completely support that decision and often I am the one recommending they avoid eating it. I may also do a food-sensitivity test and find it is a positive allergen for them.

Table 7.7. Net Carbohydrates in Dairy Products

Dairy Product and Serving Size	Carbohydrates, in grams
Cheese—1 ounce	1
Coconut Cream—2 tbsp	1
Cream Cheese—2 tbsp	2
Dairy Cream—2 tbsp	1
Daiya Cream Cheese—2 tbsp	4
Kroger plain unsweetened yogurt—6 ounces (1 container/170 g)	6

But for those patients who choose to eat dairy and do not seem to have any negative consequences doing so, I am okay with them eating it. The low-carb diabetic diet is already very restricted. If there is no reason for a person to avoid a food on it, I will not be adamant about removing it. Table 7.7 shows net carb amounts for various dairy products.

There are a couple of dairy items to avoid, however, particularly the ones that are more liquid or loose, as those contain higher levels of lactose, which can raise glucose levels, including regular milk and cottage cheese. But any hard cheese is okay for a diabetic patient, and even a little cream cheese is okay.

Unsweetened low-carb alternative milks are acceptable: coconut, almond, flax, soy, macadamia nut, hazelnut, hemp, and so forth. I recommend patients avoid rice milk due to its carb content. Cream is okay, both regular dairy or coconut. Also, cheeses other than cottage cheese are allowed. Cow, goat, or sheep milk cheeses are fine, and raw or organic cheeses are ideal, but they are hard to find. I would like patients to avoid highly processed artificial dairy products, like pasteurized processed cheese foods such as American cheese and Velveeta. You can try Daiya cheese, Kite Hill, or other nondairy cheese brands if you wish to be dairy free. But watch the carbohydrate totals in them.

Yogurt has to be eaten carefully; it may raise glucose in some patients. You need to check to see if eating yogurt is okay for you. Yogurt should be plain, and without any fruit added. Higher protein Greek yogurts work for some patients. You may wish to try Kroger's CARBmaster yogurt if you can find it. You can eat cow, goat, sheep, plain soy, or plain coconut yogurt.

Eggs. There are two key words to look for on your egg carton: organic and omega-3. If the eggs are organic, you know the chickens were not fed GMO feed or antibiotics, and had more space to roam. Crowded chickens packed into a room require antibiotics to prevent infections. The omega-3 means the chickens either ate their normal diet of insects and worms, or were fed flax or chia seeds. There is no medical association between eating these eggs and raising one's cholesterol; in fact, the American Heart Association now does not limit the amount of eggs people can eat. People often eat a lot of chicken and beef but avoid eggs due to worries about the cholesterol they contain. Actually, organic eggs are super healthy—full of lecithin (which is not in chicken or beef!), which helps to lower cholesterol, aid memory and mental focus, and prevent gallstone formation when weight loss is occurring. The yolk is also high in vitamin D, carotenoids, vitamin E, and vitamin B_{12}.

Protein powders. Aside from soy protein isolate, I feel protein powder is fine for patients. Some patients love the speed and convenience of making healthy smoothies containing protein powder in the morning. That's great! The protein powders I like are pea protein, rice protein, whey protein, and egg protein. Pea and rice sound like they would contain carbs, but they do not; they're just straight proteins enzymatically extracted from those foods. Patients may want to use beef protein powder, but it seems that is made from all the nasty leftovers of beef from the slaughterhouse. Hemp is a great protein powder, but most people do not like the flavor. Many protein powders have added sugar (especially chocolate flavors) or other added carbohydrates, so make sure you read the ingredients of any product you wish to use, and get one that is very low in carbohydrates.

Protein Powder Smoothie

Serves 1

MAIN INGREDIENTS

1½ cups (12 ounces) very clean water

1 to 3 tablespoons ground flax or chia seeds

RECOMMENDED INGREDIENTS

Unsweetened alternative milk (coconut, almond, etc.)

1 to 3 tablespoons all-natural nut butter

1 teaspoon to 1 tablespoon coconut, walnut, or flax oil

Stevia, monk fruit, xylitol, erythritol, or Truvia to taste

OPTIONAL INGREDIENTS

1 large handful (at least 2 cups) dark leafy greens (kale, collard greens, spinach, chard, etc.)

Small bunch of cilantro

Small bunch of parsley

¼ whole avocado

1 teaspoon to 1 tablespoon green powder

Protein powder (rice, pea, whey, egg, or hemp; avoid soy protein isolate)

Instructions: Blend the main ingredients together in a high-powered food processor or blender, with as many recommended and optional ingredients as you like. Many people also like adding ice to their smoothie. Pour into a glass and enjoy right away.

Beverages

While water is the healthiest drink, most people like a little variety. However, there are quite a few beverages a person with diabetes should not drink:

Regular soda pop. Obviously, soda pop is too high in sugar. Also, avoid sweetened energy and electrolyte drinks.

Diet soda pop. Why is diet soda pop on this list? Diet soda pop contains unhealthy chemicals used as sweeteners. These sweeteners can harm your mood, cause headaches, cause thyroid problems, and worse, are associated with promoting weight gain. These chemicals do not signal your brain that you have ingested calories, so people drinking these types of sodas often overeat and gain weight.

Fruit juices. Fruit juice is too high in fructose, a fruit sugar that contains a lot of calories and causes fatty development in the liver, as well as insulin resistance.

Vegetable juices. Some are fine. But some vegetable juices have added sugar in them, and some, such as carrot or beet juice, even if they are unsweetened, have enough sugars in them naturally that diabetic patients should avoid them. Read vegetable juice labels carefully for their total carb content.

Milk. Milk contains lactose, a milk sugar that raises glucose levels.

Here are the beverages that are okay for any diabetic patient to drink:

Pure filtered water.

Club soda/seltzer water. A lot of my patients use home carbonator units to make their own carbonated drinks. This saves both money and landfill space, because they can reuse their liter bottles and do not have to constantly buy new plastic bottles and then throw them out or send them for recycling. Many people find carbonated water refreshing. Adding in some stevia-flavored drops, cucumber slices, or lemon juice can give the water some pizazz.

Herbal teas. Any herbal tea is acceptable.

Green or black teas. Green teas in particular have antioxidants, which are very useful to diabetic patients and are protective of the pancreas and liver.

Coffee. Although a lot of coffee can be protective and reduce the onset of T2DM, once a patient has T2DM, 1–2 cups of coffee a day should be enough. With T2DM, too much coffee may raise glucose levels, upset the stomach, and interfere with sleep.

Alternative coffees. There are several brands, such as Teeccino, Cafix, and Pero, that use chicory for bitterness and other ingredients for flavor. Some contain barley, and these should be avoided in patients who are 100 percent gluten free. Chicory is a good bitter for the liver, and it helps the liver detoxify.

Unsweetened chocolate or carob powder. It is okay to take unsweetened chocolate powder (Guittard, Ghirardelli, Hershey's), or unsweetened carob powder (Chatfield's or organic ones), add some hot water, unsweetened alternative milk, and stevia and make a cup of hot chocolate / carob that will not raise your glucose and may contain some antioxidants.

Vegetable juices. As noted above, vegetable juice falls in the "maybe" category. Read the ingredients of all processed vegetable juices to check for both carbohydrates and salt levels, neither of which should be high. Even healthy ones like Suja Twelve Essentials contains 7 grams of carbs in 8 ounces, but having 4 ounces may be okay with a meal. Adding greens into low-carb smoothies is always okay.

Unsweetened alternative milk. (As discussed in protein dairy category.)

"Healthy" soda pops. There are several brands, such as Zevia, Virgil Zero, and Rob's, that are sweetened with stevia and erythritol.

Alcohol, specifically wine, and distilled liquors such as whiskey and vodka. Alcohol contains calories, so overweight T2DM patients who want to lose weight should use caution. The main myth about alcohol is that it turns into sugar; it doesn't. Alcohol breaks down into aldehydes (if some refined sugar product is not added to it, or it is not made from grains, like beer). Alcohol reduces the liver's capacity to engage in gluconeogenesis or glycogenosis, two biochemical pathways that enable the liver to make glucose. Thus, having a glass of wine at supper will usually *lower* a diabetic patient's fasting glucose number. That doesn't mean you should feel compelled to drink every night, however! Also, if you have a fatty liver, you should completely avoid alcohol, as a liver damaged by any condition, even something as reversible as fatty liver, is always significantly aggravated when it has to detoxify alcohol. Types of alcohol to avoid include mixed drinks that include soda pop (e.g., rum and coke), port wines, most beers (except for Michelob Ultra), and sweetened mixed cocktails.

Sweeteners

Refined sugars are processed carbohydrates that have the most devastating effect on raising glucose. Of course, refined sugars need to be avoided by all patients with diabetes. The average American ingests 155 pounds of refined sugar a year; sugar is obvious in overtly sweet foods—candies, cookies, pastries, soda pop—but is also hidden in so many other foods, from ketchups and salad dressings to granola, and nearly every other processed food people have in their refrigerator and pantry.

SUGARS TO AVOID

The list of sugars to avoid is long: sucrose, glucose, fructose, dextrose, maltose, corn syrup, corn syrup solids, high-fructose corn syrup solids, honey, maple syrup, brown rice syrup, barley malt syrup, evaporated cane juice, organic cane juice, turbinado sugar, brown sugar, raw sugar, coconut sugar, yacon syrup, and agave. Although agave supposedly has a low glycemic index, it is exceedingly high in fructose, higher than high-fructose corn syrup, meaning it turns into fat in the liver, causing insulin resistance, and should be avoided.

People who are diabetic should also avoid the artificial chemical sweeteners, such as saccharin, Equal/aspartame, and Splenda/sucralose. These sweeteners have never been proven to be safe in people, and there are many concerns about ingesting them. Aside from a very occasional use, I ask patients to avoid them as much as possible. There are a couple of companies, including Walden Foods and DaVinci Gourmet, that produce certain fake foods containing sucralose or Splenda such as vanilla syrup or barbecue sauce. For occasional use of specialty products I am okay with patients using one of these products, but by no means do I want them to be eaten daily, or even frequently.

Sugar alcohols, also called polyols, can occur naturally in foods, like mannitol, but mostly they are made from sugars that are chemically altered to alcohols. Sorbitol and mannitol are problematic for most people; they are partially absorbed and can turn to glucose, thus raising your glucose levels, and the rest that is not absorbed can cause gastrointestinal distress, such as gas, bloating, and diarrhea. These are often found in "diabetic" foods in supermarket aisles, or in sugar-free chocolates in chocolate stores. They should not be eaten.

DIABETIC FRIENDLY SWEETENERS

Sweeteners that patients with diabetes can regularly use include stevia, sugar alcohols such as xylitol and erythritol, Just Like Sugar, monk fruit, and combination products containing two of any of those.

Stevia comes in both liquid and powder form. For powdered, look only for organic stevia, which does not contain maltodextrin, a corn-based filler. Stevia drops come in many different flavors. Stevia can be used both raw and in cooked foods. Some people find stevia a little bitter, but stevia from different companies may taste different. Studies show that stevia may even help heal the pancreas.

As for xylitol and erythritol, most people absorb these sugar alcohols well; they are not metabolized and are excreted unchanged, with no effect on your glucose. Some people, however, do not absorb them well, and these sugar alcohols may upset their stomachs. There are some concerns that they may increase glucose levels, but that is not common. Xylitol and erythritol can be used in both uncooked and cooked foods. Some companies make xylitol candies, and sometimes it's nice to have a little oral fixation. I recommend Dr. John's kosher sugar-free xylitol sucking candies, even if you are not Jewish. The kosher candies do not have the chemical colors that the nonkosher candies have; they contain natural colors and flavors. Spry sucking candies and gum are also tasty and use xylitol. Similarly, PUR Gum is a xylitol healthy gum made without any bad ingredients. The gum flavor does not last long, but it is an acceptable gum.

Just Like Sugar is made mainly, along with a few other ingredients, from inulin from chicory, the same chicory that I mentioned above in the fake coffees. There is a product for tabletop use and one for baking. It appears to contain massive amounts of carbohydrates, but it is also from the root fiber, so it should not affect your glucose. But make sure of this by checking your glucose after trying it in a food. Inulin is also considered a prebiotic, a food that feeds the beneficial bacteria in intestines, so it is very good for your microbiome.

Monk fruit, also known as lo han guo, is the fruit of a perennial vine in the gourd family, whose extract is two hundred and fifty times sweeter than sugar, though it is essentially carb free. Many patients prefer this sweetener when stevia is too bitter for them, as monk fruit is not bitter at all.

Helpful Diet Accessories

There are a number of helpful websites to use for particular diets. These are great resources (if you use them) to help you figure out just how much carbs, proteins, fats, fiber, calories, salt, and nutrients you are getting in your diet.

Many adult patients use My Fitness Pal (www.myfitnesspal.com) or Carb Manager (www.carbmanager.com), either online or through phone apps to record their diets and analyze them to ensure they are meeting low-carb dietary target goals. Doc's Diet Diary is another phone app where one can record a diet diary and then email it to one's physician; there is a Doc's Diabetes Diary app, too.

The USDA SuperTracker website (https://supertracker.usda.gov) is designed for adults, but it can also be used for pediatric patients. On this diet analysis site, a person can analyze their intake of micronutrients, such as calcium, magnesium, omega-3 oils, vitamin E, and so forth.

Another helpful website is www.nutritiondata.self.com, which provides patients with a quick guide to the nutritional breakdown of each food per quantity eaten.

Last, there are some good Facebook forums for emotional and culinary support: Low Carb Diabetes Association; The Vegetarian Low Carb Diabetic Healthy Diet Society; and Dr. Bernstein's Diabetes Solution Advocates. There are also Pinterest, Instagram, and all other sorts of social media platforms where diabetic patients can feel supported, learn new recipes, and be successful eating a low-carb diet.

Combination products—such as Truvia, Swerve, Super Sweet Blend, and so forth—abound, usually mixing stevia and erythritol together.

I want to alert patients with diabetes to watch out for hidden sugars! Low-fat and nonfat foods are usually higher in sugars than full-fat products, to make up for the loss of the fat flavor. Remember, fat does not raise your glucose and is very safe for you to eat; sugar is the key problem. Read ingredient labels on any product advertising it is low-fat or fat-free to see how many total carbs it has.

Spices and Condiments

All unsweetened spices are fine to eat. Some of them, such as garlic powder, onion powder, turmeric, cinnamon, and basil, are excellent to help flavor food and reduce glucose levels.

Condiments such as mustard and mayonnaise are fine. Salsa and guacamole can also be okay, although do not eat a pint of salsa. Some companies, such as Nature's Hollow, make barbecue sauce, ketchup, and even maple syrup with xylitol. Otherwise, those foods in any conventional form need to be avoided.

— CHAPTER EIGHT —

Diabetic Low-Carb Diet Options

The last chapter discussed the components of a low-carb diet. This chapter will cover how to put all the foods together into different dietary options. Different diets will work equally well for patients with diabetes to get their glucose under control extremely well. Whichever one a patient wishes to follow is fine with me. In this chapter, I will be discussing the intricacies of all these diets, and their pros and cons, including the Mediterranean diet (for those who are prediabetic), Ma-Pi2 diet (an unusual high-carb outlier diet for those who are diabetic), omnivore low-carb diet, vegetarian low-carb diet, vegan low-glycemic diet, low-carb and high-fat ketosis diet, and the paleo diet.

Type 2 Diabetes Prevention: Mediterranean Diet (for Prediabetes)

What makes up a Mediterranean diet? Most Americans just think it means using olive oil exclusively in their kitchen. That is only one small part of this diet. In general, a Mediterranean diet is a wonderful, healthy omnivore diet, consisting of fresh fruits and vegetables; whole grains; nuts, seeds, and legumes; olive oil; cheese and yogurt; seafood; eggs; lamb, beef, and chicken; and wine in moderation: simple, fresh, unprocessed, whole foods. If we can get the eighty-nine million Americans who are prediabetic to stop eating fast foods and processed foods, and get back to a healthy omnivore diet, we could save millions of people from becoming diabetic.

In fact, a four-year study of prediabetic patients showed that middle-aged and senior patients with a risk of cardiovascular disease who ate a Mediterranean diet reduced their occurrence of diabetes by 52 percent. That is a significant result! Two types of Mediterranean diet were used; neither had a caloric restriction, but one advised one liter of olive oil a week, while the other advised eating 30 grams of nuts a day instead. These were compared to a low-fat diet as the control group. Both of the Mediterranean diets were more effective at preventing diabetes onset than the low-fat diet.

The Diabetic High-Carbohydrate Outlier Diet

Although my focus with diabetic patients is on low carbohydrates, I do wish to make note of the Ma-Pi2 diet, also known as a macrobiotic

Table 8.1. Hematologic and Biochemical Variables in Diabetic Patients at Onset and Termination of 6-Month Ma-Pi2 Dietary Intervention

Variable	Onset		6 Months		*P* value
	Mean	Median	Mean	Median	
Hemoglobin (g/dL)	13.38	13.40	12.39	12.05	0.02329
Total proteins (g/L)	77.73	77.45	74.79	76.15	0.2979
Albumin (g/L)	41.26	41.00	41.57	41.00	0.6601
Creatinine (μmol/L)	62.69	64.00	63.06	59.00	0.8908
Total cholesterol (mmol/L)	5.37	5.46	4.49	4.55	0.002279
HDL cholesterol (mmol/L)	0.45	0.46	0.89	0.85	0.000480
LDL cholesterol (mmol/L)	3.52	3.90	2.72	2.81	0.002145
Triglycerides (mmol/L)	2.97	2.40	1.87	1.91	0.001092
Glycemia (mmol/L)	14.03	12.55	5.08	4.70	0.000214
HbA1 (%)	12.60	12.00	5.73	5.70	0.000481
C-peptide (ng/mL)	2.15	2.21	2.43	2.47	0.3052

high-carbohydrate diet. Yes, high carbohydrate! Two well-done studies have shown that the Ma-Pi2 diet can be amazingly helpful to diabetic patients. One study, for example, focused on poorly controlled diabetic patients (with A1Cs higher than 8.5 percent) from Cuba, China, Italy, and Ghana. The study lasted six months, during which 70 percent of patients' total daily caloric intake came from carbs (including brown rice, barley, millet, and many vegetables), 12 percent from protein, and 16 percent from fat. Patients also ate seaweeds and drank bancha tea. They also ate around 2,200 calories per day, so it was not a low-calorie diet.

The results were astounding (see tables 8.1–8.3). Eating this high-carb diet significantly lowered glucose and A1C values, and lowered lipids and cholesterol. Patients lost weight, but their lean mass was maintained; that is, patients lost fat, but did not lose protein or muscle mass. Their BMIs

Table 8.2. Lipoproteins and Cardiovascular Risk in Diabetic Patients at Onset and Termination of 6-Month Ma-Pi2 Dietary Intervention

Variable	Cut-off Values		Onset		6 Months	
			n	%	n	%
Total cholesterol (mg/dL)	Desirable	≤ 200	5	31.25	13	81.25
	Borderline	200–240	8	50.00	3	18.75
	High	≥ 240	3	18.75	0	0
LDL cholesterol (mg/dL)	Acceptable	≤ 130	7	43.75	14	87.50
	Borderline	130–160	4	25.00	1	6.25
	High	≥ 160	5	31.25	1	6.25
HDL cholesterol (mg/dL)	Desirable	> 62	0	0	5	31.25
	Acceptable	34–62	0	0	5	31.25
	Undesirable	≤ 34	16	100.00	6	37.50
Triglycerides (mg/dL)	Acceptable	≤ 200	5	31.25	15	93.75
	High	200–500	10	62.50	1	6.25
	Very high	≥ 500	1	6.25	0	0

Table 8.3. Physical Variables in Diabetic Patients at Onset and Termination of 6-Month Ma-Pi2 Dietary Intervention

Variable	**Onset**		**6 Months**		***P* value**
	Mean	Median	Mean	Median	
Weight (kg)	69.28	69.40	63.03	59.90	0.001470
Waist circumference (cm)	89.79	86.30	83.75	80.50	0.004101
Hip circumference (cm)	98.93	96.55	93.86	92.60	0.003478
Triceps skin fold (mm)	26.81	23.00	20.31	21.50	0.000317
Subscapular skin fold (mm)	32.88	30.00	24.94	25.50	0.000439
Biceps skin fold (mm)	16.19	14.50	14.63	14.00	0.1313
Suprailiac skin fold (mm)	31.88	28.00	22.94	22.00	0.001511
BMI (kg/m^2)	27.97	28.41	25.43	25.10	0.000255
Fat (%)	41.82	41.51	37.78	39.54	0.000723
Lean body mass (%)	58.18	58.49	62.22	60.46	0.000481

decreased. Moreover, all patients got off insulin (although some still needed to be on a sulfonylurea).

Yet, this diet still confounds me. While a low-carb diet is the key diet for T2DM, this high-carb Ma-Pi2 diet was very effective. Despite its effectiveness, the diet would be difficult for many to implement. It was a very clean diet, with no animal products, and the food was all prepared for the patients. On the negative side, all people in this diet had noticeably lower vitamin B_{12} levels after six months, so supplementation of vitamin B_{12} would be required. What's most confusing is that when one of my diabetic patients eats rice or another high-carb grain, their glucose numbers always elevate. While this diet seems like a mysterious outlier, I think that when I discuss the acid and alkaline effects on glucose later in the chapter, I may be able to point out some theoretical associations for the Ma-Pi2 diet's success.

The Different Low-Carb Diabetic Diets

Before we discuss the various low-carb diet options, a few things need to be mentioned. The different diets below have some similarities and one main difference. The similarities are that all the diets are low in carbs and should contain the same amount of vegetables. All oils recommendations are the same. All condiments and spices are fine among them (there is vegetarian mayonnaise, if desired). The beverages are the same among them. The main difference is the choice of protein. Some will allow all the protein choices discussed in chapter 7, and some will only allow some or a very few. All of the below diets are appropriate for T2DM or T1DM patients, and for pediatric or adult patients (although caution should be used for pediatric patients in one diet, as I'll discuss).

The Omnivore Low-Carb Diabetic Diet

The original omnivore low-carb diet was developed by Dr. Richard Bernstein, who paved the way for patients and physicians to realize that a low-carb diet is the best diet for diabetic patients. I have adapted it for my patients; I am not quite as strict as the eminent Dr. Bernstein, and I still see my patients doing very well.

An omnivore is someone who will eat any type of protein, from both animal and vegetable sources. The omnivore low-carb diabetic diet follows what I discussed in chapter 7 regarding what proteins a person can and cannot eat in their diet. What one can eat are all appropriate healthy animal proteins (meat, poultry, fish, dairy, eggs) and protein powders, nuts, nut butters and flours and coconut products, and soybeans. These are mixed with vegetables, and maybe, at lunch, if it can occur without glucose elevation, a few berries.

This is the main diet I've used with patients to get them in good control and to prevent the development of diabetic complications. It is also the way most Americans eat, so they are familiar with it and can more easily implement it into their lives. There are innumerable recipes in books and on the internet, so a lot of variety is possible to make the diet enjoyable. Eating out is easy, as this diet is quite adaptable to many types of restaurants.

Diet Examples for an Omnivore Low-Carb Diabetic Diet

BREAKFAST OPTIONS

- Organic three-egg omelet with onions and green peppers
- Can of sardines and pistachio nuts
- Eggs and turkey sausage with low-carb crackers or almond or cauliflower bread
- Nut granola with unsweetened macadamia nut milk
- Protein powder smoothie with kale, unsweetened almond milk, nut butter, and half avocado

LUNCH OPTIONS

- Salad greens with scoop of chicken, tuna, salmon, or egg salad
- Almond bread with salmon salad, and fresh veggies (celery, cauliflower, etc.)
- Salad with feta cheese and walnuts
- Oopsie bread (a roll made from eggs and cream cheese) sandwich with turkey, lettuce, tomato, and sprouts
- Lettuce wraps with mayo, mustard, tomato, cucumber, sprouts, onions, and turkey bacon, bacon, or roast beef slices

DINNER OPTIONS

- Stir-fry with chicken or ground turkey and vegetables
- Stir-fry with shrimp, curry sauce, vegetables, and shirataki noodles
- Broiled fish with cream sauce and grilled veggies
- Lamb chop with roasted Brussels sprouts and red bell peppers
- Side dishes like almond muffins, cauliflower rice, or cauliflower mashed potatoes, or avocado ice cream for dessert

Diet Examples for a Vegetarian Low-Carb Diet

BREAKFAST OPTIONS

- Two-egg omelet with cheese, onions, and mushrooms
- Smoothie with plain Greek yogurt and pea protein, and a handful of kale
- Belgian waffles made with coconut and almond flour, shredded coconut, acceptable sugar substitute, salt, eggs, coconut oil, and alternative milk (blueberries optional)

LUNCH OPTIONS

- Green bean and tofu salad, with olive oil, almonds, pepper, salt, and soy sauce
- Egg salad with Cheddar Bay Almond Flour Biscuits made with almond flour, shredded cheddar cheese, salt, baking soda, butter, eggs, garlic, Old Bay seasoning, and dried parsley
- Stir-fry with avocado oil, tofu, onion, red pepper, bok choy, kale, squash, green cabbage, broccoli, carrots, salt, pepper, onion, and garlic powder

DINNER OPTIONS

- Steamed veggies with coconut curried almonds (1 egg white, 2 cups of almonds, shredded coconut, sugar substitute, curry powder, kosher salt, white and cayenne pepper)
- Cauliflower risotto with roasted mushrooms (porcini mushrooms, salt, and pepper, olive oil; onion, garlic, cauliflower, low sodium vegetable broth, white wine vinegar, salt, and pepper)
- Creamy brodettato soup (2 cups water, 2 tbsp salted butter, 2 chicken bouillon cubes, minced garlic, 2 eggs, lemon juice, salt and pepper) with an almond muffin served on the side

This is a familiar, safe, effective diet for patients with diabetes. The vast majority of my patients choose this as their low-carb option. I make it clear that I do not want any patient eating animal protein three times a day, every day, but vegetarian options, nuts and seeds, soybean, protein powders, and even fish, need to be included regularly. Just because a patient can eat meat in their diet does not mean that it should be the only category of protein they choose.

Vegetarian Low-Carb Diabetic Diet

A vegetarian low-carb diabetic diet relies on eggs, dairy, nuts and seeds, soybeans, and protein powders for proteins. I do not believe it is innately any healthier than including some good omega-3 fish, such as wild salmon or sardines, or even some organic grass-fed and grass-finished meat, but vegetarians have chosen not to eat those foods, and I always respect a patient's food choice in that regard. It is a very effective diabetic diet, so that counts, too, although due to eating a lot of cheese, cholesterol levels may rise.

Ensure the eggs are omega-3 organic eggs, and regarding dairy, it would be good to buy organic cheeses and yogurts, as well as some goat milk and sheep milk products and not just cow milk products, as much as possible. Soy should also be organic, and nuts, seeds, and foods made from alternative "grains" should be eaten in variety.

This can be a healthy, egg and dairy heavy, ovo-lacto vegetarian low-carb diet, but it is more restrictive and may not fit with the diet of one's family, and limits one's options when eating out. It is necessary with this diet to ensure a variety of different proteins. Eating eggs and dairy three times a day, 365 days a year, is not healthy.

If a patient has a moral or spiritual or other reason they do not wish to eat other animal products, this diet is a tasty, safe, acceptable low-carb diet. All the menu suggestions are also acceptable, of course, for a patient eating a low-carb omnivore diet.

Vegan Low-Glycemic Diabetic Diet

The term *veganism*, referring to a diet that includes no animal products whatsoever, was created in the 1940s and first used in vegetarian discussions in

1947. No native cultures have been shown to eat a vegan diet, as by their very nature, vegan diets are entirely deficient in vitamin B_{12}. Prior to the invention of a vitamin B_{12} supplement, following a vegan diet would have wiped out any people who attempted to follow it.

A vegan diet relies exclusively on beans, peas, legumes, and nuts and seeds for protein. A diabetic application of veganism needs to remove almost all the beans, peas, and legumes (except for peanuts), leaving only nuts, seeds, and soybeans.

Although above I noted I do not recommend a low-glycemic diet in general, the term here is used very specifically to define a limited number of foods that fit into this diet plan. Many vegan diets can consist of many grains, but with this diet, the carbohydrate intake is due to vegetables, nuts, and soy, and those carbs have a negligible glucose effect.

What is the benefit of eating a vegan, nonanimal-product diet? Discussing the acid versus alkaline nature of food may be helpful in understanding this. Foods break down into either metabolic acids or metabolic alkaline substances and have either alkaline or acidic effects on our body. Our body serum pH is between 7.35 and 7.45, based on a basic chemistry scale where 7.0 is completely neutral, like water, below 7.0 is considered acidic, and above 7.0 is considered alkaline. Acidosis of our serum occurs when our pH is below 7.35. However, we are not talking about our serum, but rather what is happening inside our cells. In our cells, the pH can range from 6.0 to 7.4. Minor changes to an ideal cell pH can cause a significant health crisis.

There is science showing that a diet too high in foods that break down into acidic metabolites can affect cells and be problematic for patients with diabetes. Dr. Joe Pizzorno, one of the most respected naturopathic physicians and researchers in my profession, gave an excellent lecture on acid and alkaline facts at a medical conference I attended in 2014. I credit his lecture for some of the information below.

When foods break down into acidic metabolites, there is indeed a minor internal acid change in the cell. The standard Western diet is associated with a low-grade chronic metabolic intracellular acidosis. Eating a diet that causes the body to become too acidic sets it up for the development of many conditions, from osteoporosis to diabetes. Dr. Pizzorno reported that the two most acidic foods we eat are salt and sulfur amino acids—methionine and cysteine—from animal protein intake. Thus, acid foods are sodium chloride (salt) and beef, pork, lamb, poultry, bison, eggs, fish, dairy, as well as phosphoric acid–containing soft drinks. Soybeans and brazil nuts have a lesser acidic effect.

Our historical diet was exceedingly high in potassium and exceedingly low in sodium; in our modern diet, it's the exact opposite. The vast majority of our ancestral diets were more alkaline, while in a typical American diet, there is a significant acid production. High salt intake comes from bread and rolls, packaged deli meats, pizza, soups, fast-food sandwiches, frozen dinners, vegetable juices, canned vegetables, marinades and flavorings (e.g., soy sauce), spaghetti sauce, salty snacks, and poultry.

Refined sugar, refined grains, and coffee also have acidic associations.

Nonfood causes of cellular acidity include things that impair renal excretion of dietary acid load: NSAIDs (nonsteroidal anti-inflammatory drugs, such as ibuprofen, naproxen, and aspirin) and other medicines such as ACE-inhibitors and ARB medications, which are frequently given to T2DM patients and may be problematic. Other causes of acidosis include diseases like renal disease, diabetes, diarrhea, fever, androgen deficiency, and lupus; anaerobic exercise; and medications producing lactic acids (statins, for example); and phosphoric acid–containing soft drinks.

The kidneys lessen but cannot eradicate a diet-induced acidemia. As the years progress with the kidneys exposed to increased acidity, they can become damaged and lose their ability to function. There are buffers in our body to help balance the acid, but these can also be overwhelmed by a continually acidic diet. One buffer is calcium in our bones, and bone calcium can be lost in the urine attempting to buffer the acidity.

Cellular acidity is very problematic for diabetic patients. Acidity can cause the following:

- Reduced insulin sensitivity and increased onset of metabolic syndrome
- Increased glucocorticoid secretions
- Decreased IGF-1 concentrations
- Increased fasting blood glucose, A1C, and triglycerides
- Decreased glutathione synthesis (a major antioxidant in the body)

- Encouragement of tumor cell growth (and diabetic patients have an increased risk of cancer)
- Bone loss and increased renal stone formation
- Impaired mitochondrial function, which means less energy production
- Reduced immune system functioning, particularly of lymphocytes

Poor control of one's diabetes can also increase systemic acidity, which sets patients up for a number of these problems.

What type of diet makes our cells more alkaline? According to Dr. Pizzorno and the studies he cited, one can make a diet more alkaline by increasing the amount of fruits and vegetables, especially citrus fruits (although these are not low in carbohydrates). Fruits and vegetables create bicarbonates from potassium salts and magnesium citrate, the two most alkaline minerals we can eat. Eating a high-potassium diet, including lots of vegetables and avocados, is very helpful.

To be more alkaline, one should also eat a low-sulfur protein diet, which means eating mostly nuts for proteins and eating a low-salt diet. This is perhaps the connection to the Ma-Pi2 diet (and to the vegan low-glycemic diet). Could it be that removing all animal products and salt so reduces cellular acidity that the patient's insulin resistance is reduced significantly, allowing all the positive diabetic results seen in the studies? Perhaps so! At least, it makes sense.

Supplementing potassium citrate and magnesium citrate, or potassium magnesium citrate, can help restore a more alkaline internal system, especially if the diet is also more alkaline. Eating bacon for breakfast, chicken for lunch, and pork for supper will not allow those simple supplements to have much effect. However, adding in those supplements to anyone's daily intake will not cause harm and may indeed help. For diabetic patients eating a high-animal-protein diet, these supplements may help reduce cellular acidity.

How do we assess our bodies for acidosis? There is no perfect, gold-standard methodology, but the best way to measure is through a twenty-four-hour urine collection sent to a lab for analysis. First-morning urine or salivary measurement using a pH test strip, a fad among many people, is *not* a good measure of total acid load and is not predictive of what the twenty-four-hour urine collection will show.

One concern with interesting implications about low-carb diets is that when diabetic patients reduce their carbohydrates and eat too much animal protein, they may form—and may strive to form—ketone bodies. Many patients on a low-carb diet, particularly the low-carb, high-fat ketosis diet discussed later in this chapter, interpret the presence of ketones as meaning they either are losing weight and burning their own fat from cells or are using the fat they eat for their energy source.

Ketone bodies can apparently intensify acidosis in the body, which may then promote insulin resistance and potentially some of the other concerns listed above. However, we do not generally see people initiating ketosis on a low-carb diet having these complications. If someone does, it may be that their body is particularly susceptible to cellular acidosis. Supplementing with potassium and magnesium citrate may be helpful.

The vegan low-glycemic diet for diabetes is a very strict diet. One is not allowed to eat any animal products. It is permissible to eat nuts and seeds (although some nuts have sulfur in them, overall they have much less than any animal product), organic tofu, berries (in moderation), vegetables (sulfurous vegetables, such as the cruciferous ones—broccoli, cauliflower, kale, Brussels sprouts, radishes, and cabbage—are allowed, as again, they contain much less than animal products), and oils.

This diet produces very little glucose and puts little strain on the body to process glucose. It is quite common that when a newly diagnosed pediatric T1DM patient is put on this diet, they can stop using insulin and enter into a honeymoon period lasting months to years. In fact, this is absolutely the best diet with which to initiate and maintain a honeymoon period in a newly diagnosed pediatric T1DM patient.

One problem with this vegan low-glycemic diet is that some kids do not get enough protein, and thus their growth is impeded, so monitoring the growth of a child on this diet is vital. If a child shows no growth over three to six months, they are likely protein malnourished, and that child needs to have animal protein added in to their diet, because growth hormone (like all hormones) requires protein for production. Monitoring protein intake is

The Difference between Ketosis and Ketoacidosis

Ketone bodies are end products of fatty acid metabolism. Ketosis is the metabolic state where most of the body's energy supply comes from ketone bodies in the serum. It means the body is burning fat and not glucose or starch. Ketone bodies can be measured in the urine or via the glucose/ketone meters I mentioned earlier: Nova Max Plus and Precision Xtra, both of which measure both glucose and ketones. If your meter does not measure ketones, there are also urine ketone test strips, such as Ketostix, that you can buy at a typical drug store. People losing weight or eating a low-carb, high-fat diet will find ketones in their urine or blood. That is perfectly safe

Ketoacidosis is the metabolic state associated with high concentrations of ketone bodies, causing uncontrolled extreme ketosis; when this extreme ketosis combines with dehydration and high blood glucose levels (due to not enough insulin), it forms a deadly triad. Ketoacidosis is indicated by a decrease of the blood pH into a more acidic state, increased acetone in the urine and breath (making the patient's breath sweet). It is caused by the body not producing enough insulin and shifting to burning fat for energy. It is seen in T1DM patients due to insulin deficiency, hyperglycemia, and dehydration, and can occur during stressful situations such as illness and trauma. It can be life-threatening.

A person in ketosis is not a person in ketoacidosis; being in ketosis is a safe way to use body energy and keep one's glucose levels substantially lower. Being in ketoacidosis is a medical emergency, and any patient in this state would need to call their physician or head to the emergency room.

important for pediatric patients on this diet, and keeping a log (such as on https://supertracker.usda.gov) is helpful.

I have also seen children become iron anemic on this diet, and vitamin B_{12} and vitamin D_3 deficiencies are huge risks. Any child or adult on this diet

Diet Examples for a Vegan Low-Glycemic Diet

BREAKFAST OPTIONS

- Granola made from nut flours, nuts, coconut flakes, oil, and flax seeds, with unsweetened alternative milk
- Protein smoothie including vegan protein powder, veggies, coconut or flax oil, unsweetened alternative milk, and stevia
- Almond flour pancakes
- Chia seed and sunflower nut butter hot cereal

LUNCH OPTIONS

- Pecan bread with nut butter, fresh vegetables
- Vegetables with various nuts
- Salad with nuts
- Many soup options

DINNER OPTIONS

- Almond muffins with stir-fried vegetables
- Tofu and vegetable stir-fry
- Roasted vegetables with almond tortillas
- Avocado ice cream

will need appropriate nutritional supplementation of the vital nutrients that it lacks.

Adults with diabetes (both T1DM and T2DM) who go on this diet will have better glucose control and require significantly less insulin, and may be able to reduce their oral medications as well. Weight loss is also possible, which is great, no doubt, for the T2DM patient but may not be needed for the T1DM.

Dan and Sally Roman (https://healthesolutions.com) are experts at using the vegan low-glycemic diet, and they promote its use for any diabetic patient.

They are not physicians but rather are parents who were able to get two of their children healed from an apparently very early transition into diabetes by initiating a vegan low-glycemic diet. The Romans have written an incredible amount of information on how to incorporate this very kitchen-heavy diet, including excellent cookbooks I regularly suggest to my patients. Their programs make the transition easy with step-by-step instructions. I make their nut granola recipe all the time for breakfast. I strongly recommend that any patient, or anyone reading this book who is interested in eating this way, connect with the Romans for truly helpful advice and support on how to implement it.

The vegan low-glycemic diet can be considered a healthy diet. It contains a lot of vegetables, reducing glucose and insulin needs significantly. I have seen many T1DM children eat this way and they grew well, were active in sports, and were very happy.

However, a person on this diet would need to take a good multiple vitamin with minerals, a calcium supplement, omega-3 fish oils, and vitamin D_3. Someone on this diet may find it difficult to eat at restaurants or in other peoples' home. It does take a lot of work in the kitchen as well.

When a newly diagnosed T1DM child goes on the vegan low-glycemic diet and within days enters a honeymoon period, staying there for quite some time, even years, it is very exciting for both the child and the parents, and I've seen that occur many times. That type of insulin-free glucose control can really motivate and inspire the family to continue eating this way. Having seen this diet be successful in significantly reducing glucose levels and need for medications, I will continue to suggest this diet as an option for patients.

Modified Vegan Low-Glycemic Diet

After patients have been on the vegan low-glycemic diet for a short or long while (depending on the family), most wish to start adding in some animal protein. The strict vegan diet may be very difficult for all family members to follow, and may be tiresome to some, though it is not fair for the diabetic patient to eat this way and watch everyone else in the family eating differently. And, if the child is not growing, animal protein is medically necessary.

The first animal proteins most commonly added are wild salmon and organic omega-3 eggs. Some patients then, over time, also add in organic poultry or grass-fed and grass-finished meat, and then the diet basically becomes an omnivore low-carb diet.

It is very understandable that many families are not excited about starting the vegan diet; it is very restrictive. The modified diet can still achieve glucose and insulin-lowering benefits, is pure and healthy, and is easier to live by. I find many patients are happier doing a modified diet with some salmon or eggs thrown in a few times a week.

The concern for a T1DM patient entering a honeymoon period is whether or not loosening the diet's restrictions will end that honeymoon period. If a lot of animal products are reinitiated, it is very likely that, yes, the honeymoon period will end and insulin will need to be started again. However, a little salmon or a few eggs here and there, a few times a week, may keep the honeymoon period going. Each family will need to figure out their own right balance between enjoyment of the diet and good glucose control for the child with diabetes.

Low-Carb, High-Fat Ketosis Diet

The low-carb, high-fat ketosis diet (also referred to as the ketogenic diet) was originally devised around one hundred years ago to help control seizures in children with epilepsy. The diet is designed to have people burn fats for energy instead of carbohydrates. When there aren't carbohydrates in the diet to metabolize into glucose, the body will metabolize fats into fatty acids and ketone bodies, and the ketone bodies can pass into the cells and be used as energy. In the last few decades, eating a ketogenic diet has been discussed for its value in weight loss, glucose control, and reducing lipids. The low-carb ketogenic diet is now being used with cancer patients to remarkably lower glucose levels in order to prevent the cancer cells from feeding and growing.

Dietary oils are usually long-chained or medium-chained, though some are short-chained—the medium-chained oils turn into ketones easier. This occurs because they are more easily absorbed from the intestine and rapidly taken to the liver via the blood, not the lymphatic system, through which other oils travel.

In one good study about the long-term use of a ketogenic diet in obese patients, patients ate only 20–30 grams of carbs a day, with a protein requirement of 1 gram per kilogram of body weight; oils ingested were 80 percent polyunsaturated and 20 percent saturated. The results were that the patients experienced significant weight loss and lower BMI; decreased total cholesterol, LDL cholesterol, and triglycerides; and increased HDL cholesterol.

There was also a four-month study on using a ketogenic diet in T2DM patients. In this diet, allowable carbs totaled less than 20 grams per day. Patients ate unlimited meat, poultry, fish, shellfish, and eggs. They also ate 2 cups of salad a day; 1 cup of low-carb veggies; 4 ounces of hard cheese; and unlimited amounts of cream, avocado, olives, and lemon juice. This was also a positive study. The diabetic patients had significant weight loss, losing around 3 percent of their body fat. They also saw decreases in heart rate; their fasting glucose levels lowered 17 percent; and their uric acid and triglyceride levels decreased. Most patients lowered their A1C by around 1 percent and were able to reduce or discontinue medications.

As mentioned earlier in the chapter, ketone bodies can be easily measured via urine, using Ketostix strips, or via blood (Precision XR and Nova Max Ultra meters). With urine test strips, ketones are graded from beige/cream (no ketones), light pink (trace or small ketones), light purple (moderate ketones), and dark purple (large ketones). Using ketone meters can be costly, as the test strips are expensive; too expensive to be used for a daily ketone check, they are typically used for T1DM patients who feel they may be in actual ketoacidosis. So, checking urine is best to ensure you are still making ketones. The goal is to have a purple urine test strip.

The ketogenic diet has a macronutrient breakdown of 70 percent (or higher) fat, 20 percent protein, and 5–10 percent carbs. So, someone with an 1,800 calorie intake would eat 1,260 calories of fat, 360 calories of protein, and 180 calories of carbs. In general, eating 5 grams of carbs per 100 grams of food is a simple, easy-to-remember ratio.

The low-carb, high-fat ketogenic diet consists of:

- Meat, fish, seafood, poultry, eggs, pork, bacon, sausage, bison, game, fermented soy, protein powders
- Full-fat dairy: heavy cream, full-fat sour cream, hard cheeses, plain unsweetened whole milk yogurt
- Nuts, except for chestnuts and cashews

- Above-ground vegetables: no potatoes, sweet potatoes, yams, corn, or parsnips
- Natural fats: butter, oils, beef/chicken/duck/lamb/pork fat, mayonnaise, olives

These diets are very high in fat, dairy, meat, and eggs. Low-carb, high-fat recipes include making cheese "chips" from parmesan cheese and rolls made from eggs, cream cheese, salt, baking powder, and fiber. They are very satiating, using a lot of butter and cream, salad dressing, and other tasty fats to dress up the protein and vegetables. Probably the most famous ketogenic meal is "bulletproof coffee" made by adding 1–2 tablespoons of grass-fed butter and 1 tablespoon of organic unrefined coconut oil to coffee and mixing it in a blender for breakfast.

Obviously, this diet is meat and dairy heavy, but it does call for decent amounts of vegetables every day. The benefits of this diet include its ability to lower glucose levels; the satiating effect of its high fat and protein intake; and that it can lower one's weight, A1C, lipids, and cholesterol (although it will raise lipid and cholesterol in some patients, so these should be monitored). Problems with this diet include that it's very restrictive and very high in animal products, which can be prohibitive if a patient cannot afford to eat organic, grass-fed, and grass-finished animal products. The very high fat content may affect gallbladder function over time; is scientifically associated with causing intracellular acidosis; and may be pro-inflammatory if too high in omega-6 or saturated types and not balanced enough with omega-3 oils. I would definitely recommend potassium and magnesium citrate supplements, among other daily supplements, for anyone on a low-carb ketogenic diet. Finally, patients may become constipated on this diet. Unless a diabetic child has refractory seizures even on medication, I would not suggest this diet for them, due to its intensity. People can also become fatigued of this diet. The diet may become tiresome to people, with so many animal products and high-fat sauces.

Honestly, few of my patients choose to follow this diet. But for those who do, there is science supporting its value and I would support their dietary choice.

Typical Meals on a Ketogenic Diet

DAY ONE

Breakfast

- 2 eggs cooked in butter, with 2 ounces onions
- 3 slices cooked bacon
- Coffee with heavy cream

Lunch

- ¼ pound chicken breast deli slices
- 1 cup sliced summer squash sautéed in butter or oil
- 3 cups mixed greens with cheese shreds and full-fat dressing

Dinner

- 6 ounces ribeye steak
- 1 cup mushrooms and broccoli sautéed in butter
- Heavy cream sauce to cover steak and veggies

DAY TWO

Breakfast

- 4 ounces ground beef, mixed with spices, 1 ounce chopped onion, 1 ounce low-carb vegetables fried in butter or olive oil
- Unsweetened spiced tea with heavy cream

Lunch

- 4 ounces baked halibut with dill butter sauce
- 1 cup cauliflower sautéed in butter or olive oil
- 1 cup salad greens with blue cheese and full-fat dressing

Dinner

- 6 ounces pork chop baked in garlic cream
- 2 cups shredded cabbage sautéed in butter
- Salad greens with full-fat dressing
- Coffee with heavy cream

This diet is the complete opposite of the vegan low-glycemic or the Ma-Pi2 diet, and yet it can work equally well. There are many leading researchers advocating this diet for diabetes control.

Paleo Diet

I admit I am not an advocate of a Paleo diet in general, and I do not agree with the supposed science attempting to justify Paleo food choices. The Paleo diet removes grains, beans, peas and legumes, potatoes, starchy vegetables, refined sugar and junk food, processed foods, soy, dairy, and most alcohol. Paleo eaters can eat grass-fed meats, fish and seafood, fresh fruits and vegetables, eggs, nuts, seeds, and healthy oils. It is not a diabetic diet per se, as it is designed to be used by anyone.

Of course, removing all the sugar, junk, and highly processed foods is something I heartily believe in and is invaluable for any person, especially a diabetic patient. But, for people who are not diabetic patients, eating beans and legumes is amazingly healthy, and probably the healthiest protein choice there is. Also, I do not feel nondiabetic patients need to avoid all grains, such as brown rice, or starchy vegetables.

For patients with diabetes who do not have any negative reaction to dairy, removing it from the diet can be an unnecessary limitation. Also, the Paleo diet winds up very meat heavy, like the low-carb ketogenic diet, so I'd want to ensure all that meat is very high quality.

In reality, it seems a Paleo diet is similar to a low-carb ketogenic diet, though it also removes dairy and alcohol (low-carb alcohols can be used on a low-carb ketogenic diet). However, if a patient wishes to follow this diet, it is certainly an acceptable low-carb diet.

Choosing Your Diet

One of the most interesting things about medicine is that it is not always cut-and-dried. There are many low-carb diets (plus one high-carb diet) that have shown significant benefits for attaining glucose control, weight loss, reduction in medications, and lipid regulation, despite being very different from each other. It's easy for diabetic patients, and medical practitioners, to get confused about all this.

People have different bodies, minds, families, life schedules, and desires to spend time in the kitchen. All these factors have a huge impact on which diet a diabetic patient is drawn to and wishes to commit to. Everyone needs to find the diabetic diet they resonate with best and want to incorporate into their lives. Not every low-carb diet option will work for every person. It's important to choose one that is right both for you and for your family. I've seen patients on all of these diets, and they have all been successful. As a physician who specializes in diabetes, I am happy to work with any patient using any of these diets, and I am confident all of them will enable a diabetic to have significant success in reversing or controlling their diabetes.

Other Diet Ideas

In addition to the diets themselves, there are other ideas that can help inform what and how diabetic patients eat.

Testing Food Sensitivities

The main integrative lab test I do with patients is an IgG (immunoglobulin G) serum food-sensitivity test. However, I do not do it regularly with diabetic patients.

What do I mean by "food sensitivity"? Most patients are familiar with having their back scratched with needles at an allergist's office. MD allergists focus on the IgE immune system that sets up patients for immediate acute reactions, such as pollens making your eyes red and itchy and peanuts causing your lips to swell. That makes sense for environmental allergies, but most people with food reactions do not have an IgE reaction, but an IgG reaction, which is called a "delayed food reaction." The IgG sensitivity is associated with being an etiologic factor in many chronic diseases, such as psoriasis, asthma, migraines, GERD (and other gastrointestinal problems), chronic ear or sinus infections, and autoimmune diseases. Removing a delayed reaction food sensitivity can be curative in those conditions. We diagnose IgG sensitivities using a blood draw or finger stick.

When patients present with autoimmune diseases, there are several things for naturopathic or integrative practitioners to investigate: celiac disease, vitamin D_3 levels, IgG food sensitivity, gut bacterial imbalance, and environmental toxicity. Not all of these tests are performed with all autoimmune patients; a good physician can figure out which seem most logical to perform on any individual patient.

The classic method to discern food-sensitivity problems in medicine is the elimination/challenge protocol. That is, we eliminate foods, watch symptoms and signs clear up, and then add foods back in one at a time to discover which food(s) bring the symptoms and signs back into existence and are thus the reactive foods. A food-sensitivity test helps to narrow the range of foods to eliminate, which is very helpful, as there are many foods we all eat, and having a more precise starting point for elimination speeds up the process considerably. There are several good labs that perform high-quality food-sensitivity testing in the United States, including Alletess, US BioTek, and Immunolabs. I recommend patients avoid labs that do cytotoxic testing, such as Alcat or MRT Leap testing, as research has shown their methodology to be faulty.

Another good reason to do food-sensitivity testing is to analyze a patient's gut status: if it is healthy (has only a few reactions on a test of ninety-six foods), or if it has leaky gut (more than ten to fifteen foods are positive). Leaky gut, also known as intestinal permeability, means that the integrity of the lining of the patient's small intestine is not wholly healthy, thus foods are able to sneak through the tight junctions, tubes between small intestine cells, instead of actually being absorbed through them. Some people believe that any positive food test indicates leaky gut, but I am more confident of this diagnosis when more allergies are present. There are two additional tests a physician can run to more specifically diagnosis leaky gut, and I'll note them in chapter 9. An allergy panel with an indication that leaky gut exists means we need to heal up the gut, which for many patients only takes a couple of months. The intestinal lining is highly vascularized, meaning it has a lot of blood flowing to it, which enables it to heal quickly.

When I am working with a patient with positive food sensitivities, I recommend removing positive foods for one to two months in what is called the elimination stage, healing the gut at that time with certain supplements like probiotics, L-glutamine, and digestive enzymes. As a result of this process, we expect to see a clearing up of the presenting condition, or at least a huge improvement. Then the patient adds the foods back in one at a time during the challenge stage, to learn which specific food(s) may indeed be a real problem to the patient; that is, to see which food reintroduction brings a return of symptoms or signs. Patients can always add in the vast majority of positive foods once their gut has healed, without those foods causing a medical reaction. The patient is usually only truly sensitive to between one and three foods that will cause symptoms.

Still, I do not recommend food-sensitivity testing otherwise with T1DM or T2DM patients, if there is no other health problem, for two main reasons. First, their diabetic diet is already very restricted, and to keep removing more foods may make eating very difficult and cause depression or stress in the patient. Second, it does not cure their diabetes or even lower their glucose more to remove foods to which they are sensitive. You might think it would, but from my experience, I can clearly state it does not. Gluten, a common food allergen, is already removed on their grain-free, low-carb diet.

No Grazing

Now that I've discussed all the different dietary options, I want to talk about not eating. A person with diabetes should eat three meals a day and not snack. Each meal should be planned so that it provides enough energy and satiation to take the person to the next meal without a need to eat in between.

As a naturopathic physician, I was taught that health begins in the intestinal tract by what we eat, how we chew, how we digest, how we absorb, how we process and excrete, the quality of our microbiome, and how our digestive enzymes and organs work. Having all of those individual systems work well is exceedingly important not just to maintain and promote our gut health, but also to maintain our systemic health.

Resting the gut and not stagnating it by overeating or eating too often is very important. There are many mistaken ideas about eating and "grazing," that is, that it's best to eat every two or so hours. There is nothing more unhealthy than grazing, and I always strongly recommend that my patients eat three meals a day and do not graze and do not snack in between meals (of course children, growing adolescents, serious athletes, and young people in construction or other active careers usually need to snack, but most people do not).

For insulin-dependent diabetic patients, snacking and grazing add the danger of stacking insulin and increasing the risk of a hypoglycemic episode. "Stacking" insulin means that more and more insulin is added bit by bit, for a meal, for a snack, for another snack, for another meal, and so on. It seems obvious that so much insulin continually added in would increase the occurrence of low glucose episodes, and it does.

Another benefit to eating only three times a day is to promote intestinal movement. *Peristalsis* is the term used when discussing the movements made by the large intestine (the colon) to push food through to form and pass a bowel movement. The migrating motor complex (MMC) is the nerve complex that is active in the upper gut; it empties the stomach and energizes the small intestine. The MMC enhances movement of food out of the stomach and through the twenty feet of the small gut. The MMC starts working two hours after eating stops, so two hours after you are done eating breakfast, your stomach and gut move the food through your intestine to maximize digestion and absorption of nutrients. If you decide to snack between meals, you will temporarily shut down the MMC, and the movements of your gut will slow or stop.

Each of us should allow four to five hours to pass inbetween meals. If you eat good protein (animal or plant-based) and oils at a meal, your food can easily support your energy levels for those hours. There may be times when this type of plan needs to be altered, such as if you eat lunch and then after work go to the gym and need a little food for energy for working out. You and your physician can make those small adaptations for your specific diet. You can also drink between meals, of course, though ideally noncaloric beverages such as water, herbal or green tea, and stevia lemonade.

Not eating between meals and having a long fast from supper to breakfast is a wonderful way to enhance gut health, movement, nutrient absorption, and stool formation, to enable you to wake up in the morning ready to have a bowel movement and begin a new day of maximized digestion. It also helps lower calorie intake and glucose levels. It is a kind of "intermittent fasting," which I will be discussing below.

In summary, I ideally want most patients to eat three meals a day, fasting from supper to breakfast, with no midmorning, afternoon, or after-supper eating.

Intermittent Fasting (IF)

Intermittent fasting takes resting the gut to a higher level—it means significantly reducing frequency of eating, reducing daily calories, or even fasting from calories entirely. It is a type of diet that has been shown in studies to help promote weight loss, so it's something overweight or obese diabetic patients might consider.

Intermittent fasting means reducing calorie intake but maximizing nutrient intake, and is sometimes referred to by the acronym CRON—calorie reduction optimal nutrition. There are several ways of doing IF, and science supports its benefits. IF in animal studies showed animals who fasted were healthier and lived longer. In humans, IF can burn fat, reduce insulin resistance, initiate improvement in lipid and glucose profiles, and decrease inflammatory cytokines TNF-a and IL-6, the two main cytokines involved in causing and promoting insulin resistance.

Sixty hours of fasting—two and a half days—has been shown to decrease plasma glucose by 30 percent, decrease serum insulin by 50 percent, and significantly increase lipolysis (burning of fat). One other benefit is enhancement of the function of the migratory motor complex.

I do not recommend all patients immediately begin a low-carb diet *and* start intermittent fasting. That might be overwhelming for some people. First I start with eating correctly, and then, when that new diet is established, for T2DM patients who need to lose weight, I ideally initiate some sort of intermittent fasting protocol. If a patient can begin both at the same time, I will counsel them on how to do so.

Let's talk about the different ways of doing intermittent fasting.

Protocols for Intermittent Fasting

There are many options for how to apply intermittent fasting in one's life. Some I recommend more than others. However, whichever protocol best resonates with and be committed to by any individual patient works for me.

HARDER METHODS

These first three methods are a little harder for people to commit to, for understandable reasons.

The first method suggests people fast for sixteen hours a day, and then wake and eat three meals all within eight hours—breakfast; four hours later, lunch; four hours later, supper—and then fast again for sixteen hours. For most people that is a difficult protocol; one is very hungry after a sixteen-hour fast, and eating using this method can interfere with normal family meal planning and socialization.

Another difficult option recommends eating normally for five days a week but then two days a week fasting completely, eating no food at all. Again, most people do not wish to engage in this protocol, at least not over the long term.

A third problematic intermittent fasting option is fasting all day long and then eating a fairly massive supper—so a person is eating only once per day, and it is a very big meal—then fasting the rest of the twenty-four hours, except for being allowed to have some raw fruits or vegetables, or veggie juice, or a little protein. I really do not agree with this choice, and I strongly urge patients not to do this.

In general, I like protocols that are more moderate in nature. I suggest the type of protocol that can be absorbed into a lifestyle that does not terribly ruin the capacity for family meals and socializing and enjoying one's life and diet; also, I don't think people have to be hungry all the time to regain health and stay healthy.

GOOD STARTING PROTOCOL FOR INTERMITTENT FASTING

Here are more moderate but still effective methods of intermittent fasting. As noted earlier, the most common method I introduce to patients regarding IF is to eat breakfast, lunch, and supper, without any snacks inbetween, and then fast entirely from supper to breakfast for at least twelve hours. This process of having patients learn to eat meals that support energy throughout the day, and then have at least a twelve-hour fast daily—that is, for half of each twenty-four-hour day one does not eat—is a great way to introduce IF in a feasible manner for patients. It is not too extreme or inhibitive of socializing and family meals but is doable and sensible. In this way I feel glucose metabolism, fat burning, reduction in inflammation, reduction in insulin resistance, appetite control, and increased gut functioning can all occur in a fairly painless manner. If people can fast for even longer, up to fourteen hours, that is even better.

A person should wake up hungry. If they do not, then there may be some liver stagnancy occurring, where the food did not process well in the gut and liver and was not able to enter into the system for good metabolic use. Eating dinner and fasting for at least twelve hours usually enables the body to process the food effectively, lower the glucose and insulin resistance, and cause a person to wake up ready to eat a nourishing low-carb breakfast.

A second option is a variant of the eat-five-days-then-fast-two-days protocol; instead, the regimen is to eat normally for five days and then significantly reduce calories for two days a week, down to around 500 calories. Some protocols have patients eat normally one day and the next day reduce caloric intake to 500 calories per day, and continue that rotation day by day all week long, but I feel that is too extreme. Eating normally five days and then eating less for two days is certainly a more acceptable way for most people to try IF.

No matter which low-carb diet you and your physician choose, make sure that most of the day you are not eating it. Starting in this pragmatic manner is a good introduction to IF. If you wish to try a more extreme version of IF, that's fine! However, even staying with this simple protocol is an excellent way to rest your gut, lose weight, and maximize your health. Intermittent fasting is a valuable tool that I strongly encourage all patients to master to some degree.

Fasting Mimicking Diet (FMD)

This type of diet, developed and patented by Dr. Valter Longo at the University of Southern California, is one last option for diabetic patients. In his protocol, Dr. Longo found people reduced their weight and abdominal visceral fat, and lowered the inflammatory marker c-reactive protein. That's good; it is what we are looking for when working with diabetic patients.

Dr. Longo views his protocol as reaping the benefits of fasting without actually fasting. The protocol consists of eating normally for twenty-five days of the month, and then significantly reducing one's food intake for the remaining five days. For example, based on Dr. Longo's recommendations, if a patient typically eats 1,800 calories for the twenty-five days, her caloric intake would reduce to 825 calories for the first day of the FMD diet, and from days two to five it would reduce further to only 600 calories. This cycle is repeated three to four times.

Dr. Longo's diet recommendations consist of food from fat, carbs, and plant-based proteins. No animal protein is allowed (egg, fish, poultry, meat, or dairy). Allowable beverages are water, herbal tea, black tea, and unsweetened dairy-alternative milks (coconut, almond, etc.). The focus is on eating many veggies, some oil, and a little protein.

I agree with the basic form of Dr. Longo's protocol, but not with the dietary specifics. For my diabetic patients, I ask them to stay with their low-carb diet plan during the low-calorie days, if they choose to adopt this protocol.

Diet Summary

The recommended low-carb diets for patients with diabetes have quite a range—from vegan low-glycemic to omnivore low-carb to high-fat, low-carb ketogenic—and there are passionate advocates for all of these dietary protocols. All will lower your glucose and insulin needs, allow weight loss, lower your A1C, and get you in much better diabetic shape than the typical American diet you have been eating or the higher carb diet you were instructed to consume by a nutritionist in a conventional diabetic medical setting.

The application and success of any dietary protocol depend on many factors that you and your integrative medical practitioner should closely analyze and discuss. Your physician will need to present clearly all diet options, with excellent recipes and books for guidance, and give his or her opinion on what is best for you, seeking your agreement, and then you will need to be compliant with the diet you choose. I suggest establishing a team mentality between you and your physician. It will not be helpful to go to a physician and have her demand that you eat a very high-fat diet if that diet is not attractive to you.

Making sure you bring your diet diary and glucose graph to your visits is also important; only through those tools can a medical practitioner understand what you are eating with any accuracy, to determine how that diet is affecting your glucose levels.

You and your physician will need to understand what you like to eat and how that can be transformed into a positive diabetic diet. How do you live your life? Are you a stay-at-home mom, do you travel every week for work, or do you work twelve-hour days six days a week? All of these might have a huge impact on how you can or want to fashion your diet.

Do you like to cook? The amount of time one has to prepare food may be the ultimate key to which diet is best. How much time a person can, or wishes to, spend in the kitchen making their food is pertinent to consider in ensuring a diet plan is successful.

Can you pay for a personal chef to make your meals or order meals off the internet, delivered to your home? A diet is not just what you eat, but also the methods of preparing it, too.

Food variety is important. The human body thrives on variety. People can get sick of eating just eggs for breakfast or eating only almond flour "grains" or salad for lunch every day. Ensuring that the chosen diet has loads of recipes that a patient loves to eat, with a multitude of foods, is vital for long-term success—physically, mentally, and emotionally—and it's much healthier. The more variety in a diet, the healthier the intestinal bacteria.

With children, I am avid about monitoring the link between nutrient density and growth and development, especially when a child with T1DM is on a vegan low-glycemic diet. I've seen many kids thrive on that diet and develop fantastically well, but a few of my pediatric patients require more solid protein for their hormones to kick in properly, and growth hormone is the first one we can clearly identify as a problem when a child does not grow. With kids, monitoring their intake using the USDA's SuperTracker website is extremely useful; from it we can see how many macronutrients and micronutrients a restrictive diet is providing the child, and their growth can be noted during every office visit.

Cost can be a factor, too. Eating organic omega-3 eggs and organic grass-fed and grass-finished meat and poultry can be expensive. On the other hand, these diets save money by avoiding fast foods, processed foods, desserts, high-carb snack foods, and all the other junk foods people regularly spend their hard-earned money on. Moreover, your health is worth spending money on. Getting your diabetes under excellent control saves money both now and in the long term by avoiding complications. However, buying nuts and nut flours in bulk can save money, and other ingredients like organic soy are not expensive, so there are ways to make a low-carb diet work and keep one's budget balanced.

How food relates to socializing and enjoyment is something I've mentioned several times. A diet is designed to nourish you, return you to health, and maintain that health, but eating is also an enjoyable time to be with friends and family. What type of low-carb diet would your family like to share with you? If your family eats an omnivore diet and doesn't want to eat vegan all the time, then for you to adopt the vegan low-glycemic diet may cause unwanted stress in your family or among your friends. It's not that you should not stand out from family and friends if you are committed to changing your diet, but know that you will have to be extra sure, extra strong, and extra capable to ignore negative words and opinions or people not being cooperative (and serving pasta and cheesecake when you come by for dinner) in order for you to be successful.

For T2DM patients and adult T1DM patients, I find most prefer the omnivore low-carb diet, which means people have, for example, eggs and veggies for breakfast, a salad and some nuts for lunch, and wild salmon and stir-fried veggies at supper, with maybe a nut muffin. It is a diet they are familiar with, just minus grains and potatoes! It can easily be adapted to work, home, and travel circumstances. For newly diagnosed T1DM pediatric patients, I recommend the vegan low-glycemic or omnivore low-carb diet with more emphasis on plant-based proteins. However, I have patients on all of these diets and unless I see that they cannot comply well or the diet is not working for them with regard to weight loss or blood work changes, I am happy to keep them on their chosen diet. As different people have different tastes, cultures, lifestyles, kitchen skills, and metabolisms, I cannot say that everyone has to follow one particular diet.

A good medical practitioner knows all the options and works individually with patients to choose the right diet. Guidance from a knowledgeable physician is necessary for patients to ensure that they are getting enough nutrients, antioxidants, variety, quantity, and quality of all the different acceptable categories of low-carb foods.

The medical practitioner will then do comprehensive follow-ups with patients, proving the diet's effectiveness. Through this methodology, excellent diabetic nutritional care can occur.

— CHAPTER NINE —

Essentials Two through Six:

Exercise, Sleep, Stress Management, Healing the Gut and Microbiome, and Environmental Detoxification

Of The Eight Essentials of a comprehensive diabetic protocol, I've already discussed the foundational aspect of diet and the complex reality of medications. In this chapter I am going to discuss five more of the essentials. Regular exercise, sleeping well, engaging in stress management, having a healthy gut and microbiome, and environmental detoxification are aspects of healing that cannot be ignored for diabetic patients and need to be fully understood. Let's take them one by one.

Exercise

The benefits of exercise to a patient with diabetes are immeasurable. Exercise is also, for many patients, the most difficult practice to habituate. The Low Carb Diabetes Association's focus is on developing and enhancing cardiorespiratory fitness, not just showing up at the gym for thirty minutes to stroll on a treadmill. Our motto is *Be Fit. Be Strong.*

Glucose is mostly burned in muscles, which of course are used during both aerobic and resistance exercise. Moreover, the more muscles you develop, the more you burn glucose even when you sit and watch television, as muscle cells need to be fed even when you are at rest.

Regular exercise is preventive of diabetes. Established exercise regimens like the Diabetes Prevention Program, which is set up for people who are prediabetic to exercise and lose weight, reduce risk for the onset of diabetes. For those with diabetes, exercise has profound effects on numerous systems. Effective exercise can do the following:

- Decrease insulin resistance and lower insulin levels
- Decrease lipids and increase HDL cholesterol
- Aid in weight loss
- Help reverse fatty liver
- Decrease high blood pressure
- Increase cardiac muscle mass and efficiency
- Increase disposal of metabolic wastes
- Increase activity in mitochondria, the energy production units in our cells
- Increase fat burning
- Increase lean muscle mass
- Help lower one's appetite
- Improve sleep
- Improve circulation
- Increase metabolism
- Build bones and muscles
- Increase balance, agility, and flexibility
- Decrease anxiety, stress, and depression

Exercise also enhances blood flow, oxygenates tissues, and causes us to sweat. Sweating is a marvelous way to detoxify the body, as heavy metals and environmental pollutants can be excreted through sweat. Exercise can also slow down the aging process; people who exercise regularly can slow the degeneration of their chromosomes, helping to delay the changes commonly seen in people as they age. That is a great collection of benefits to anyone, let alone a person with diabetes!

Some important questions to consider before embarking on an exercise routine include:

Do you belong to a gym? Gym memberships can be very reasonable; some require no down payment and only cost $10–$20 a month for endless use of the gym.

Do you have any home exercise equipment? Many patients have treadmills, weights, elliptical machines, or stationary bikes—not to hang clothes on, but to use regularly! I find it extremely helpful to have a good Precor Elliptical in my study. At any time, I can hop on it for a thirty to forty minute session and then hop off, shower, dress, and get back to work. I encourage patients to get a piece of equipment they are drawn to. Of course, buying an outside bicycle is great, too!

What time of day is best for you to exercise? Don't forget the weekends—exercising on Saturday and Sunday means there are fewer days during the workweek you need to find time to exercise.

Can you exercise alone or do you require the company of a friend or a class? Answering this can help you figure out what type of exercise will be most successful for you. I am a solo exerciser, but many people love working out in classes or with a best friend. Getting that all organized in advance is helpful for patients.

When did you last buy new sneakers? Good sneakers are important to ensure no foot, knee, or hip pain develops with exercise. Sneakers should be new every ten to twelve months, depending on what type of exercise you use them for. If foot, knee, or hip pain develops even while wearing new sneakers, orthotic insoles can be helpful, particularly for middle-aged and older patients.

To achieve cardiorespiratory fitness (CRF), it is important to maximize three main aspects of health: cardiovascular fitness, strength, and the trio of agility, flexibility, and balance. There are simple tests medical practitioners can do in office that measure those three vital components of CRF in patients. Grip strength on a hydrolic hand dynamometer measures the strength of muscles in a body very accurately. In fact, a stronger grip is associated with a significantly reduced risk of developing diabetes. Step tests, such as stepping up and down a step and measuring pulse can easily be done in an office to measure fitness. Also, measuring how quickly a patient walks is a great sign of CRF. Agility, flexibility, and balance can be measured by standing on a single leg with one's eyes closed, sitting down and standing up without using one's arms, and a half sit-up test. Within five minutes, all these analyses can be done in a medical practitioner's office to get a baseline understanding of every patient's CRF. Joining the Low Carb Diabetes Association allows one to see videos and, for medical practitioners, to download helpful handouts on enhancing CRF in patients.

If you have not exercised for a long time and are an overweight or obese person with diabetes, you should consult with your physician to see if a cardiovascular workup might be indicated. That would mean going to a cardiologist and getting an EKG, a stress test, or other exams the cardiologist needs to analyze your cardiac function and to clear you as being able to exercise safely.

Also, if you're just starting out going to a gym and you plan on using free weights or weight machines, sign up for one or two (or more) sessions with a personal trainer. That way, you can learn the proper ergonomics of using the machines, and they can help you develop an exercise protocol to follow. This is very valuable to prevent injuries and maximize your workouts. Trainers are also excellent for support and motivation to achieve worthwhile goals.

If you want to continue using a trainer, that's wonderful, but costs can add up, which may or may not fit into your budget. At least learn the safe and effective ways to use the machines, and get the initial support to set and achieve your goals. It would be frustrating to decide to exercise and then, soon after beginning, injure yourself and have to stop to recover, or to not know what you should achieve by putting in your hard work.

How much should a person exercise? The answer depends on the patient's cardiorespiratory fitness and their individual needs. However, there are some general guidelines. For the purposes of weight loss, exercising one hour a day, five days a week is suggested. For weight maintenance, thirty minutes a day of good exercise (doing laundry does not count as exercise!), five days a week is recommended.

When should you exercise? One study showed that exercising first thing in the morning, before breakfast, burns more fat, especially if one's diet is high in fat and calories. However, not everyone has the energy to exercise without eating, so that may not work for many people. And, of course, I don't want people overeating, either!

On the other hand, another study showed that exercise after a meal for thirty minutes reduced the postprandial glucose response in both T1DM and T2DM patients.

The key is that it's important to find the time to exercise, whether that's before or after breakfast, after other meals, in the middle of the day, or after work; anytime is a good time if it works for you.

Before one does any exercise, it is good to do some stretching, which can prevent muscle tearing and strains. Stretching enhances one's flexibility and increases one's range of motion. It circulates blood to the muscles, enhances muscle coordination, and after working out can help with relaxation, posture, and a sense of well-being. A good stretching book I recommend is *Stretching* by Bob Anderson. It has simple yet helpful stretches to do before beginning many forms of exercise.

If you are stuck in a rut of not wanting to exercise (and so many people unfortunately are!), you should discuss this with your medical practitioner or even a counselor. Creating new habits can be hard to do; look at all the New Year's resolutions that are forgotten and abandoned days after the holiday. Common reasons patients give for not exercising include that they are too busy; work twelve-hour days; lack money to join a gym or buy exercise equipment; do not like exercise; do not like to sweat; and do not have anyone to exercise with. It is important to troubleshoot these problems with compassion and understanding, which are key relationship components an integrative physician should have with their patients.

Remember that in wintry weather you can walk in malls; there are DVDs and free YouTube videos to use to work out at home; exercise phone apps can be downloaded; and hotels usually have gyms for use when you travel.

One thing to also acknowledge is what is not considered exercise—putting a load of clothes in the washer or standing and watering some flowers in your garden, for example, although I do like patients doing anything aside from sitting and watching TV or being on their computer.

I often tell exercise-resistant patients that there are 148 hours in the week, and all they need to do is exercise for 5 hours (1 hour five days a week) or 2.5 hours (30 minutes five days a week) of them. That leaves them 143–145.5 hours a week, out of 148, to do whatever they wish! When patients see the reality of time needed for exercise, it can help put it in a better perspective.

So, let's hope you are now committing to get on the exercise bandwagon.

Aerobic Exercise: Cardiovascular Fitness

There are two main types of exercise: aerobic and resistance. Aerobic exercise, also known as "cardio," is the kind of exercise that requires the body to use oxygen for energy generation. Examples of this type of exercise include walking, hiking, jogging, swimming, cycling, and—in gyms—using the treadmill, elliptical, stair stepper, rowing machine, or skipping rope. Playing soccer, basketball, or racquetball counts. I am a hiker and consider hiking to be one of the most enjoyable forms of aerobic exercise, as I get away from crowds and into nature while also getting intense workouts. But, I can only hike one day a week, so I use my elliptical machine at home several days a week and add in resistance exercise twice a week.

Cardio increases one's heartbeat, and although it is not scientifically proven, there is a general rule for figuring out the maximum rate your heart should beat during exercise. You can find this rate by subtracting your age in

Table 9.1. Target and Average Maximum Heart Rate Goals, according to Age

Age	Target HR Zone 50%–85%	Average Maximum Heart Rate, 100%
20 years	100–170 beats per minute	200 beats per minute
30 years	95–162 beats per minute	190 beats per minute
35 years	93–157 beats per minute	185 beats per minute
40 years	90–153 beats per minute	180 beats per minute
45 years	88–149 beats per minute	175 beats per minute
50 years	85–145 beats per minute	170 beats per minute
55 years	83–140 beats per minute	165 beats per minute
60 years	80–136 beats per minute	160 beats per minute
65 years	78–132 beats per minute	155 beats per minute
70 years	75–128 beats per minute	150 beats per minute

Source: http://www.heart.org/HEARTORG/HealthyLiving/PhysicalActivity/FitnessBasics/Target-Heart-Rates_UCM_434341_Article.jsp#.WH6H32VMrow years from 220, then multiplying that result by 0.7. Multiplying by 0.7 results in a heart rate that is 70 percent of the maximum for your age, a frequently used safety standard. So, if you are fifty years old, your heart rate goal during exercise should be 119 beats per minute.

Many people feel this formula is inaccurate and also creates lower than necessary heartbeat goals. The American Heart Association has its own general guidelines based on age, shown in table 9.1.

I prefer using this AHA table to the 220 equation because it allows for higher heart rates, and I think that if safely done—slowly increased as the patient's fitness increases—this allows for more aerobic benefits to the whole body. According to these guidelines, the same fifty year old has a much wider range of acceptable pulse responses to exercise, up to 145 beats per minute at 85 percent, rather than the only 119 beats per minute allowed by the 220 equation.

There is also a third formula you can use. Dr. Phil Maffetone discusses on his website (www.philmaffetone.com) exercising in a way that promotes lower heart rates and workouts for the long-term safety of the body and heart. New studies show that pushing your heart rate too fast is dangerous, that going above the maximum heart rate, especially for extended periods of time, may increase risk of cardiovascular disease, just as not exercising at all does. So following guidelines like the AHA's makes really good sense for physicians and patients.

Dr. Maffetone discusses his formula, called the 180 Formula: Subtract your age from 180. Modify this number by selecting from the following categories the one that matches your fitness and health profile:

- If you have a major illness or are recovering from a major illness (heart disease or any operation or hospital stay) or are on any regular medications, subtract an additional 10.
- If you are injured, have regressed in training or competition, get more than two colds or bouts of flu per year, have allergies or asthma, or if you have been inconsistent or are just getting back into training, subtract an additional 5.
- If you have been training consistently at least four times a week for up to two years without any of the problems just mentioned, keep the number the same.

- If you have been training for more than two years without any of the problems listed above, and have made progress in competition without injury, add 5.

Some seniors over age sixty-five who are in shape may add up to 10 beats to their score. This formula does not apply to athletes under sixteen years old.

Which formula should you use? Things seem to be getting complicated now! Your physician (and perhaps cardiologist) can help you analyze your exercise history, current health presentation, and other factors to help you set up your heart rate goal when exercising. Also, be aware that taking certain hypertensive medications, which is common among T2DM patients, lowers your maximum heart rate range, so you may not be able to reach a higher target pulse. You and your physician can decide on your maximum heart rate range to ensure you feel successful with your exercise intensity and resultant heart rate.

Of course, when a person is in good athletic shape, she can attain higher pulse rates when exercising without getting completely out of breath, and her resting heart rate is lower than a typical rate. Achieving those goals may not be what you need to do, but getting at least some exercise is.

Regular and High-Intensity Interval Training

There are two main types of aerobic exercise: regular and high-intensity interval training. Regular aerobic exercise means walking, jogging, cycling, or hiking at a good solid pace consistently for the time allotted to exercise. It is the best way for those who have not exercised throughout their lives to get started. It requires oxygen and is fueled by stored fat. Moreover, steady-state aerobic exercise is the foundation for most activities in life. Aerobic exercise that is easy on the joints includes swimming and elliptical machines, both good places for older patients to start.

High-intensity interval training (HIIT) is currently very popular. It is an exercise strategy consisting of alternating segments of short, intense exercise periods with less-intense recovery periods. In the intense period a person exercises at 80–100 percent of their maximum heart rate, and in the recovery time, they continue to exercise at 50–70 percent of their maximum. Many professional athletes regularly engage in this type of aerobic exercise because in shorter exercise times a person can have a significantly beneficial cardiac and fat loss result. One can build more mitochondria for better energy production. A person could do all HIIT workouts, but even one HIIT session along with four aerobic exercise sessions per week is helpful.

There is no one set cycle of intensity and recovery established for all people. You need to work with your medical practitioner or trainer to figure out a HIIT scenario that is safe and effective and not too initially overwhelming for you.

A typical session of HIIT starts with a warm-up before the actual exercise. Here are a few typical examples:

Beginning ratio. Jog at a normal pace for four minutes, then run as fast as you can for thirty seconds; repeat four to six times.

Middle ratio. Cycle at a normal pace for two minutes, then cycle as fast as you can for thirty to sixty seconds; repeat four to six times.

Advanced ratio. Thirty to forty seconds of hard sprinting with only fifteen to twenty seconds of recovery; repeat for five minutes total.

However, studies have also been performed on ratios of sixty seconds high intensity with seventy-five seconds recovery; twenty seconds high intensity with ten seconds recovery; sixty seconds high intensity with sixty seconds recovery; and two minutes normal intensity with twenty seconds high intensity, with entire exercise sessions lasting from four to twenty-four minutes. It seems that any split between normal and intensive exercise that works for you is acceptable.

So, which exercise is best—regular aerobic or HIIT? One study examined young college students doing aerobics, HIIT, and Tabata, another HIIT-like form of exercise. In the study, students did either twenty minutes of straight aerobic biking at 90 percent of their ventilator threshold; HIIT biking for twenty minutes and thirty seconds at 100 percent, then sixty seconds at recovery rate; or Tabata biking for four minutes and twenty seconds at 170 percent maximal oxygen consumption, followed by ten seconds recovery. They all did a warm-up and warm down.

All three exercise methods were equally effective in increasing students' fitness. The basic aerobic exercise was liked the most; Tabata was liked the least. Tabata was so intense students could not function well afterward. They could not go to class, needing a longer recovery time. These were young college students, so middle-aged and senior out-of-shape diabetic patients probably would not fare well, either!

For older patients, this obviously means that starting with regular aerobic exercise is valuable, effective, easier, and more enjoyable. It is what people are more familiar with and is not scary. It is easier to do with friends, too. It's definitely how patients should start out. I do not expect any patient just beginning exercise to leap into the intensity of HIIT. Once a diabetic patient is doing well with basic aerobic exercise, and is becoming more cardiorespiratory fit, then I might suggest beginning a gentle HIIT exercise session once a week, if that patient is willing to try it. Taking that first step can also be the first step to regaining and maintaining your health!

Managing Aerobic Exercise with Your Medications

There are no specific regulations on adjusting medications when patients with diabetes begin exercising. People with diabetes should measure their glucose before, during, and after exercise. Glucose changes due to exercise are based on:

- Length of exercise
- Intensity of exercise
- What one ate before, during, and after exercise
- How long ago one ate before exercise
- Type of medication(s)

In patients without insulin dependent diabetes, exercise decreases insulin levels and stimulates increased glucose secretion from the liver and free fatty secretion from fat cells. In patients with insulin dependent diabetes, if they come to exercise with *high* insulin levels, it will increase their muscle glucose uptake and prevent free fatty acid or hepatic glucose release, which may cause hypoglycemia. In patients with insulin dependent diabetes who come to exercise with *low* insulin levels, they can have an increase in glucose production and free fatty acid release and wind up with hyperglycemia. These results can occur in endless ways, so if you are beginning exercise or increasing the length or intensity of your exercise regimen, keep in close contact with your integrative medical practitioner. Different people have different nuances to their diabetes, their metabolisms, their exercise regimens, and their medications, so each patient has to be worked with individually.

It is easier to exercise if one is on oral medications and non-insulin injectables, though closer care is needed for patients on sulfonylureas, GLP-1 injections, and SGLT-2 inhibitors. A good physician, keeping close contact with her exercising diabetic patient, should not have problems dealing with those medicines and reducing them when glucose numbers require it. The problem is watching for hypoglycemia with those medications and ensuring patients check glucose numbers regularly and have glucose tabs and gels with them to immediately address any lows. However, diabetic patients should not constantly have lows while exercising! If that happens once or twice, your physician should give you effective treatment advice to help ensure it doesn't happen continually.

The following section deals with patients on insulin who are exercising, which is more difficult to organize and arrange, but is certainly achievable.

Aerobic Exercise Safety Guidelines

There are glucose ranges that will maximize energy during exercise—a person should be in the 70–170 mg/dL range ideally when beginning to exercise. Below 70 mg/dL means you have too much insulin in your system and not enough glucose for your cells, and you will have poor performance, you will sap your energy, and likely you will struggle to exercise. Beginning above 170 mg/dL there is enough glucose in the blood, but there may not be enough insulin to foster entrance, and you may struggle as well. Above 200 mg/dL, you will not be at your best, but you can start exercising, but over 250 mg/dL, it is generally not a good idea to exercise until glucose numbers come down. So, starting between 70 and 170 mg/dL is what I recommend, and even better is between 90 and 140 mg/dL.

Table 9.2 helps clarify how glucose numbers can affect athletic performance.

If you are below your glucose initiation goal at the beginning of the exercise, take a glucose tab, or tabs, to raise it to the target number. You may need to wait up to forty minutes, which is the maximum length of time it can take a glucose tab to work. Repeat the process if you are still not at your goal

Table 9.2. Effects of Blood Sugar on Insulin and Glucose Action and on Athletic Performance

Blood Sugar	Insulin and Glucose Action	Effect on Athletic Performance
< 70 mg/dL	Usually a result of too much insulin injected; hypoglycemia and not enough glucose to enter cells	Frustrating, fatigued, poor capacity to exercise
70–170 mg/dL	Insulin levels seem good; glucose can easily enter cells	Maximum athletic capacity
> 170 mg/dL	Insulin level may be low or adequate; glucose entering cells depends on insulin status	Athletic capacity may be good or subpar
> 250 mg/dL	Insulin is too low; glucose cannot enter cells and will increase due to adrenal hormone output	Fatigued, frustrated and poor capacity to exercise Do correction dose of insulin Do not exercise until glucose is lower and can enter cells

number. If that still doesn't work, you may have too much insulin in your system to exercise safely right then and there.

If you are an insulin dependent patient, always be around others when doing a long, intense bout of exercise, and alert the other person or persons that you are diabetic in case some crisis occurs. Also, wearing your medical ID and carrying glucose tabs or gels to treat lows is very important, as is ensuring you have enough water to drink so you do not become dehydrated. Carry a glucagon shot, especially if you are hiking or camping far away from immediate emergency care. Check your feet before and after exercise to ensure they handled the workout without any injury or lesions. Ensure your shoes fit well. Avoid exercising in extreme heat, humidity, or cold. In heat above 84° F and cold below 34° F it's best to ensure your insulin is in an insulin carrier to keep it viable.

You may need to take a glucose tab every fifteen to sixty minutes when first getting started, so keep checking your glucose regularly. You will need to check your glucose right after exercise and at least every hour for a few hours to make corrections.

Frequently checking your glucose levels during long, intense exercise and for hours afterward is required in order to understand how your body adapts and uses glucose and how insulin may need to be adjusted. For a light workout of less than thirty minutes, you may or may not need to have a small snack of several glucose tabs. For more intense and prolonged exercise, you may need up to 15 grams of carbohydrates every thirty to sixty minutes. Keeping good records of your exercise and your glucose before, during, and after will help you and your physician learn how much snacking you may need if you need it at all. Most non-insulin dependent T2DM patients do not need to snack at all during exercise; many T1DM patients (and possibly T2DM) on insulin may need to.

If you have gastroparesis, you may need to use glucose gels instead of tablets, as they can work better at increasing your glucose quicker, being better absorbed through your mouth lining.

If you inject insulin, do not inject it in the limb that will be involved in the exercise—for example, do not inject into the thigh before running a half marathon. Use of the muscle will cause the insulin to enter your system more rapidly, which will put you at risk of going too low at first and then too high as the insulin is used up quicker. Be alert to signs and symptoms of hypoglycemia and act upon them right away.

Table 9.3 shows how many grams of carbohydrates are typically burned in an hour of activity by a typical person based on the length of exercise, the type or intensity, and the patient's weight.

Your system may or may not mesh exactly with these numbers; a couple of exercise sessions will allow you and your physician to figure that out.

In terms of adjusting carbohydrates, if you are a T1DM patient and doing a moderate activity for less than thirty minutes, you may need a small carbohydrate snack, even just one glucose tab. If you are a T2DM patient, you probably will not need extra glucose, but it depends on what medications you are on. For prolonged or intense exercise, any diabetic patient may need up to 15 grams of carbs every thirty to sixty minutes. You also may need carbohydrate supplementation after exercise for a while, too.

For my athletic, insulin dependent diabetic patients who, for example, hike twelve miles or run a half marathon, the basal dose *before* exercise may need to be lowered, and the meal bolus dosing *before*, *during*, and *after* the exercise

Table 9.3. Grams of Carboyhdrates Burned per Hour of Exercise, by Patient's Weight

Activity	Grams of Carbs Burned an Hour— 100 pounds	Grams of Carbs Burned an Hour— 150 pounds	Grams of Carbs Burned an Hour— 200 pounds
Bicycling 10 mph	35	48	61
Downhill skiing	52	72	92
Moderately vigorous basketball	35	48	61
Raking leaves	19	28	38
Swimming slow crawl	41	56	71
Vigorous dancing	28	43	57
Walking 3 mph	30	45	59

Source: http://www.diabetesnet.com/node/237

for some hours may also need to be reduced; the basal dose after exercise may need to be reduced as well. Those are many variables to consider. It is easier for a patient on a pump to make basal adjustments, as he can reduce or turn off basal insulin, as well as increase or turn it on; the pump can be used to specify insulin needs step by step. When a patient is injecting basal insulin once or twice a day, he cannot change what was already injected.

Adjusting insulin for exercise is difficult at first, but it can be figured out with calm, rational analysis of how things went for the patient during a few workouts. Insulin adjustment depends on insulin dosage, which type of insulin is being used, which types of other medications are used, the timing of exercise regarding peak insulin action, and intensity and duration of exercise. It is vital for the exercising diabetic on insulin or even aggressive oral medications to be precise, recording their glucose numbers accurately for analysis and medication adjustment.

If glucose continually rises after exercise, you probably need to inject a little insulin before exercise begins. Exercise stimulates the release of cortisol, which makes the liver secrete glucose. Muscle does absorb glucose, but if the insulin is a little low in your system, the secreted glucose cannot enter cells as efficiently and may cause a rise in glucose after you exercise. Sometimes this will stay up, and sometimes over an hour or two it will come down on its own. This is why excellent charting of food, insulin, and exercise is so vital.

For moderate exercise in insulin dependent patients, insulin may need to be reduced by 20–30 percent. For intense and prolonged exercise, both basal and bolus insulin may need to be reduced by 50–80 percent beforehand, and insulin may continue to need to be reduced for up to one to two days after a long, intense exercise, such as running a marathon. This is the same for all patients, whether injecting insulin or using pumps.

Bolus dosing for moderate or strenuous exercise that lasts less than ninety minutes, or that begins within ninety minutes after having eaten a meal, should be reduced, and it may need to be reduced for a meal or two after the exercise is over, as well. For strenuous exercise lasting longer than sixty minutes or moderate exercise lasting longer than ninety minutes, in general, it would make sense to skip the bolus dose and even reduce the basal dose prior to exercise, and likely reduce or skip both afterward, as well. Again, it is better to wind up with glucose that's a little high while learning how to achieve precision glucose control than to suffer a scary low. It usually takes me around three patient workouts, all similar in duration, type, and so on, to figure out how to get the insulin dosed with precision.

Aerobic exercise insulin guidelines, summarized:

- A patient may need to lower their basal dosing the day before strenuous or prolonged exercise. I usually start with cutting pre-exercise basal in half for long athletic events.
- A patient usually needs to lower premeal bolus if exercising at length or intensely within ninety minutes after the meal. I usually cut bolus insulin in half before a long athletic event.
- A patient may need to lower postexercise basal and bolus insulin.
- A patient will need to check glucose frequently and record levels.
- A patient will need to be aware of the possibility of hypoglycemia and correct immediately upon occurrence.

I once had a T1DM patient who hiked sixteen miles up into the mountains. In order to do this, she needed to cut her previous basal dose in half

Case Study: Beth's Half Marathon

Beth is a T1DM patient who wanted to start running marathons. I live near Phoenix, which hosts a very popular PF Chang Half Marathon (13.1 miles) each year. Beth woke on the day of the marathon with a glucose level of 60 mg/dL. Per my directions, she ate breakfast and injected half her normal bolus dose. She was on a pump, so I instructed her to lower her basal to 0.35 units per hour (half her typical basal dose). She then ate some trail mix and crackers before the race (not my recommendation!) and did not inject, so at starting time her glucose had shot up to 250 mg/dL. That was not good, but she decided to begin anyway. She did not feel very good jogging at first, which was to be expected, but she kept hydrated, and her numbers slowly came down. She did not experience any hypoglycemia throughout the race, and checked her glucose every couple of miles. Her glucose stayed between 80 and 90 mg/dL and she took three or four glucose tabs throughout the race. She ended the race at 126 mg/dL and felt great after the first couple of miles when her glucose lowered.

Beth ate a normal lunch and injected less bolus for the meal than was indicated. However, we erred at increasing her basal dose to normal levels after the race, and then she injected her normal supper bolus dose. She wound up having lows in the evening and throughout the night, into the next day. We adjusted her dosing so that she kept her basal at half dosing the rest of the day after she did long runs like that, and she used only half a supper bolus dose as well. With this protocol, Beth had no more hypoglycemic events after running other races. As with a patient who likes to hike, insulin needs to be reduced for quite a long time after intense exercise is over.

Having a diabetic patient carefully record their glucose during exercise gives a medical practitioner the information they need to help, in the shortest amount of time, get the insulin dosing appropriately matched to the patient and her glucose needs.

the night before, start the hike with her glucose around 200 mg/dL, turn off her basal during the hike, keep it at half dosing after the hike until the next morning, skip her bolus dose at the first meal after the hike, and use only half the bolus dose indicated for her food later that evening. It took us three hikes to figure all that out to prevent hypoglycemia after the hikes. You can see that serious hiking had a profound effect on lowering her insulin needs. Most patients need to have a significant decrease in insulin dosing when doing extended exercise.

Don't worry or feel discouraged by this complexity. I've worked with many patients, and it works out well for all of them. It is amazingly helpful when patients are on a low-carb diet, since matching food, insulin, and exercise are much easier than otherwise.

Moreover, it is also very helpful if patients exercise at the same time daily and if their eating, sleeping, and other habits are similarly routine. Regular routines make managing medications a lot easier. If you are just hopping on a treadmill for thirty minutes, four days a week, and are in the middle of your heart rate range, it is unlikely any serious low will occur, which makes managing your medication much easier than for those who exercise longer and more intensely. Yet, even those lighter exercise sessions are a definite benefit to glucose control.

If you wish to use a Fitbit or other such technological aid while exercising, that is a fine idea to help learn how far you walked or how high you raised your pulse rate. Using a CGMS and getting immediate glucose readings is a huge boon to diabetics who are active.

Resistance Training/Strength Training/ Weight Training: Strength

The other main type of exercise is resistance exercise, which is of equal importance to if not more important than aerobic exercise for patients with diabetes. It is also called strength training or weight training. Resistance exercise uses weights or calisthenics to push a muscle group to its level of fatigue. Muscles contract against an external resistance, which increases their strength, tone, mass, and endurance. The benefits of resistance exercise include that it:

- Burns nineteen times more glucose than aerobic exercise! If a diabetic patient could only exercise for twenty minutes a day, choosing resistance over aerobic might make sense. Intensely using up glucose and building muscle strength is incredibly advantageous for glucose control.
- Prevents muscle loss with weight loss. This is very important because—especially as they age—when people begin losing weight, muscle mass loss can be significant, and the goal is to preserve muscles and only lose water and fat. Resistance exercise can prevent loss of muscle mass and ensure weight loss is only fat loss.
- Builds bone.
- Increases your metabolic rate.
- Creates more insulin receptors on muscles, making them more insulin sensitive.
- Helps to burn free fatty acids.
- Lowers glucose both immediately and long term.
- Sculpts your body to give it tone and definition.
- Enhances your sports performance.

As with aerobic exercise, your physician should clear you for resistance exercise. It's important to ensure a diabetic patient has a healthy heart, does not get dizzy, and has stable blood pressure (that does not get high or low), especially when working out, and doesn't have a joint, tendon, ligament, or muscle injury that would be aggravated by weight training.

Resistance exercise can include the use of free weights or weight machines. A strength-training program of muscle development ideally should consist of (at least) two nonconsecutive days a week. The focus is on major muscle groups, with eight to ten exercises devoted to each. Common resistance exercises include bench presses, using barbells, push-ups, pull-ups, body weight lunges, and leg extensions.

There are many variations of resistance training involving the number of repetitions (reps), the number of sets, the tempo, and the weight used. In general, based on the weight used, a patient does between one and three sets of between eight and twelve repetitions, resting two to three minutes between each set. Typically, you should choose a weight that causes fatigue in your muscle in eight to twelve lifting repetitions and continue to repeat the exercise two to three times. When you are used to that weight, and can do the exercise without muscle fatigue, increase the weight or the repetitions, or rest less between each set. Doing this type of exercise for eight to ten separate muscle groups—say upper body muscles Monday and Wednesday and lower body muscles Tuesday and Thursday—is a typical method for resistance exercise.

As noted in the introduction to this chapter, I recommend that a patient work with a trainer at a gym to learn the machines or free weights the patient will use, have the trainer establish a protocol to follow, and show the patient the correct ergonomic way to position themselves to prevent injuries, give support and motivation, and set up goals to track progress. There should be an upper body workout and a lower body workout, and these should be done on different days to allow recovery and growth of muscles.

There is also high-intensity interval strength training (HIIST) to consider. This type of training focuses on slow, controlled movements, keeping muscles under constant tension for many seconds, through the whole range of motion, without locking your joints. Moreover, HIIST strives to achieve momentary muscle fatigue in the target muscle so that the muscle trembles and burns during the last repetition. The key with HIIST strength training is having your muscles be in full contraction for longer periods of time while also monitoring the weight and number of repetitions.

Here is an easy, step-by-step guideline to HIIST training:

1. Do warm-up exercises, including cardio and stretching.
2. Use a weight that allows you to reach momentary muscle fatigue within eight repetitions of the exercise, and take six to eight seconds to move the limb through the exercise.
3. When you are able to do this more easily, in future workouts you can increase the number of repetitions, reaching a maximum of fifteen.
4. Once you can do fifteen repetitions at that weight, increase the weight by 5–10 percent and start over again.
5. Only change one factor—weight, repetitions, or total time under tension—at any individual workout.

6. Allow ninety seconds to rest between repetitions at the beginning, but you may need less rest in the future.
7. Allow at least forty-eight hours between sessions to allow the muscle to recover fully.
8. Cool down after the workout for five to ten minutes, including some aerobic exercise.

Any competent trainer at a gym can walk you through this type of protocol, starting you off slowly, steadily, and safely. I highly encourage getting professional help at the beginning to ensure you understand how to apply HIIST strength training to avoid injury and to get the maximum benefit.

As with aerobic exercise, resistance exercise can easily cause hypoglycemia due to the intense amount of glucose the targeted muscles are absorbing. Monitoring one's glucose before, during, and after is vitally important, as well as recording when insulin or other diabetic medications were taken, and how long and intense your strength training routine was. Basal and bolus insulin may need to be reduced before, during, or after your weight training, especially if you are spending considerable time and intensity (over thirty minutes) in resistance training. Tell your physician if you are planning on starting this type of exercise and ensure extensive glucose graph records are sent to him or her for follow-up analysis of glucose regulation.

Do research studies on exercise actually show improvement in diabetes? Absolutely! Studies have shown that aerobic exercise reduces the risk of T2DM onset, and with more exercise, more reduction in risk. Studies have shown that endurance and resistance exercise lowers the A1C in T2DM patients, and that even moderate intensity walking can reduce glucose after meals. Exercise has been shown to improve glycemic control in T2DM patients using insulin. Doing low-impact endurance and resistance exercise for five months caused a significant decrease in fasting glucose and A1C values. Other studies showed that an eight-week circuit-training program increased muscle strength and decreased body fat, waist and hip circumference, caliper measurements, A1C level, and fasting glucose. Exercise can even help prevent diabetic complications—one study showed that walking briskly four times a week significantly reduced the onset of neuropathy in diabetic patients (versus diabetic patients who were sedentary). Yoga has

Soft Exercise: Agility, Flexibility, and Balance

Aside from aerobic and resistance exercise, there are also slow movement exercises that have enormous benefits for the body and the mind, sometimes referred to as "soft exercise." Yoga, Tai Chi, and Ki Chung, for example, are three common types of exercise that increase blood flow, focus, and strength, and that equally relax and calm a person. They can be specifically beneficial for diabetic patients.

Taking a yoga class or doing Tai Chi outdoors in an early morning class each week is an excellent way to balance the more intense movements of aerobic and resistant exercise. Most gyms and community centers have classes in these, and other, slower, ancient and valuable exercises.

Pilates is another popular type of soft exercise that can help improve flexibility and develop a strong "core," meaning central strength in the abdomen. It can help improve balance and coordination, which for seniors may lead to a reduction in falls. This is another type of exercise that can be added to a weekly schedule of movement.

been shown to reduce oxidative stress, reduce BMI, and improve glycemic control in T2DM patients. Tai Chi has also been shown to reduce A1C levels.

Summary of Exercise Safety Guidelines

With any type of exercise—aerobic, resistance, or soft—there are some safety guidelines all diabetic patients should follow. It's a long list but they are all equally important:

- Exercise regularly—aerobic, resistance, and soft—to gain and maintain excellent cardiorespiratory fitness.
- Exercise at the same time each day, and eat at the same times, too.
- Set up and manage an exercise program with an integrative medical practitioner who is skilled at regulating diet, exercise, and medications.

- Exercise safely in the ways that best suit you, your stamina, and your motivation. Getting analyzed by a cardiologist may be a good idea. Slowly adding intensity to exercise is a great idea.
- Exercise four to six days a week, for a total of at least one hundred and fifty minutes, whether at home with your own equipment or at a gym.
- Set achievable goals and work toward attaining them.
- With your medical practitioner, decide what your ideal pulse rate should be during exercise.
- Exercise with an informed partner, or if alone, tell a family member where you are or tell someone at the gym, in your exercise group, or a race organizer that you have diabetes.
- Know your training level and stay within your exercise capacities.
- Measure your glucose numbers diligently—before and numerous times during and after exercise.
- Drink fluids frequently before, during, and after exercise to prevent dehydration.
- Inspect your feet visually and tactilely before and after exercise.
- Wear appropriate footwear and clothing.
- Carry a medical ID if you are on insulin.
- Avoid exercising during peak insulin action.
- Direct insulin away from working limbs if exercise is within thirty minutes of injection.
- It is safer to reduce postexercise insulin and be a little high than to inject normal doses and suffer a serious low.
- Always carry glucose tabs and gels.
- Avoid exercising in extreme heat, humidity, or cold, and protect your insulin.
- For your first time doing moderate or strenuous exercise after beginning a low-carb diet regimen, it may be helpful to take a glucose tab every fifteen minutes, but check glucose levels to verify need.
- Be alert for signs and symptoms of hypoglycemia, especially when exercising longer and with more intensity, both during the exercise and for many hours afterward.
- Have a glucagon shot available.

- Record your glucose during exercise.
- Work with your medical practitioner to ensure all variables are analyzed and appropriate changes are made.

The key to exercise is going out and using your body. Your body is a system of pulleys and levers and is designed for movement, blood flow, oxygenation of tissues, and sweating. Exercise is necessary on a comprehensive diabetic protocol. Following these guidelines and working with a good physician can ensure any diabetic patient who wishes to commit to regular exercise will have a safe, effective, fun experience, under excellent glucose control.

So, what are you waiting for? Get up and exercise!

The Value of Sleep

Most people need between seven and nine hours of sleep a night, and how much you sleep can affect your appetite and weight. Held to this benchmark, Americans are chronically sleep deprived.

The National Health and Nutrition Examination Survey from 1982 to 1984 showed the effect of sleep on weight and body hormones. Getting fewer than seven hours of sleep a night was correlated with increasing rates of obesity, and getting more than seven hours of sleep a night was correlated with decreasing rates of obesity. Most shocking was the fact that those who were thirty-two to forty-nine years old who reported getting only two to four hours of sleep a night were 235 percent more likely to be obese. Those getting five hours of sleep a night were 60 percent more likely to be obese, and those getting six hours of sleep a night were 27 percent more likely to be obese than subjects who got seven hours of sleep a night.

Sleep deprivation can contribute to developing obesity through the following mechanisms:

- Decreasing leptin, a hormone that decreases appetite
- Increasing ghrelin, a hormone that increases appetite, especially for carbohydrates
- Increasing cortisol, a hormone that can increase glucose levels and reduces insulin sensitivity, causing insulin resistance and poorer control of glucose levels

Sleep is exceedingly important to each of us, but for patients with diabetes who are already insulin resistant, getting a good night's sleep is vital.

There are some notable sleep interferences. Caffeine is a leading one, even if you drink only a cup or two early in the morning. Not everyone detoxifies caffeine effectively. Caffeine can prevent some people from falling asleep but often it affects the system so that a person falls asleep well but then wakes up in the middle of the night and feels wide awake. According to the twenty-four-hour body organ clock of traditional Chinese medicine, the liver time is between 1 a.m. and 3 a.m. Since the liver's role is to detoxify caffeine, a person may wake up during that time and find it hard to return to sleep for an hour or so if the liver is not working effectively. If you're having difficulty sleeping, avoiding caffeine entirely is a good idea to see if even that one cup in the morning, before 9 a.m., is a problem. If you drink coffee in the morning, and then diet pop and iced tea later in the day, it might surprise you to learn how much caffeine you're ingesting. If cutting off your caffeine intake all at once gives you a headache, it's because caffeine is a drug your body is addicted to, and it should definitely be reduced or avoided. No one should wake in the morning *needing* a cup of coffee; our energy should be good from the get-go. If your energy is not good, the reason why needs to be figured out so that caffeine is not a necessity but rather an occasional enjoyment.

Some medications can also affect the liver and cause you to wake up in the middle of the night. If you are not consuming caffeine but wake up around 3 a.m. every morning, your physician may wish to evaluate your medications.

Especially in patients who have genetic single-nucleotide polymorphisms, or SNPs, B vitamins can also prevent a very small minority of patients from falling asleep easily, especially if they are taken in the evening.

Alcohol, which interferes with the onset of rapid eye movement (REM) sleep—our deepest, most refreshing sleep, can cause difficulty sleeping or waking.

Imbalanced emotions, such as anxiety or depression, can often prevent the onset of sleep or wake a patient up in the middle of the night.

Physical reasons, such as frequent urination or defecation, or menopausal night sweats, may need to be addressed so they do not continue to impact negatively on sleep. Physical ailments such as restless leg syndrome, heartburn, or arthritis can wake a person up during sleep.

Elevated cortisol at night can interfere with sleep onset, because it prevents the output of serotonin, a relaxing, calming neurotransmitter from which melatonin is made. A saliva cortisol test can uncover if this is a problem, and there are natural ways to reduce an elevated nighttime cortisol.

It should be part of a physician's workup to ask diabetic patients about the quality and duration of their sleep. Sleep hygiene—protocols regarding enhancing good sleep—is required to ensure patients with diabetes get the best sleep possible. Here is how I direct my patients to get ready for sleep as night occurs:

Turn down most of the lights in your home starting around 8 p.m. Melatonin, the hormone designed to help us fall gently asleep, starts to be secreted as it grows dark. When you leave all the lights on in your home throughout the evening and into the night, you may be hindering the signal for melatonin to be secreted. Therefore, turning down lights considerably as evening progresses will help your body be able to produce melatonin for sleep. Use lamps, but turn off the big overhead ceiling lights.

Do not watch unhappy, violent, depressing shows on television at night. It amazes me that so many people come home from a hard day's work, watch unsettling television shows or news media, and then turn off the television and expect to easily fall asleep. If you watch television at night, it should be entertaining, educational, or humorous. That is it. It should be TV that relaxes the mind, and pulls it into reducing tension and discord from the day.

Go to bed at the same time each night. It's better for the body to have a set time of sleep that you regularly follow. This keeps your biorhythms in good working order.

Make sure your bedroom is completely dark. Many people enjoy having televisions in their bedrooms, but it is better not to. Your bedroom should be dark and should have the least amount of electromagnetic fields near where you sleep, as these fields can subtly affect your sleep. A lamp and an alarm clock are okay on your night table, but it's best to not keep your cell phone by your bed, and to not wake up to check it during the night.

Don't use your computer or cell phone for at least an hour before bed. The blue light rays emanating from the television, cell phone screen, tablet screen, and computer screen activate the brain and reduce the capacity to fall asleep. The effect might be less with television, as we tend to sit farther away from it than we do from other screens. It is best to turn off the technology and read a book before bed, which can elevate your intellect and also start slowing your brain down so entering sleep may be easier. If you need to use technology, it can often be helpful to wear amber glasses, which block the blue rays from affecting your brain. You can buy inexpensive amber glasses on the internet. Uvex amber glasses are highly rated for blocking nearly all the blue light from screens. Also, software such as f.lux can be installed on computers and phones, which darkens the screen to help prevent blue light emittance as evening rolls around. Some phones even come with preinstalled settings for nighttime use.

Maintain good glucose control. Of course, ensuring blood sugar is under good, steady control during the night can help sleep. Hypoglycemia during sleep will often wake a diabetic patient, and it needs to be treated. Working with a physician who sets up a comprehensive protocol that helps you keep your glucose level constant during sleep will certainly lead to much better sleep.

There are also many helpful sleep aids to enhance falling asleep, staying asleep, and returning to sleep if one does wake up. A hot bath is a great way to calm down, relax, and get ready for bed. Maybe add some Epsom salts, one or two cups per bath, as your body will absorb the magnesium, which will help it relax. As mentioned earlier, reading is a great way also to let the day go, relax, and have one's brain fall asleep. Please do not read about zombies, the apocalypse, or serial killers! Also, praying and journaling are other ways to slow down and welcome sleep. Regular exercise helps people become calmer, and can also tire people out at the end of the day so that sleep comes easier. Many people notice that beginning an exercise routine helps them sleep better. In general, though, do not exercise right before bed; for many, exercise can energize them and keep them awake. Finally, many supplements are safe and effective for most people, but make sure your physician knows about any you are taking to help with sleep, and helps you choose safe doses. A sleep formula may include these ingredients:

- Melatonin, the sleep hormone, works well for some.

- Neurotransmitter precursors like tryptophan, 5-HTP, GABA, and glycine are commonly used substances to help initiate sleep. Nutrients like calcium and magnesium are minerals that can help relax the body and mind when taken before bed.
- Botanicals like passion flower, valerian, skullcap, chamomile, hops, wild lettuce, kava, and L-theanine can be helpful.
- Phosphatidylserine, ashwagandha, magnolia, and *Rhodiola* are used by integrative physicians to reduce elevated cortisol at night.
- For patients with anxiety, phobia, or depression keeping them from having an excellent night of sleep, taking their homeopathic "case" can be invaluable for helping to heal those emotional imbalances and allowing sleep to occur.

Sleep is vital to a healthy constitution and also for lowering glucose numbers and controlling one's appetite. Working in a comprehensive way can uncover blocks to sleep and help a patient get those wonderful eight hours of peaceful sleep.

Obstructive Sleep Apnea

Obstructive sleep apnea (OSA) is the most common sleep disorder. Forty percent of OSA patients have T2DM, and estimates are that 23–58 percent of T2DM patients have either OSA or some other type of sleep disordered breathing. Diabetes can cause OSA and OSA can lead to developing diabetes.

Many overweight metabolic patients develop obstructive sleep apnea, a condition where a person stops breathing frequently throughout the night, interrupting good rest and making the patient very tired during the next day. Other symptoms of OSA can be a morning headache, dry throat, problems thinking or staying focused, mood changes, sexual dysfunction including decreased libido and impotence, and gastrointestinal reflux. Sleep apnea is also associated with causing weight gain, diabetes, cardiovascular disease, and other serious conditions.

If you are overweight or obese, feel tired throughout the day and don't sleep well, or your sleeping partner notices you have an odd breathing rhythm during sleep or that you stop breathing, snore badly, or wake to gasp or to choke, you should discuss this with your physician. In fact, when an overweight or obese patient notes that he snores regularly, that is usually enough for me to want to send him for a formal sleep study, checking for OSA. Snoring is the first easy-to-notice symptom of this serious and dangerous condition.

Obstructive sleep apnea is diagnosed via a sleep study, where you go to a sleep lab and they hook you up with wires to measure your breathing as well as your eye and chin movements, heart rate and rhythm, respiration rate, leg movements, and oxygen and carbon dioxide levels in your blood during sleep. A technologist is present during the test. Obstructive sleep apnea is defined as your breath stopping for at least ten seconds during sleep; how many times this occurs per hour is important and is referred to as an apnea-hypopnea index (AHI). An AHI of 5–15 is mild obstructive sleep apnea, 15–30 is moderate, and 30 or higher is severe.

There are also home sleep tests, sometimes called "unattended sleep studies," whereby the patient gets sensors to apply to his body that measure key biologic parameters to help rule OSA in or out. The evaluation is done for one or two nights. It does not collect as much information as the official in-lab sleep study; however, it is three times cheaper than the patient going to a laboratory setting at a sleep center and, of course, it is more convenient. A home sleep test may be helpful, but if the result is unclear, then a formal sleep study will need to occur.

Both types of tests can be covered by insurances. Your medical practitioner will decide which test seems best for you.

OSA can be treated in numerous ways:

Losing weight. For many patients, losing abdominal weight can cure the apnea.

CPAP machine. This is a machine that a person wears over his nose, with hoses attached to a machine. The machine initiates a positive airway pressure that allows you to breath regularly throughout the night. Drawbacks include patients disliking to wear it during sleep, having to travel with it, and the need to do regular cleaning to prevent mold development.

BiPAP device. A device very similar to a CPAP machine.

Dental device/oral appliance (also known as a mandibular advancement device or tongue retraining device). Some dentists can create an oral device that you put into your mouth at bedtime and wear during your sleep. It adjusts your oral cavity to allow for proper breathing during sleep. One big drawback is jaw pain, as it puts pressure on the jaw to redefine its normal shape.

Surgery. This is a last considered option, as surgery in your mouth is unpleasant, and it is only used when other options are ineffective.

OSA is a serious medical condition, and if there is any chance you have this condition, it is imperative to get a sleep study and initiate successful treatment.

Poor sleep quality and less efficient sleep are significantly correlated with worse glycemic control and higher A1Cs. Under- or oversleeping leads to higher A1Cs. Using a CPAP has been shown to improve glucose control in T2DM patients with OSA. Diabetic patients with restless leg syndrome have higher A1Cs due to poor sleep, so all conditions negatively affecting sleep need to be addressed, not just OSA.

All in all, it's vital for all medical practitioners to ensure their patients are getting a great night of sleep each and every night. It's especially important for diabetic patients. Clear discussions on sleep need to occur regularly among patients and medical practitioners, to enable glucose levels and A1Cs to lower, to help control appetite, to prevent carbohydrate cravings, and to create good energy throughout the day.

Stress and Diabetes

It would be wonderful if we all went through life never feeling stressed, overwhelmed, sad, anxious, frustrated, or any of the other emotions that darken our moods. However, it is uncommon for a person to traverse the years of their life and never have a down time.

There are two ways of looking at mental health—as the absence of mental illness or as the ability to feel fulfilled, happy, spiritually connected, and that one is a responsible and beneficial addition to the planet. What enables a person to have a positive outlook about themselves and life? The ability to take responsibility for one's actions, flexibility to adapt, a high tolerance for frustration, an ability to accept the uncertain aspects of life, involvement in activities of social interest, courage to take appropriate risks, serenity to accept what one cannot change, acceptance of handicaps, the capacity for self-control, loving and friendly relationships with self and others, one's spirituality or religion, kindness and concern for others—these are all qualities that define a mentally well person.

This recipe is a tall order, though, for all of us to achieve every day, through all the events of our lives. Feeling stress is inevitable at times, and that is okay. What we do not want, though, is for people to live in a stressful state all the time, and develop mental or emotional problems as a result. To make matters worse, stress can have devastating effects on our physical bodies, as well, and can affect glucose control.

Stress can play a role in both the development and the management of diabetes. Although I'm using it as a catchall phrase here, I advise my patients not to use the word *stress* to describe how they feel; it is much more important for patients to state the exact emotion they are experiencing or struggling with. Americans tend to not want to identify when they are sad, or angry, or frustrated, and so patients use the terms *stressed* or *overwhelmed* as broad, vague terms to cover up their actual feelings. Once patients stop, pause, think, feel, and state and acknowledge their specific feelings, healing and rebalancing can begin.

Research has shown that stress may lead to developing diabetes, can aggravate diabetes control, and can lead to difficulties with diabetes self-care. So, checking in on a diabetic patient's life and how it is affecting them needs to be part of every office visit; time has to be made for the mental and emotional lives of patients, alongside going over labs and discussing diet and exercise.

General Stress

Stress can be related to finances, job, career, family relationships, friend relationships, deaths and other tragedies, politics, health conditions, past traumas, and many other factors.

Feeling stress is a problem for all of us at times, but if it is short-lived and we return to emotional balance and joy, it's not too concerning. It is a much larger problem when it leads to chronic unhappiness that results in a drug prescription. Don't we all know someone on an antidepressant or an antianxiety medication? The statistics are very sad: One in ten Americans takes an antidepressant, and among women in their forties and fifties, the figure is one in four.

What is *stress*, really, and how does it affect us with regard to diabetes? When someone feels stress or is threatened by unwelcome events in his life, his brain sends out vasopressin and CRH, a hormone that stimulates the adrenals to produce cortisol. Vasopressin initiates water retention in his body, a physiologic response to help keep him alive if he loses blood. Cortisol has been shown to increase the glucose levels of T2DM patients. Cortisol counters insulin by promoting higher blood sugars and signaling the liver to produce more glucose and release it into circulation. Cortisol decreases insulin release and interferes with the production of melatonin (a sleep promoter and antioxidant), leading to insomnia. Cortisol also decreases the functioning of our immune system, and it can be pro-inflammatory to the lining of our intestine if there is too little or too much of it.

Both caffeine and alcohol can promote higher levels of cortisol secretion from the adrenals. So, both drinking caffeine to counter the effects of poor sleep due to stress and drinking alcohol as treatment for stress can wind up producing more of the hormone that makes you feel stress!

One last, powerful adrenal hormone related to stress is epinephrine. Epinephrine can be elevated when a person feels anxiety or has an anxiety or panic attack. It raises the heartbeat, causes sweating, causes shakiness, and is our basic fight-or-flight hormone, also designed to raise our glucose levels. It is problematic if it is secreted regularly without some actual life crisis occurring. Many people suffer from anxiety and panic disorders and epinephrine levels rise during those events.

Stress comes from life, but it also comes from having diabetes. Developing T1DM when young, or T2DM or LADA when older, can come with a world of stressful associations: dietary restrictions, all the medications and supplements, financial costs, dealing with using insulin, having to live one's life around checking one's glucose all the time, lack of support, people nagging you, disease progression and complications, the struggle to lose weight, all the injections, mastering pump technology, and worrying about hyperglycemia and the damage it can cause to your body and hypoglycemia and how poorly you feel during a low. All of these stresses can work against maintaining one's steady happiness, especially when one is using conventional care and one's disease is not well controlled.

Working on the emotional level with diabetic patients is just as necessary as working on diet and other lifestyle aspects. It is very understandable that someone with diabetes will at some point become overwhelmed with their condition and need help. One book I recommend to patients is *Diabetes Burnout: What to Do When You Can't Take It Anymore* by Dr. William Polonsky, who runs the Behavioral Diabetes Institute (BDI) in San Diego. The BDI is devoted to helping patients with diabetes maintain a positive mental and emotional equilibrium with their condition. This is an informative book for patients and also has some journaling exercises to help patients learn more about themselves, leading to a new, fresh outlook on their condition. Patients of all ages, from a twelve-year-old T1DM patient to a senior T2DM patient, have read this book. It is a very helpful tool.

Dr. Polonsky, whom I have interviewed for the Low Carb Diabetes Association, also created an innovative etiquette card, which is very helpful for patients to give to others who do not have diabetes but who have taken on the role of "diabetic police" around them. Patients with diabetes can experience inordinate stress from "helpful" others who feel compelled to question, judge, and too closely watch and comment on how the person with diabetes should manage their condition. I highly recommend my diabetic patients buy the etiquette cards from BDI's website (behavioraldiabetesinstitute.org) if they have people in their life who create stress by regularly crossing boundaries.

The etiquette card has ten rules people without diabetes should follow in relationship to those who do have it:

1. **DON'T** offer unsolicited advice about my eating or other aspects of diabetes. (It is not nice to give advice when it is not asked for, and some of your views on diabetes may not be scientifically accurate.)
2. **DO** realize and appreciate that diabetes is hard work. (Diabetes is a full-time job that I did not want and cannot quit—I have to constantly think about what, when, and how I eat, where my glucose is, how exercise, medication, or stress may affect me and my glucose, and this is a 24-7 responsibility.)

3. **DON'T** tell me horror stories about your grandmother or other people with diabetes you have heard about. (Stories like this are obviously neither helpful nor reassuring, and my focus is to live a long, healthy life with my diabetes under good control.)
4. **DO** offer to join me in making healthy lifestyle changes. (It is great to feel I am supported and not alone in managing this condition.)
5. **DON'T** look so horrified when I check my blood sugars or give myself an injection. (I do not particularly like doing these things, either, but I must be in good control. Making me feel bad or ashamed makes managing my diabetes much more difficult.)
6. **DO** ask how you might be helpful. (I appreciate you asking me how to help and letting me guide you in ways that are most beneficial to me.)
7. **DON'T** offer thoughtless reassurances. (It is not helpful to tell me it could have been cancer, instead, which infers diabetes is no big deal. It is a big deal.)
8. **DO** be supportive of my efforts for self-care. (I welcome working with you to set up an environment of success regarding my diet, exercise, and other aspects of this complicated condition. Moreover, most of all, do not tell me "one cookie" would be okay; keep me away from temptations that I need to avoid.)
9. **DON'T** peek at or comment on my blood glucose numbers without asking me first. (My lab results and glucose checks are private; if I want to share them, I will. Moreover, if you do see them, unsolicited opinions about them can greatly upset me.)
10. **DO** offer your love and encouragement. (Knowing that you care is the most important part of my having diabetes. Just being there for me, supporting me, and motivating me will make my journey easier and more fun).

For teenage diabetic patients, there is a unique etiquette card that applies specifically to them:

1. **DON'T** stop trying to scare me with diabetes statistics. (Bugging teens about the risk of complications is not a good way to encourage

good diabetes control. It is better to motivate a teen with an important thing that happens right then, not way in the future.)

2. **DON'T** assume I've done something stupid when my blood sugars are high (although I may have). (Work with the teen to figure out want went wrong and do not just accuse him of screwing up.)
3. **DO** please acknowledge when I am doing something right, not just when I've messed up. (Positive support is vital for teens, instead of just focusing on when numbers are not good.)
4. **DON'T** always be in my face about diabetes, but don't leave me completely alone with it either. (Teens need things to be well balanced, have some independence with their diabetes, but also know that if they have any troubles or problems, you will be there to help.)
5. **DO** make the effort to understand diabetes from my point of view. (Diabetes is unfair, inconvenient, a lot of work, and it sucks. Just listen when a teen complains or needs to vent.)
6. **DON'T** tell everyone about my diabetes, especially not during the first minute you meet them. (That is very embarrassing to teens when their goal is primarily to fit in, not stand out. The teen should be allowed to tell others about their diabetes when they are ready.)
7. **DO** recognize that I am never going to be perfect with my diabetes care, no matter how much you want this. (It is nearly impossible to manage diabetes perfectly every moment of every day; your teen is doing the best she can but also needs to have a good life outside diabetes.)
8. **DON'T** limit my activities based on diabetes. (A teen does not want to be considered weak, fragile, or physically sick, or for it to seem that something is terribly wrong with them. Allow him to do what other teens are doing and maintain good socialization and sports.)
9. **DON'T** be the food police. (Teens might not eat perfectly all the time, but watching everything they eat all the time is a way to get them to start avoiding you when they eat.)

I encourage all patients with diabetes to buy etiquette cards from the BDI, and give them, when necessary, to pertinent people in their lives. They are a great start for nondiabetic friends and family to realize the day-to-day actualities of having diabetes and to learn to pull back from the nagging and instead give the respect and support a diabetic patient needs and deserves.

Emotional Eating

Using food for emotional support is a common reaction to the lows of life, and most people do not choose to eat carrots and kale when they feel emotionally out of balance. Emotional eating or overeating can also be a remnant from childhood habits and how your parents or grandparents lovingly used food around you.

The impulse for emotional eating—craving specific foods that one feels they must eat immediately—can come on suddenly. It can easily lead to mindless eating, whereby the calories and amount of food you eat are way beyond what you need. Emotional eating also doesn't satiate the way a good healthy meal does, because emotional eating is driven not by the stomach but by the mind.

Emotional eating triggers a vicious circle of problematic eating. When life is difficult and a person uses food as an escape, release, reward, or combination of these to achieve a temporary improvement in mood, the food often can have a negative effect on her neurotransmitters, and lower her energy, so that it becomes easy to feel bad again. However, of course, eating food does not solve the problems she is experiencing in life that are causing the stress, and usually, what she is left with is guilt, shame, or regret for eating badly or overeating, resetting the cycle of feeling the need to eat for temporary relief.

You may be eating emotionally if you:

- Eat more when you are feeling stressed
- Eat when you are not hungry, and may even be full, but still feel the need to eat a particular food
- Eat to feel better when you are upset
- Reward yourself with food
- Eat regularly until you are stuffed, or feel stuffed and you leave the table but then come back soon to eat more
- Feel food is a friend and is there for you when others may not be
- Feel powerless or out of control around food

It is important to recognize what triggers initiate the automatic habit of grabbing food when life is not ideal. Emotional eating destroys people's self-empowerment and leads them to feel even more helpless; they seem out of control when opening the fridge in a bad mood. This book is designed to educate and support everyone so that they feel totally empowered regarding their diabetes and getting it under control.

Ironically, following a strict diabetic diet can also lead to moments of emotional eating in some, especially when others around them are eating what they cannot. Emotional eating can also result from not eating well-balanced meals and not keeping glucose levels steady and even. Ensuring your diet is balanced with macronutrients, micronutrients, and oils is important; nutrient deficiencies can harm appetite control. This is another value to keeping a diet diary so that any nutrient imbalances can be seen and corrected.

A good physician should not solely focus on your physical body and lab results, but should also help you feel comfortable discussing your life, your personality, where you are happy and fulfilled, and where you are stressed or unhappy. Your physician should work to enable you to establish new habits that control your emotional hunger, and take positive steps through the low times. Also, a referral to a counselor if necessary may be helpful if improper eating habits are long-standing or hard to overcome on your own.

Keeping an emotional eating diary can be very helpful. The idea is to note when you overeat or feel compelled to eat your compulsive food, and take a moment to figure out what triggered the urge each time it occurs. Write down the following: the food you ate, what mood you were in, the episode that triggered the eating crisis, and how you felt before, during, and after eating. Working with a good physician or counselor, patterns can emerge that can help you identify people and situations that affect you the most and cause the emotional eating. That is the first great step to learn how to disrupt this habit and institute positive changes.

Ways to Deal with Stress

Life is life, both the highs and lows, the beauty and the difficulties, the joy and the sadness, the celebrations and the tragedies. An integrative physician cannot change your life, but he or she can help you learn how best to journey through the stressful times in ways that are more beneficial to your mind, emotions, soul, and also your blood glucose. You want to find a physician who discusses this with you in a sympathetic, empathetic way, and understands that diabetes itself—even in a stable and happy life—can wear down a person's mood with its endless needs to watch food, glucose, weight, and labs.

Stress management can help a patient with diabetes reduce their A1C level, even up to 0.5 percent. It is very important for a patient with diabetes to strive to remove or reduce daily stress, to learn to change his response to stress, and to modify the long-term effects of stress on his body and mind.

We know there are many people in the world who have an emotional center of joy and balance. It is not beyond anyone's capacity to feel solid in his path through life and not break when the winds of life blow strong.

How can a person work toward feeling happy again? Let's talk about all the ways you can process stress well and become much more emotionally resilient to it.

Saliva Lab Test

This is one lab many integrative physicians do when stress has been part of a patient's life. As noted, cortisol levels can be raised in people who are stressed. In this test, which is done at home, patients collect their saliva in little plastic vials four times a day: morning, noon, evening, and night. Those vials are then analyzed at a specific lab that measures their DHEA and cortisol levels. This is a valid test of cortisol production, and can help a medical practitioner know how much of an impact cortisol is physiologically having on a patient who is stressed. Cortisol may be low, normal, or high when someone is stressed. Those hormones and the adrenal gland that secretes them can be rebalanced back to normal levels, if need be.

Turning Off the Noise

Texting or using Facebook, the phone, the computer, and watching or listening to the news—these all contribute to mental noise. It is well known and now scientifically proven that when people pull back from being Wi-Fi connected, they become happier and less stressed. If you find yourself endlessly checking your emails, texts, Facebook posts, and so on, and walk around with your phone in your hand all the time or eat meals with friends with your phone in your hand all the time, yes, you are too plugged in. When eating with someone else, I suggest looking at and talking to them, not watching your phone feed. Reducing your Wi-Fi connected time will definitely soothe your brain and reduce your stress. Avoiding violent TV, movies, and books and substituting educational, easy, or humorous entertainment, in addition to helping one's sleep, is much better for stress management.

Being Grateful

I highly recommend that all patients keep a gratitude journal each night. That is, at the end of the day, write in a journal about all that you are thankful for. On days you had a fender bender, you may still have kissed your healthy child goodnight; on days you were overwhelmed at work, you still came back to a warm home filled with food. When we develop an attitude of always knowing that every day we have things to be truly and significantly thankful for, it can reset our minds to see the daily mundane difficulties as the minor events they are. Seeing the big picture—the love you have in your life, the pets you adore, your child's smile, the food, clothes, home, the health of those you love, the connection with friends, the fun you have—is a wonderful way to be emotionally healthier, and this has been proven through medical studies. No one can say for certain why you have diabetes, but life is still full of hope and blessings. Being grateful is one way of constantly recognizing that.

Eating a Healthy Diet

Within days of starting one, a low-carb diet reestablishes excellent appetite control by nearly immediately decreasing insulin resistance. Remember, insulin resistance keeps body cells from taking in glucose, but it also affects the neurons in your brain. Insulin signals the neurons to reduce appetite and cravings, and it is very common after initiating a low-carb diet for patients to come back even in a week and state their appetite is decreased and they find it is easy to eat an appropriate diet without having cravings. Seeing glucose numbers drop is a great source of positive feedback for patients and is a great method for raising self-esteem and hope. Eating a healthy diet also contains good oils, like omega-3, which are needed by your brain cells to produce happy neurotransmitters, which make you feel satisfied, calm, and content. It does not contain sugars, processed foods, and chemicals that can play havoc with the brain and make moods unstable. Eating well will make you feel better both physically and emotionally.

Exercise/Yoga/Tai Chi

Exercise produces endorphins and enkephalins, hormones that make people feel better, happier, content, and calm. A person beginning an exercise program should feel proud for exercising. Many people develop good self-esteem as they routinely exercise. As noted above, not all exercise has to be aerobic or resistant—yoga, Tai Chi, and Ki Chung, for example, also promote health physically, mentally, and emotionally. If a slower exercise resonates with you during the week, putting your mind into a calm, peaceful state, fitting in that type of movement is highly valuable.

Humor

Did you know there are over 350 scientific research papers on laughter? Even forced laughter has been shown to be a powerful, readily available, and free method for people to reliably boost their mood and psychological well-being. Your mood is more positive, you can handle pain better, and you are more fertile if you laugh when trying to conceive via in-vitro fertilization; laughter lowers cortisol and epinephrine, boosts your immune system, improves relationships in ailing couples, lowers depression and anxiety, improves insomnia and sleep quality, reduces skin allergy reactions, and oxygenates body cells. Laughter can lower glucose levels and help with weight loss; it's even more important to laugh with friends and family and share that bond of camaraderie and fun. Bringing humor and laughter into your life on a daily basis is a marvelous, fun, free way to regain health and stay healthy.

Spirituality

Spirituality, whether separate from or as part of a religion (institutionalized spirituality), can give a person a purpose in life and also help a person feel connected to the immensity of existence as a whole. Studies show that people who are spiritual and religious, who engage in regular religious services, who participate in social activities with like-minded people, or who make prayer and a connection to God a part of their lives have more positive moods, lower suicide rates, and better medical prognoses. Delving into, discovering, or rediscovering one's religion or spirituality can be a very helpful way to minimize stress reactions. If one is an atheist or agnostic, searching for ways you can bring more fulfillment into your life and increase your connection to others and your community is still pertinent.

Creativity and Hobbies

Most people have a creative side, whether it is writing, painting, crafts, sewing, photography, dancing, music, games, or any of the other innumerable activities that help our brains blossom, focus our minds, and increase our confidence. Spending some time each week in an inspired and productive creative endeavor is something we should all have as a standing habit. Another part of cultivating this is joining groups where you meet others who have your same interests. In these groups you can socialize with others in positive ways, and indulge in your hobby, interest, or creative endeavors.

Nature

Spending time in nature is one of the most peaceful activities one can enjoy. Getting out of the house, away from technology, and entering into the beauty of the earth has consistently been shown to be a worthwhile, relaxing, stress-reducing activity. The green color of tree leaves and grass has even been shown to reduce adrenal stress reactions. Whether you are going for a hike in the wilderness, walking along a nature trail to a waterfall, or even walking around the park in your neighborhood, directly encountering trees and wildlife is a way to clear the mind, deepen the breath, and relax. Even getting into your backyard and doing some gardening or planting some flowers, touching the earth, is a simple and effective way to connect with nature.

Support Groups

When my cat died, I entered into a severe depression, but finding a support group of other pet owners who had lost their pets and could understand what I was feeling and not disdain it was very valuable to me and helped me recover much quicker. There are support groups for all types of conditions and tragedies in life. If something has put you in a rut, and you do not feel others can comprehend why it has affected you so terribly, seeking out a support group of people in a similar place in life is highly recommended. It's great to have family and friends be supportive, but there is something special about being around others who feel the same as you, do not make you feel defensive or weird, and have guidelines for moving through that particular stress.

Meditation

Meditation has been practiced around the world for thousands of years and has also been scientifically proven to reduce anxiety, tension, and worry and to reestablish daily peace of mind. Meditation puts a person into a deep state of relaxation and produces a tranquil mind. Meditating can typically result in enhanced emotional and physical well-being; this state lasts not just during and right after the meditation session—the same calm, peaceful frame of mind can extend for hours or days. Meditation has many benefits: improvement in processing stressful situations, increasing self-awareness and focus on living in the present, and reducing negative emotions. Meditation has been shown to be useful in anxiety, asthma, cancer, heart disease, high blood pressure, pain, and insomnia; for diabetics, meditation has been found to have an enhanced clinical effect on improving glycemic control. There are many forms of meditation, but the key to most of them is to focus your attention on a word, prayer, mantra, or other focal point and eliminate the constant flow of hectic thoughts that can crowd a mind and cause stress. You can do it for five minutes or fifteen; whatever time you can allow. One specific form is called "guided meditation," where a pleasant voice guides you through deep breathing and relaxing your body part by part. Any type of meditation is helpful, so find what best resonates with you.

Massage/Travel/Culture

Finding time for yourself by getting a regular massage or pedicure, going to a spa, going shopping, seeing a movie, traveling to a beach, seeing a play or opera, or having a date night with your spouse or partner is beneficial. Getting away from the mundane routine of life, and treating ourselves to things that we enjoy is highly rated to reduce stress and improve our lives.

Volunteering

Those who volunteer have been shown to live longer, healthier, and happier lives. Giving back to others in the community is a win-win situation for all involved. Whether it is helping out at a food bank, in an art museum, or at an animal shelter—wherever, doing whatever—getting outside our own lives to work to better another's, human or animal, does us a world of good.

Counseling

If a person has a deep-seated or acutely intense situation of stress, getting professional counseling might be useful. I am not talking about seeing a psychiatrist and immediately being prescribed medication; as much as possible we want to avoid adding medications. What I recommend to patients is going to a psychologist, social worker, counselor, or mental health therapist and sharing one's story to learn techniques on how to move forward. There is less stigma now about getting counseling than there has been in the past, which is wonderful, and many people at some point in their life find this kind of guided support invaluable to their growth and fulfillment.

Homeopathy

As a diplomat of the Homeopathy Academy of Naturopathic Physicians, which shows that I have a certain expertise in this modality, I hold homeopathy in high regard. While I could write a whole essay on the validity of this misunderstood and underappreciated medical modality, I'll instead refer you to the most commonly recommended book for lay people on what homeopathy is and how it works: *Homeopathy: Beyond Flat Earth Medicine* by Dr. Timothy Dooley. This book is free to read on the internet. I always suggest to my patients new to homeopathy that they spend an hour or two reading the book and come back to the office with any questions. I have used homeopathy successfully to heal patients from anxiety, panic disorder, grief, and depression, among other mental or emotional imbalances.

Other Mental and Emotional Techniques

Whether seeing a therapist for EMDR (eye movement desensitization and reprocessing) or getting an Alpha-Stim machine for anxiety, there are many other methodologies for helping patients achieve lasting peace of mind, so many that I do not have room to list them all here. Ask your physician for recommendations for the many other options available.

Supplementation

Many newly diagnosed diabetic patients, especially those with T2DM, have probably not eaten well for a long time, so they usually are deficient in omega-3 oils, and they may also be low in B vitamins, zinc, magnesium, and chromium, among others. Nutrients are used to make neurotransmitters, to help us detoxify, to give us energy, and to help us produce hormones; when we eat right and take some extra nutrients, it can make a huge difference. Which forms of nutrients to take specifically for diabetes, and at what dosage, I'll discuss in chapter 10. However, here are some specific supplements to consider for reducing stress and helping to balance the adrenals, and to give a person more strength in order to not have any type of breakdown when under stress for a long time. Botanical medicines shown by research to help reduce stress include *Rhodiola*, ashwagandha (also known as withania), magnolia, *Phellodendron*, *Eleutherococcus*, and *Panax ginseng*. These are called adaptogens and they help the adrenals and the body as a whole process stress better physiologically and emotionally. Nutrients like extra B vitamins (especially vitamin B_6), and extra vitamin C are helpful, as well. Finally, nervines and calmatives are supplements that help a person feel more calm, feel less tense, and rest better, and they include tryptophan, GABA, valerian, passion flower, hops, L-theanine, wild lettuce, kava kava, Jamaican dogwood, wild oats, skullcap, and chamomile. Note that these are very similar to the nutrients that help a person fall asleep.

Whether nutrients, botanicals, or nutraceuticals will be best depends on the individual. A good integrative medical practitioner will be able to recommend products either in tea, tincture (an alcohol-based liquid form of herbs), glycerites (a glycerin-based liquid form of herbs), or capsules specific for ingredients, and at doses, particular to your body, situation, and stress response.

Working on decreasing stress is important in a comprehensive regimen to control diabetes. Each office visit with your physician should include checking in about life stresses and finding out if any stress is interfering with good compliance of the entirety of a diabetic protocol. The medical practitioner must provide support and validation, allowing a patient to feel safe sharing her struggles. Then it's important for a brainstorming and troubleshooting session to occur, to help the patient move forward out of the stress and find solutions.

I often talk to patients about calling stressful situations "problems," which are solvable, instead of "issues," which are more amorphous and are hard to encompass and fix. Words have power. My aim is to help a diabetic patient heal a life problem, so they can move forward into a life full of happiness and hope.

The key to stress is to not give up. It may take a consistent effort to retrain your mind and emotions, but like everything else about the human experience, change can occur, and you were made for healing and health. Working with an integrative physician who is always on your side, who does not rush through your visits, who has time to sit and listen to you and your life story will be a great boon to you and all patients.

Supporting the Microbiome

The term *microbiome* refers to the comprehensive collection of thousands of species of bacteria, archae, fungi, and viruses that live in our intestinal tracts, both the ones that are normal and nonharmful to our intestines (those that live in symbiosis with it) and those that are (at least potentially) pathogenic. There is 1.3 times the amount of bacteria in our intestines than there are cells in the whole rest of our body. In fact, 60 percent of the dry mass of your stool is made up of gut microorganisms.

Our gut microbiome is established by the time we are two years old. It consists of between five hundred and one thousand different species, though the vast majority belong to thirty or forty species. The most common bacteria in our intestines include *Bacteriodes*, *Clostridium*, *Eneterococcus*, *Bifidobacterium*, *Lactobacillus*, *Escherichia*, *Enterobacter*, *Klebsiella*, *Staphylococcus aureus*, *Proteus*, and *Pseudomonas*. The most common fungi are *Candida*, *Saccharomyces*, *Aspergillus*, *Penicillin*, *Rhodotorula*, *Trametes*, and *Pleospora*.

The intestinal microbiome fosters an incredible amount of health benefits: It acquires nutrients from our food; decreases our toxic and carcinogenic burden by catabolizing them, and even makes nutrients and helps the absorption of nutrients. When the microbiome is normal and balanced it also keeps the lining of our intestines healthy and functional. A good microbiome helps regulate our immune system, both the part that fights infections and the part that can become autoimmune and attack our own cells. Good bacteria also increase levels of interleukin-10, a protein that reduces inflammation and reduces the development of autoimmunity. A healthy microbiome regulates how much energy we absorb from our food, setting our glucose metabolism and our weight. It can affect our moods, whether we are happier or more anxious and depressed.

Intestinal bacteria ferment fiber to produce short-chain fatty acids (SCFAs), the food of the colon cells, and without SCFAs, colon cells can atrophy in days. These SCFAs also stimulate GLP-1 secretion, which, if you remember, has been made into a non-insulin injectable medication used to help control elevated glucose levels, reduce appetite, reduce the inflammation response, and promote weight loss. Intestinal bacteria also stimulate peptide YY, which helps suppress the appetite. It seems almost as if every day we are learning about new influences our gut bacteria have on our health.

Integrative physicians use the term *dysbiosis* to refer to dysfunction in the microbiome. Dysbiosis means that instead of the normal microbiome existing in the small and large intestine, changes have occurred that either lowered beneficial bacteria or increased problematic bacteria or fungi.

What can harm the microbiome? Unfortunately, many things:

Birth by cesarian section. Though a necessary procedure for many women, babies born via C-section miss out on exposure to helpful bacteria (both ingested and on the skin) in the birth canal that is part of vaginal birth.

Bottle feeding instead of breastfeeding. Bottle-fed babies have a different microbiome than infants fed breast milk.

Antibiotics. Of course, it is well known that these life-saving drugs, which are immensely overused both in people and in animals fed to people (such as cows and poultry), can wipe out healthy microorganisms. Giving antibiotics to an infant can also increase the risk of that child becoming overweight.

Proton pump inhibitors. These commonly used drugs for gastroesophageal reflux disorder cause malabsorption of protein and some nutrients, and can cause negative changes in the microbiome. Due to their lowering of stomach acid, they can also increase the risk of food poisoning in people taking them daily.

Non-steroidal anti-inflammatory drugs (NSAIDs). These medications for pain and inflammation, such as aspirin, ibuprofen, naproxen, and their prescription counterparts, have been shown to cause terrible intestinal inflammation and leaky gut. People take NSAIDs frequently for this or that pain or ache, but these medications are not safe, harm the intestine, and should be avoided as much as possible.

Food poisoning. Most people have had an episode or two of food poisoning. That one day of stomach flu is usually actually food poisoning, and feeling nauseous, vomiting, or having diarrhea between four and twenty-four hours after a meal are the signs and symptoms of food poisoning.

Poor diet. A diet high in sugar, refined grains, lacking fiber, lacking fermented foods, lacking vegetables, high in animal protein, and featuring regular overeating, can cause detrimental changes to the microbiome.

Genetically modified organisms. As described in chapter 7, GMOs seem to cause harm to the intestine and may lead to dysbiosis.

Obesity. The gut microbiome is problematically different in obese people than in nonobese people; it contains higher levels of a type of bacteria that absorbs more energy (calories) and can cause more insulin resistance in the body.

When the microbiome is changed negatively it can cause many problems, including gas and bloating, indigestion, constipation or diarrhea, irritable bowel, and many systemic reactions related to food sensitivities (as discussed in chapter 7). An increase in insulin resistance and autoimmunity, including the risk of developing T1DM, is associated with intestinal permeability.

A dysbiotic gut can cause inflammation of the lining of the intestine, causing it to become damaged and develop intestinal permeability, or "leaky gut." Small intestine cells have alleyways between cells called "tight junctions."

These alleyways contain gates that regulate what is and is not allowed to pass through into our circulation. Leaky gut means that the gates are no longer tightly regulating what gets through into the bloodstream, and therefore food antigens, bacteria, and bacterial toxins might get through, causing harm, and some nutrients might not get through, causing deficiencies.

Leaky gut can cause the release of inflammatory chemicals and begin the process of confusing the immune system, setting it up to attack its own cells (in this case, the pancreatic beta cells) but other autoimmune conditions can develop as well, such as Hashimoto's thyroiditis and rheumatoid arthritis, among others.

Children with T1DM were noted in a study to have negative changes in their microbiome, decreases in bacteria that make SCFAs and increases in others. Interesting studies have been done in children who are "prediabetic for T1DM." These children have positive diabetic antibodies but no clinical expression of diabetes for many years. They have found that these children who are pre-T1DM have leaky guts that seem to precede the clinical onset of the disease, and this condition may be leading to the development of their autoimmunity. In one study, 339 pre-T1DM patients were measured for zonulin, a protein that initiates leaky gut in those tight junctions; zonulin was detected in 70 percent of these patients. Children already diagnosed with T1DM were also found to have elevated levels of zonulin.

Intestinal enteroviruses, rotaviruses, and coxsackie viruses may help cause T1DM or be a result of T1DM. Coxsackie B virus seems to be the most concerning. This virus has been found in the pancreas of newly diagnosed patients with T1DM. It is found in siblings who developed T1DM, but not in siblings who did not. And, it has been found in mothers who had a child develop T1DM.

T2DM is associated with the gut microbiota, as well. Negative changes in the diabetic intestine can produce more bacterial endotoxins, leading to more inflammation, causing insulin resistance. Negative microbiota changes can lead to more inflammation in a fatty liver and are also associated with promoting the development of diabetic complications, such as retinopathy, nephropathy, atherosclerosis, hypertension, and even foot ulcers. On top of all that, the diabetic microbiome, in general, has been shown to produce less vitamin B_{12} and vitamin K, two key nutrients.

What is the best way to analyze a patient's microbiome? Unfortunately, not even the best integrative labs can fully analyze the entirety of one's microbiome for clinical use. On top of that, the small and large intestine have very different environments and need completely different analyses to interpret them. Conventional investigations, such as a colonoscopy or an esophagogastroduodenoscopy, mostly analyze structural changes, such as ulcers, polyps, and hiatal hernias, but cannot analyze the individual microbiome. There are national labs, like uBiome, using DNA-sequencing technology to analyze the microbiome. I have not yet started using those types of labs.

The most common tests used to understand the microbiome include:

DNA analysis of microbiome, as conducted by uBiome.

Stool analysis. A stool analysis only analyzes the colonic, or large intestine, microbiome. It does not reflect what is going on in the small intestine. A stool analysis can show the levels of important beneficial bacteria, overgrowth of bacteria normal to the gut and pathogenic bacteria, normal and pathogenic overgrowth of fungi, and parasites. Depending on the lab, a stool analysis can be analyzed via culturing and a MALTI-TOF analysis, or by PCR DNA procedure.

Comprehensive stool analysis. This test includes the stool analysis listed above and adds analysis of food and digestive enzyme production, checks for inflammation of the lining of the intestine, and measures SCFA levels. I generally do this expansive stool analysis with patients who have inflammatory bowel disease, but I do not believe a diabetic patient with no serious gut disease needs this full (and much more expensive) test.

Breath tests. Dysbiosis or maldigestion in the small intestine can be measured with breath tests. The small intestine bacterial overgrowth (SIBO) breath test records if you have one of three colonic microorganisms overgrowing in your small intestine. I only do this test if a patient presents with terrible, daily abdominal bloating. Two other breath tests for the small intestine include testing for lactose or fructose intolerance and are related to the failure to produce enzymes that break down those sugars.

Candida *questionnaire.* This is a two-page detailed questionnaire to help discern if the patient may have a fungal overgrowth. It was created by Dr. William Crook, an innovative MD, whose 1984 book *The Yeast Connection* brought the idea of intestinal overgrowth of yeast into the medical mind-set. Fungi are sometimes difficult to culture, so this questionnaire is another aid in discerning overgrowth.

Intestinal permeability panel. One integrative lab company has a panel that specifically tests for the proteins involved in tight junction regulation—zonulin and occludin—and also antibodies made against endotoxins produced by bacteria in the gut.

Intestinal permeability mannitol/lactulose test. A different integrative lab company has a panel that specifically measures the absorption capacity of the small intestine. A patient drinks a liquid with mannitol and lactulose in it. Mannitol is an easily absorbed sugar, and lactulose is not well absorbed by our intestines. They are both unmetabolized by our bodies and excreted through the urine. When the urine is collected hours later, it is measured for those substances. If both are present in the urine, there is leaky gut, as lactulose should not have come through. If neither are in the urine there is malabsorption and nothing is coming through the gut. If mannitol is in the urine but not lactulose, the intestinal lining is considered healthy and normal.

One concern for integrative physicians treating diabetic patients with low-carb diets is that those diets in and of themselves can have negative effects on the gut bacteria and health. Studies, both on animals and humans, show that a high protein, reduced carbohydrate, weight loss diet promotes microbiome profiles likely to be detrimental to colonic health. I think we need to pay close attention to these studies, because they make great sense. Historically, our ancestors ate enormous amounts of fiber, and we are reducing that substantially in patients by removing grains. And, grain fiber seems to have particular benefits for the gut microbiome, even if patients are eating vegetables. Getting a mixture of soluble and insoluble fibers is good. There are many good fiber powder products available that have no carbohydrate effect on the body and feed the microbiome. I typically use the Whole Food Fiber powder from Standard Process. PaleoFiber by Designs for Health is another good option.

Low-carb diets, due to their lack of grain fiber, have been shown to reduce the levels of bifidobacterium, one of the main beneficial bacteria in our intestines, and also reduce those of a bacteria called *Roseburia / E. rectale*, reductions of which may significantly reduce SCFAs. In two human low-carb diet studies, there was also a reduction in *Bacteriodes*, another main bacteria that transforms fiber into SCFA; these bacteria also help break-down polyphenols, wonderful antioxidants that are activated by gut bacteria, and may be protective against cancer. There were also more hazardous n-nitroso compounds formed, which may increase the risk of colon cancer.

So, since you are on a low-carb diet (I hope) and probably have had some antibiotics in your life, and have eaten some GMO foods and so forth, and may not have the healthiest microbiome, how can we support it and have it once again return to its most beneficial status in your intestines? In a study on rats, when scientists healed the leaky gut of some of the rats, fewer of them developed autoimmune diabetes. Does this mean that ensuring the intestinal linings are healthy in all people will prevent both T1DM and T2DM? One cannot write such a statement as fact. However, there is a growing body of evidence showing that the healthier the gut lining and the less leaky it is, the healthier the intestinal and systemic body and the mind.

Treatment of the Microbiome

A study was conducted on prediabetic and T2DM patients taking a natural product called NM504, which contains inulin (a prebiotic—it provides food for the beneficial bacteria in our gut and produces SCFA), beta glucan (a fiber that makes SCFA, and increases the mucous barrier of the gut), and anthocyanin polyphenols (an antioxidant). At a simple dose of one capsule twice a day, in just four weeks both prediabetic and T2DM patients had improved glucose levels, decreased inflammation, decreased cholesterol, and decreased appetite—just by giving a simple supplement to support the microbiome!

A high-fat diet (as seen, for example, in the low-carb, high-fat ketogenic diet) fed alongside butyrate acid, a key SCFA, to mice, prevented and reversed insulin resistance.

I prefer that my low-carb patients take fiber powder, as it enhances the microbiome, which will then make SCFA. Fiber feeds the beneficial bacteria, making them stronger and more diverse; they break down the fiber into short-chain fatty acids. Just taking butyrate, a SCFA, bypasses the stimulation of beneficial bacteria to colonize, proliferate, and help the body system. I feel all diabetic patients on a low-carb, grain-free diet should absolutely add in a fiber product.

Fiber is also helpful for diabetic patients because it lowers the postmeal excursion, through slowing digestion and absorption of food. It also helps a person feel full, and that can help control appetite. Your physician can also recommend treatments for any positive results from the lab tests mentioned above.

Which fiber? Many of them are fine. Common fiber sources include ground flax seeds, ground chia seeds, psyllium seed, pectin, guar gum, oat or rice bran, triphala (an Indian mixture of belleric myrobalan, amla and chebulic myrobalan), and prune powder. Many products have one or more of these mixed together. Of course, I prefer patients get a straight fiber powder and not something mixed with chemicals, sugars, colorings, or flavorings.

What about probiotics? Probiotics are capsules containing beneficial bacteria for our intestinal tracts. A meta-analysis of human studies on probiotics showed that probiotic supplements can help lower fasting blood glucose, lower fasting insulin, and lower insulin resistance.

Researchers are avidly studying the microbiome to specifically figure out which organisms promote obesity, which promote being lean, which promote autoimmunity, which protect a person from autoimmunity, and which prevent insulin resistance. The key, of course, is to design supplements with key microorganisms in them to specifically treat various conditions. One bacteria, *Lactobacillus gasseri*, was shown to reduce waist and hip circumference in patients. Is that the key? We don't know, really, but companies are now producing supplements with bacteria, including *Lactobacillus gasseri*. I'm sure that in the future we'll have more understanding of which bacteria are best for which person and the condition they have.

It is exciting that the health of the gut is an invaluable tool we can use to help the rest of our body be healthier and perhaps help control a patient's diabetes.

SUMMARY OF HOW TO PROTECT AND HEAL THE GUT MICROBIOME AND INTESTINAL PERMEABILITY

First, let's remove irritants:

Avoid antibiotic use. Your integrative physician can very effectively treat most typical colds, flus, sinus infections, strep throats, and bronchitis without antibiotics.

Avoid alcohol and coffee. These can be irritating to the intestinal tract—do not overdo.

Avoid refined sugar.

Avoid food sensitivities. If you have tested positive for them (especially serum-drawn IgG food sensitivities), avoid those foods for at least one or two months to heal a leaky gut, and then add them in one at a time to find the one or two that might still be problematic.

Avoid over-the-counter and some prescription medicines. For example, NSAIDs, proton pump inhibitors, and so forth.

Avoid genetically modified organisms. Remove them from your food.

Avoid junk foods. Especially fast foods and unhealthy processed foods.

Add in these:

Fermented foods. As discussed in chapter 7, fermented foods are very helpful at building and maintaining a healthy microbiome. They have been shown to reduce intestinal permeability and endotoxins going through the intestinal lining.

Ensure a good daily bowel movement. Everyone should have a good, long, sausage-like bowel movement one or two times a day.

Castor oil packs. Castor oil packs are very good at reducing inflammation and promoting lymphatic flow through the area being treated. They are simple to make and you can buy castor oil kits at many health food stores. The process includes pouring some castor oil onto a flannel cloth and then applying that cloth to your abdomen or liver (wherever your physician directs). Cover the cloth with some plastic covering and then a heating pad. Wrap a towel around all of that and let the pack sit on you for forty-five minutes (or as long as you are told by your physician). This can be done up to seven times a week.

Take supplements:

Fiber powder.

Probiotic. Perhaps containing *Lactobacillus gasseri*, among other species, which is specifically helpful for T2DM patients. *Lactobaccilus reuteri* and *plantarum* (with oat bran) were shown to reduce intestinal permeability. Infants should be given a probiotic that is either entirely *Bifidobacterium*, or at least half *Bifidobacterium*, the main species in the infant gut.

Prebiotic. A prebiotic is food directly for beneficial bacteria in the intestines. Common ones are inulin and fructo-oligosaccharides.

L-glutamine. This is the food of the small intestinal cells. It is contra-indicated in children under three years old, as it can agitate them. Glutamine can be low in patients with diabetes, and it promotes gut mucosal integrity and reduces intestinal permeability. It also lowers inflammation and oxidative injury. It is nice to combine with N-acetyl glucosamine and zinc.

Anti-inflammatories. Cucurmin, *Boswellia*, quercitin.

Demulcents. These soothe and help heal the lining of the intestinal tract: slippery elm powder, marshmallow powder, licorice root, aloe vera juice.

Digestive enzymes. If indicated, helping one's food to be digested better helps the intestine stay healthy and heal.

Colostrum. This has been shown to reduce intestinal permeability. It does contain a small amount of cow or goat dairy in it, depending on the company one gets it from.

Achieving better health for your microbiome may not initially seem to affect your glucose levels at all, and it will not undo established T1DM or T2DM. However research supports that over time, enhancing and healing your gut has systemic effects, such as helping to reduce insulin resistance, lower weight, and reduce the risk of further autoimmunity. If we could identify more pre-T1DM patients, it would be fascinating to see if focusing on healing their intestines would be a continually helpful way of avoiding T1DM or at least seriously extending the time before they manifested T1DM and had to be treated. Helping to digest and absorb nutrients, having a better immune system, having fewer gastrointestinal problems, and stimulating all the other benefits a healthy microbiome promotes in the body and emotions is certainly a worthwhile endeavor.

The Need for Detoxification: Environmental Toxins and Diabetes

Environmental toxins are chemicals and heavy metals scientifically proven to be poisonous to humans (and the world in general). They are found in air, water, food, and many of the household products we buy.

Toxic pollutants are associated with causing neurological and endocrine disturbances and damage in the human body, as well as birth defects, cancer, and many other conditions. As tested by the CDC, most Americans, including newborns, have over two hundred chemicals and their metabolites in their body!

Over one billion pounds of pesticides are sprayed in the United States each year. Moreover, that does not count the amount of toxic chemicals used by unsuspecting consumers in their home cleaning and bug eradication products. Environmental toxins lead to insulin resistance and can increase the risk for autoimmunity, key etiological factors for both T1DM and T2DM.

So, what specifically are the main environmental toxins?

Heavy metals include lead, mercury, arsenic, and numerous other toxic metals (nickel, aluminum, barium, cadmium, tin, and others). Lead, mercury, and arsenic have been shown by the World Health Organization to be etiological risk factors for developing T2DM by causing insulin resistance. Arsenic is found in the soil as a result of mining and is also used in processed wood products, such as the wood used in many backyard decks. It is also found occasionally in poultry and rice. Lead persists in the soil from leaded gasoline and leaded paint, and some old buildings still contain lead pipes.

There are three types of mercury—elemental, organic, and inorganic. Huge sources of mercury in the environment are smokestacks from coal-fired power plants, waste incinerators, and other industrial factories, which send it up into the atmosphere; via rain it comes back down into the ground and waterways that ultimately empty into the oceans. That inorganic type of mercury, the same type as is in dental amalgams, is then converted to organic or methylmercury by bacteria. While all forms of mercury are dangerous, methylmercury is the worst. Via the food chain, methylmercury enters into phytoplankton, which is the food for small fish. Larger fish and sharks eat the small fish, so the bigger fish—tuna, swordfish, shark, and others—contain higher amounts due to the bioaccumulation of mercury in their tissues. Seafood is thus the source of nearly all the methylmercury found in a human body. If we can get the Environmental Protection Agency to regulate mercury emissions from smokestacks, we can begin lowering the human exposure to methylmercury. In the meantime, it's wise, especially for children and pregnant women, to avoid eating tuna fish.

Heavy metals are associated with causing free radical activity and oxidation processes, biochemical actions that cause damage to our body cells. They are linked to premature aging, mood disorders such as depression, chronic fatigue, fibromyalgia, ADD/ADHD disorders, increased cancer mortality, depression or dysregulation of the immune system, learning disabilities, low energy, and increased risk of insulin resistance. However, heavy metals are not the only toxins to be concerned about.

Persistent organic pollutants (POPs) are toxic chemicals that also negatively affect human health, and unfortunately they are all around us. These chemicals are made for or created by the following industries: agriculture, disease control (spraying for mosquitos), manufacturing, and industry. As mentioned earlier, newborn infants have well over two hundred environmental chemicals in their umbilical cord blood and most are neurotoxins. They are called "persistent" because they are resistant to environmental breakdown, so they remain able to harm humans for many, many years. They accumulate in the fatty tissues in humans (lead, on the other hand, is stored in our bones).

Chemicals such as phthalates, all the bisphenols, DDE (dichlorodiphenyldichloroethylene), PCBs (polychlorinated biphenyls), dioxins, PBDFs (polybrominated dibenzofurans), PAHs (polycyclic aromatic hydrocarbons), and polychlorinated dibenzofurans are causing diseases all over the world. They cause developmental defects, endocrine (hormonal) and reproductive dysfunction, cancer, nervous system damage, autoimmunity, and environmental sensitivities.

The Stockholm Convention on Persistent Organic Pollutants, an international treaty signed in 2001 and implemented in 2004, was designed to eliminate or restrict the use of POPs worldwide. The convention created a list of POPs that should be removed or reduced in all countries. Unfortunately, the United

States did not sign that treaty at the time and still hasn't. The United States is still very active in producing, using, and globally selling these dangerous chemicals, although a few of them, like DDT, have been prohibited.

In multiple studies these chemicals have been clearly correlated with T2DM. They can promote fatty oxidation, increase inflammation, and cause mitochondrial damage, all leading to insulin resistance. The website Diabetes and the Environment (www.diabetesandenvironment.org) is home to facts and discussions concerning the association between environmental toxins and increasing rates of T1DM, T2DM, and obesity. Its author, Sarah Howard, who developed T1DM in her early thirties and then saw her son also develop it, is the national coordinator for the Collaborative on Health and the Environment's Diabetes-Obesity Spectrum Working Group.

In one telling study, researchers analyzed two groups of obese people; one group had T2DM and the other group did not have diabetes. They found the one main difference between the two groups was that the diabetic group contained significantly more environmental toxins in their body fat than the nondiabetic group. This clearly substantiates that the more toxins in one's body fat, the higher the risk for insulin resistance, being overweight, and developing diabetes.

A 2013 study in *Diabetes Care* showed that young adults with high mercury exposure had an elevated risk of developing diabetes later in life. There are many other studies also proving this. A study in Germany showed that air pollution was associated with developing diabetes. Therefore it is important for your physician to help determine if you are at risk of toxins in your system having, potentially, some effect on your glucose regulation. A good intake with a cognizant physician should include asking you:

- Where did you grow up? In a rural or urban environment? If rural, were you near farms that sprayed their crops with chemicals?
- What jobs have you had, and did any expose you to toxins or chemicals?
- Have you hired exterminators or have you yourself sprayed pesticides or herbicides inside or outside of your home?
- When was your house built? If new, was it made with "green," nontoxic materials?

- If older, was your house ever refurbished or renovated, and if so, were nontoxic materials used?
- What types of cleaning products do you use in your home?
- Do you experience any sensitivity around the odors of perfumes, detergents, gasoline, tobacco, new paint, new carpeting, new cars, or other chemicals, including headaches, dizziness, muscle pain, weakness, lack of concentration, rashes, or other problems?
- Do you smoke?
- Do you have silicon breast implants?
- Do you use plastic water bottles, or store or microwave food in plastic containers?

All of these questions can be used to evaluate if environmental toxins may indeed play a part in your diabetes. In addition, your diet diary can help uncover if you mostly eat processed, agri-industry food, or if you eat whole, organic foods.

Considering toxin overload makes sense for prediabetic patients, as well—to uncover all the reasons their glucose is becoming imbalanced.

I am most suspicious of environmental chemicals burdening a body when weight loss stalls. Many environmental chemicals are stored in body fat (lead is stored in bones). Losing weight means the fat in fat cells is being burned, and it is consequently releasing environmental toxins into the bloodstream. Research has shown that as a person loses weight and burns fat, their plasma pollutant levels rise. Since those chemicals can produce insulin resistance, I believe that might very well be a reason why people sometimes attain a weight loss level but then plateau, with more weight to lose, and cannot easily continue weight loss. It's a theory, but it makes sense.

Other common symptoms of the body's release of environmental toxins may include "brain fog" (difficulties focusing and concentrating), muscle pain, joint pain, numbness or tingling in extremities, fatigue, sensitivities to smells, headaches, hormonal imbalances, neurological diseases, mood changes, food allergies, behavioral problems, and others.

So, when a patient is losing weight on their comprehensive protocol and then reaches a plateau, I often consider that the increased release of environmental toxins may be interfering with their weight loss. It is logical to include a method to efficiently detoxify released toxins from fat cells as part of a comprehensive diabetic protocol in overweight or obese patients.

How do we go about diagnosing a person with environmental toxicity? There are a variety of tests, the gold standard of which is a biopsy of your fat that is sent away to a lab for investigation of all the chemicals it contains. However, a fat biopsy is expensive, invasive, and not ideal for clinical use. Integrative physicians will commonly use one or more of the following tests:

Heavy metal urine test. This test includes both a baseline urine analysis and a urine analysis after having taken a chelating agent that binds to heavy metals and helps remove them from your body via stool and urination.

Heavy metal analysis of fecal material (for children). It is best not to do a hair analysis, which uses more archaic technology than those for urine and stool.

Whole blood, serum, and urine assessment of numerous toxic chemicals.

Individual serum panels of specific types of toxins (e.g., bisphenol A [BPA], chlorinated pesticide panel, organophosphates, PCBs, volatile solvents profile). These can quickly become very expensive for patients, and if a certain panel is drawn and is negative for those chemicals, it doesn't mean the patient doesn't have other chemicals that are not tested in them.

Detoxigenomic profile. This test measures genetic enzymes involved in detoxification and sees if a patient has mutations making those enzymes hypoactive or inactive.

Genetic analysis. This inner mouth swab can be done to give a rough idea of how well, genetically, your body may (or may not) be detoxifying in certain pathways.

Environmental sensitivities. Learning if a patient is environmentally sensitive to tobacco smoke, perfumes, gasoline, new car or carpet smell, and other odoriferous effluvia ripe with toxic pollutants is a guide to toxic burden levels.

Toxins are released from the body via the bowel movements, liver, skin (via sweating), lungs, and the kidneys and bladder; if those organs are strong and supported by the patient's physician, weight loss might well proceed smoothly, without any plateau occurring. This requires that any protocol must:

Aid defecation. Ensure the patient has at least one good bowel movement a day. I do not believe a person should defecate after each meal, but every day a person should have an easy-to-pass, complete, colon-emptying bowel movement.

Aid sweating. A good sweat has been shown to release both heavy metals and POPs through the skin. It is a highly effective way to cleanse the body of toxins, and I am a huge advocate of regular sweating. People should have a good sweat four to five times a week, whether through exercising and other physical activities, or saunas. Wear enough clothes when working out to ensure you soak your top. Many gyms have saunas in them, and you can also buy one for home use, as well. The best ones are infrared, and cedar is a common wood used to make them. There are also portable infrared saunas that are quite inexpensive. Both dry and steam saunas are effective, but you must get clearance from your physician before beginning to use a sauna to ensure it is safe for you. A typical length of time in a sauna is five to twenty minutes and one needs to follow it with a thirty- to sixty-second cold shower to reenergize the body. Start at shorter times and slowly increase. Skin brushing is also a good way to keep the skin fresh and healthy so that it can detox better. Brushing removes dead cells but also stimulates the lymph nodes under the skin, and they also aid in detoxification.

Aid urination. Many toxins are excreted through the kidneys and bladder. Ensuring fluid intake is correct and urination is consistent throughout the day is important. Parsley, watermelon, dandelion leaf, and vitamin B_6 are natural diuretics. In general, a person should drink half their body weight in ounces a day, and more if some of the beverages the patient drinks increase fluid loss, such as coffee, black tea, alcohol, or soda pop. So a person weighing 180 pounds should drink 90 ounces, or around 3 liters, of fluid a day. You should also drink more if you are sweating a lot.

Aid liver support. There are numerous ways to help the liver detoxify. Removing extra toxins like caffeine, over-the-counter medications (such as acetominophen or nicotine), soda pop, alcohol, prescription medicines (if possible), home chemicals, food additives, and tobacco smoke, is a great start. Cruciferous vegetables such as broccoli, cauliflower, Brussels sprouts, kale, cabbage; sulfurous vegetables such as onion and garlic; bitter foods such as radicchio, arugula, chicory; bile promoters such as beets and artichokes—all of these help the liver work and detox better. There are also supplements that are specifically oriented to helping the liver's detoxification pathways: milk thistle, dandelion root (dandelion leaf is good for the kidneys), R-alpha-lipoic acid, N-acetyl cysteine, curcumin, and *Coriolous versicolor* are good, safe starting nutrients to take. Check with your physician before taking any of them.

Detoxification is currently trendy, and many patients are interested in detoxification protocols. There are many different ways to detoxify one's body, and it is important to work with your integrative physician to ensure that the best protocol for you is chosen—one that is safe, effective, and fits within your budget.

Of course, remember that doing a detox only to reengage in activities, food, medications, lifestyle habits, and so forth that once again bring toxins into your body is somewhat futile. For example, if you have pesticides or herbicides sprayed in your yard and, even worse, in your home—or you do it yourself—there seems to be little point in engaging in a detoxification program! However, if you decide it's time to get an organic exterminator, or just pull weeds by hand, then detoxing makes sense. It is best to commit to making serious changes before the detox, so your life is cleaner overall.

Other ways to clean up your life and reduce exposure to toxins include:

- Stop smoking!
- Learn to eat whole, organic foods and avoid processed, agri-industry foods and meats. Consult the Environmental Working Group's Clean Fifteen and Dirty Dozen lists and Seafood Watch's seafood guide.
- Consider removing metal amalgams from your mouth.

- Remove all toxic and scented cleaners, detergents, fabric dryer sheets, air fresheners, potpourris, perfumes, and colognes from your home.
- Use only nontoxic cleaners, and organic personal care products. Avoid toxic toiletries like typical makeups, shampoos, and toothpaste.
- Avoid DEET bug sprays and use healthier versions, even if you need to reapply them more often. Avoid buying clothes with DEET in them.
- Avoid all pesticides, fungicides, herbicides, and nonorganic fertilizers. Use natural methods like diatomaceous earth and boric acid. There is an organic exterminator I've used who uses concentrated peppermint oil outside my home. Do not listen to any exterminator who says what they are spraying is organic because it is made from chrysanthemums; very toxic chemicals called pyrethrins are made from chrysanthemums. They are, essentially, not being truthful about what they are spraying. Also, do not believe that popular chemicals sold in stores are safe, either, even if a landscaper wishes to convince you of that.
- Always use "green" items to refurbish or redecorate your home. Do not use volatile organic compound (VOC) paints; use green flooring such as tile, bamboo, and green carpet and carpet glue, green mattresses, and green cabinets.
- Use water filters to clean the water you drink, cook with, and shower in, and measure your water's pH to see if it is excessively acidic. For example, have a reverse osmosis filter under your sink and install shower filters; or you can also add whole home filters on the main plumbing line. I like having home filters instead of relying on endless plastic store-bought water bottles; those are an environmental waste problem, even if you put them in the recycling bin. The less plastic used, the better. *Nota Bene:* If you are using reverse osmosis, you need to add in a mineral supplement, as minerals are removed through that type of filter, too. I do not recommend using distilled water. Carbon filters are a good start.

- Use a hepa air filter in your home. The best ones to consider are Austin Air, Blue Air, and IQ Air. Also, open windows when you can; inside home air is more toxic than outside air, even in cities.
- Use reusable glass water bottles for drinking instead of plastic bottles. Do not store foods in plastic, and do not cook foods in plastic.
- Wear only natural fiber clothing: 100 percent cotton, linen, wool, or silk. Do not buy clothes that are permanent press or wrinkle resistant, as these clothes are treated with formaldehyde that doesn't wash out. Do not wear clothes with bug repellent added to them.
- Avoid buying homes under power lines, to avoid being near strong electromagnetic fields.

Patients who have already developed T1DM and T2DM sometimes ask their integrative practitioner if doing a detox protocol can reverse or cure their diabetes. Unfortunately, it cannot, but removing toxins may theoretically help *prevent* the onset of both, and it would be great for future research to study if reducing a body's toxic burden also reduces the onset of T1DM or T2DM. For patients with diabetes, removing toxins may help reduce glucose numbers and insulin resistance; enable continual weight loss; prevent the development of chronic disease, including hormonal, reproductive, or neurological diseases; reduce the risk of autoimmunity or prevent further autoimmunity diseases from occurring; reduce the risk of cancer, which poorly controlled diabetic patients are at elevated risk of developing; promote social awareness of a cleaner environment and encourage companies to be more green; and protect children (and pets!) from being exposed to chemical and heavy metal toxins. It is important to live in a cleaner home, work in a cleaner office, have a cleaner body and a cleaner world, and teach family and friends to promote the same.

Standard Detoxification Protocol

In the standard detoxification protocol practiced by many integrative physicians (including me), which was created by Dr. Walter Crinnion, a naturopathic physician, we first use the urine test described earlier to see if you require detoxification. This needs to be approved and directed by your physician. Then, the complicated, complex cleansing regimen consists of four components:

Urine test. Perform a urine heavy metal analysis test, including a creatinine clearance test.

Chelation. If positive for significant heavy metal toxicity, a chelator product is dosed, which actively grabs the toxins from cells and moves them to a channel for excretion. The main chelators used are oral DMSA (Chemet / 2,3 dimercaptosuccinic acid, a prescription drug) or DMPS (2,3-dimercaptopropane-1-sulfonate). Introvenous EDTA, ethylenediaminetetraacetic acid, is another. They are used singly or combined. At the end of each three- to five-day chelator session (or at the beginning, depending on how your physician directs), it's recommended for patients to take a liver detox promoter and then do a colonic.

Replenish. Between chelation sessions there are typically nine, plus or minus, days of replenishment. During these days a few additional supplements are added in to build up nutrients.

Repetition. The cycles of chelating and replenishing are repeated five times and then the urine analysis is repeated. Cycles and testing continue until the toxin levels come back within safe limits.

During chelation, supplements taken include chelated product, hydrolyzed whey protein, fiber product, detox support product, vitamin C, liver support (N-acetyl cysteine, milk thistle, and other multiple ingredient products). In between chelation sessions, supplements taken include hydrolyzed whey protein, fiber product, detox support product, vitamin C, liver support product, multiple vitamin mineral, extra mineral product, fish oils, and probiotics.

There are some possible adverse reactions to both the DMSA and the detox protocol, including fatigue, irritability, hive-like skin reactions, allergy, or poor detoxification reaction to the chelator. If you are sensitive to sulfurous foods or products, such as eggs, onion, garlic, or broccoli, or to foods, supplements, or medications containing sulfur, your physician will probably not recommend products containing DMSA/DMPS.

While effective for many patients, this protocol is expensive, is time-consuming, and requires much supplementation. Let's talk about other options.

Product-Supported Detoxification

If the length, complexity, and cost of the standard detox protocol is not feasible, a three-week product detoxification is a less intensive, less comprehensive regimen that is more accessible for most patients. There are many companies that produce comprehensive cleansing protocols that are designed to help patients detox for generally around three weeks. This process probably will not be as comprehensive as the above standard protocol, but it can do some good, and it can also help a patient realize the impact of environmental toxins and how to avoid them.

In this simpler protocol there is no urine testing and no chelation. The goal is to eat a pure diet, avoiding all junk food and common food sensitivities, while stimulating the gut and liver for detoxification. The diets in these protocols are very clean and clearly described and organized.

An integrative physician can guide a patient through these types of programs. UltraClear, a product from Thorne, comes with a brochure clearly describing the methodology. It combines eating diabetic-friendly meals alongside a powdered drink and then, in the middle of the program, drinking just the powder for a few days before adding food back in. I particularly like a protocol from a company called Standard Process, because it contains a lovely hardcover book, including loads of recipes and great information, a helpful explanatory brochure, a healthy shake, a nonlaxative liver cleanse product, a fiber product, and a green food powder. There is a specific methodology for using each of the products during the entirety of the detox. Designs for Health also has a fourteen- or twenty-one-day detoxification program, including a food guide, powder, and supplements.

For patients for whom the more expensive, longer, and more involved protocol is not going to work, and who are wary of fasting, these programs can set the stage for beginning a gentle but effective detoxification. All my patients lose weight on them, break bad eating habits, get new meals established in their diet, and increase their energy.

Fasting

Fasting is an ancient and incredibly effective method for detoxification. Sick pets and children, for example, tend naturally to rest and not eat. In the naturopathic profession, we believe all illness begins in the intestinal tract: what we eat and how we digest it, absorb it, metabolize it, and excrete it. If our food is poor or we overeat, or our gut is unhealthy, or our digestion is faulty, as discussed in the microbiome section, it's possible for us to develop bacterial endotoxins in our gut that are absorbed into our body. These toxins can settle in our tissues and cause damage all over our body, stimulating inflammatory pathways. Fasting, or resting the gut, can help heal the intestinal lining and allow the body to initiate healing and detoxification in cells. As a result, many conditions can be healed. I am an advocate of fasting when it is safe for patients.

There are two main ways to go about a longer fast: using water or using vegetable juice. During the fast nothing else is typically ingested, aside from herbal teas.

We discussed intermittent fasting (IF) in the diet chapter, when a person doesn't eat from supper to breakfast and reduces caloric intake or fasts for one to two days a week or several days a month. Fasting to cleanse the body has some similar benefits as the IF—lower glucose and inflammation, reduced blood pressure, weight loss—but the key with detox fasting is to do it for a longer time, usually between three and twenty-one days, to initiate cleansing of the body and healing of tissues.

Which type of diabetic patients can fast? Fasting is best for most, but not all, T2DM patients—either on only oral meds or just basal insulin—as it can break the habit of eating carbohydrates and can reset appetite and food cravings to healthier foods. It can also initiate some weight loss that can be continued after the fast on the diabetic protocol. It reduces systemic toxins and increases energy and vitality and can have a huge benefit on lowering or even eradicating high blood pressure. Any T2DM patient must be cleared to fast by his physician and must work with an accessible physician whom he can easily contact as needed. I do not advocate that anyone reading this book should engage in this type of treatment on their own!

I would not fast a pediatric patient; children should not be therapeutically fasted (unless they are sick with a fever and naturally have no appetite for a day or two). I also do not recommend fasting a T1DM patient who is on basal/bolus insulin. A pregnant or nursing woman should not fast. A fast should also not be done by someone who is anemic, has cancer, is frail, has liver or kidney failure or some other serious condition. And finally, I would not push a fast on someone who did not want to do one; it's everyone's own choice.

If you are thinking of doing a fast, the first thing to do is make sure you really want to! Then discuss it with your medical practitioner, who will advise if it is appropriate in your case and will guide you through it. Be sure to understand your protocol's specific rules and adjust your life's schedule, if necessary, so you will be successful. If doing a juice fast, invest in a juicer for home use. Use organic produce as much as possible. Lastly, and this is important, be willing to slow down your life during the fast. You cannot work full time and do all the shopping, exercise, and so forth on a fast. The key to a fast is to slow down and allow your gut to rest, so all the energy your body makes is devoted to detoxification and healing. If you continue to live life at full speed, the fast may be a failure.

The first two or three days of a fast are the most unpleasant. Signs and symptoms of detoxification can include hunger, irritability, headache, bad breath, and low energy. After the first difficult days, natural processes kick in that reduce or stop hunger and bring you energy and alertness. People start making ketones, the same fat breakdown products seen on a low-carb, high-fat ketogenic diet.

There are many benefits to fasting: detoxification; healing, rejuvenation and repair of body cells; fewer food cravings; helping the body become more alkaline; balancing of body biochemistry and hormones; reducing inflammation; increased energy; mental clarity; and emotional balance and heightened spirituality.

A key part of fasting is deciding beforehand how long your fast will be—two days, three days, seven days, ten days, fourteen days, twenty-one days, or however long you are motivated to fast. Having the psychological edge of having an end date can be helpful going into it. However, it's also important to be flexible enough to stop a fast if you or your physician do not feel it is safe anymore.

During both water and juice fasts, you usually do not need to take most supplements, but your medical practitioner will decide which ones you can stop or should continue taking. Continue taking your medications as your physician has prescribed, but you may need to reduce or stop some of them, particularly oral hypoglycemic agents, basal insulin, and hypertension medications, depending on the length of the fast and your individual response. This is why you need to get approval to fast and stay in close contact with your physician if you are on prescription medications. If you develop any unexpected signs or symptoms, please call your physician right away.

Pre-Fast Diet

It is nice to prepare the gut for the fast by modifying your standard diet. Focusing on high-fiber foods; starting better liver, gallbladder, and intestinal detoxification; and beginning to eat healthier are great ways to initiate your commitment to and excitement about the fast. Do this pre-fast diet for two to three days before beginning the actual fast, once your physician has approved it.

DAILY PRE-FAST PROTOCOL

1. Start your day with three tablespoons of extra virgin olive oil, one or two cloves of garlic (crushed or minced), and the juice of one lemon. Mix with water if desired.
2. Thirty minutes later, have one scoop of a fiber product, and one capsule of a mixture of wormwood and aloe vera with between eight and sixteen ounces of water. These very bitter herbs stimulate bile secretion, and toxins are released through the bile via the liver. The herbs then promote a gentle bowel movement.
3. Thirty minutes later, eat a breakfast of two cooked eggs or an almond pancake or muffin. Drink herbal tea and water.
4. For lunch, eat all vegetables: a large bowl of salad with lettuce, spinach, half a bell pepper, one celery stick, a small tomato, half a cucumber, sprouts, one or two green onions, and one to two tablespoons of sunflower seeds (or other nuts or seeds). For dressing, you can use oil and vinegar or lemon juice, garlic, and herbs. If you wish to use other vegetables in the salad, that is fine.
5. Before supper, repeat fiber, bitter herb capsules, and water supplementation.

6. For supper, eat all vegetables. You may repeat the lunch salad or cook some veggies, such as broccoli, cauliflower, cabbage, or Brussels sprouts.
7. Between-meal snacks can include raw vegetables, raw nuts, or protein powder with water or unsweetened nut milk.
8. You should drink half your body weight in ounces of water or herbal teas a day.
9. It is best to start this diet on a day off, not on a workday.
10. If you are too hungry to only do this low-calorie diet, you can add another nut "grain" product at meals, or eat more nuts or eggs.

Water Fasting

I do not do much water fasting with my patients, as it is quite intense and safe only to do for up to a week outside of a clinic. Most patients prefer, and can only do, three days. During this fast, you just drink water and herbal tea, and rest; you should not go to work or work out or run around doing errands or do a full cleaning of your home, among other things. Avoid news and anything violent or upsetting. You should spend your time reading; giving yourself short, gentle washes; listening to relaxing music; meditating; journaling; praying; doing skin brushing; sunbathing; or going on short walks at an easy pace. Have friends over for interesting conversation. Get a massage. Do a short sauna, followed by a brief cold shower.

I feel the maximum safe duration for a water fast outside of a clinic is seven days; I do not want my patients going any longer than that on only water. For longer fasts for sicker people, there is a clinic called True North Health Center in Santa Rosa, California (www.healthpromoting.com) that helps patients do water fasting for up to a month under close medical supervision. Water fasting can help reverse, or help gain control of, T2DM. It has proven in studies to cure hypertension and has been used to treat patients with many other chronic conditions, such as lupus and rheumatoid arthritis.

I do not do or recommend water fasting for T1DM patients, only for T2DM patients. During a water fast it is vitally important to continually record your glucose and blood pressure numbers all day every day, and to stay in close contact with your physician. Obviously, insulin and oral meds may need to be significantly reduced or even stopped. Be aware of hypoglycemic signs and symptoms

Enemas

The use of enemas, and whether or not they are necessary, is a debated issue in fasting circles. During a longer fast it is very common for bowel movements to slow down or even stop, as the gut is resting and the peristalsis movement of the colon is reduced. Patients can, of course, decide if they will or will not engage in enemas. I prefer my patients to do a lemon juice and warm water enema or coffee enema (the most detoxifying enema) each morning of a fast, but most do not choose to do so, and that is fine. It is solely their choice. Many will do an enema once or twice a week, though. It is not a deal-breaker; detoxification can still be valuable and effective without doing enemas, though many of us feel an enema enhances the fast. Do not do any enemas unless your physician allows you to do so and has done a physical exam ensuring the procedure is safe for you.

HOW TO DO AN ENEMA

1. Buy a two-quart silicone enema bag or a stainless steel enema bucket, silicone housing, and insertion tube/nozzle that is at least four inches long. You can hang it from a towel rack or door knob; hang it at least three feet from the floor.
2. Use fluid close to body temperature—fluid too cold or too hot will stimulate evacuation of enema water too soon. The ideal time to hold the enema in is between five and fifteen minutes.
3. Use olive/coconut oil, KY Jelly, or herbal salves for lubrication of the end of the speculum.
4. Insert speculum slowly and gently into your anus and release clamp on the hose and allow as much solution as possible to enter. You can hold your knees to your chest, or lie on your back or side to receive the enema fluid, whichever is more comfortable for you.
5. After the solution has entered, remove the speculum, and lie in a comfortable position, gently massaging your lower

intestine. When you feel the need to defecate, get up and do so in the toilet. You may need to defecate again soon after. Do not share your enema bag with anyone else!

ENEMA SOLUTIONS

There are many different types of enema solutions a patient and physician can choose from:

Lemon juice and water. Mix one quarter to a half cup of lemon juice in two quarts of water. This is a gentle enema that uses lemon juice to stimulate bile production.

Coffee enema (best used early in the morning and if you are not overly sensitive to caffeine). Do not use if you have angina, high blood pressure, or heart disease. Ensure your physician approves using this enema. The coffee enema is a well-known detoxifying enema, made famous by the Gerson cancer therapy. Coffee is absorbed by the veins in the colon and goes to the liver, which stimulates bile production, enhancing detoxification through the liver. The recipe uses four tablespoons of ground organic light roast coffee beans (not instant) and one quart of water. Put the water in a pan and bring to boil, then add the coffee and let boil for five minutes. Let the water cool down to tepid, so you can comfortably touch it with your finger. In fact, it's good to prepare it at night and let it sit overnight for use in the morning at room temperature. Strain it through a coffee filter into a two-quart container. From that container pour into the enema bag. With the coffee enema, you can insert it all at one time and hold it ideally for ten minutes and then release on the toilet. However, another effective way is for you to insert half the bag and then clamp it off. Hold it as long as possible, at least five and up to fifteen minutes, and then use the toilet. Lie back down and then insert the second half for the same process again.

Lactobacillus acidophilus *enema.* Mix two tablespoons of plain yogurt (dairy, goat, or soy) or one hundred billion probiotic blends, into two quarts water.

Wheatgrass enema. Mix one to two ounces of fresh wheatgrass mixed into two quarts of water.

Colonic. One may do a colonic during a fast. However, ensure that your physician approves of you doing a colonic (you should have a medical exam beforehand), and ensure you and your physician trust the place and colon therapist where you would receive it.

Again, enemas are optional. If you choose to only do one, or you don't do any, the fast is still worthwhile.

and ensure you feel confident in dealing with any hypoglycemia before beginning any fast. Also, be aware of blood pressure reducing—at times, dramatically. If you feel dizzy or light-headed standing up, your blood pressure may be getting too low. Sometimes this is a reason to end the fast in some people.

Vegetable Juice Fasting

If approved by your physician, you can fast for up to three weeks on the juice fast, and continue to live your life in pretty much the same manner—you can work and go about your life, but cutting back on activities, especially avoiding intense exercise, is still important. Don't work twelve hour days six days a week on a fast! It would be good to have some quiet time each day for rest, relaxation, contemplation, and introspection, and to avoid noisy, crowded places, disruptive people, and violent or disturbing media, as well as phones, computers, email, and other electronic devices. Going for walks or doing yoga or Tai Chi fits in quite well with a fast.

Juice fasting consists of drinking vegetable juices, water, and herbal teas for as long as you are motivated to and feel physically strong. You will be drinking up to five liters of vegetable juices a day, but none with any citrus or tomato juices or with added sugar or chemicals in them. Excellent resources for juice recipes include *The Juicing Book*, by Stephen Blauer, and *The Fasting Diet*, by Dr. Steve Bailey, and many websites have helpful juice-fasting recipes. I've seen patients on two hypertensive medications get off both during juice fasts of ten days, and one year later they were still normotensive. A couple enjoyed the fast so much they decided to do a one-day juice fast regularly each month.

I will repeat, as it is just as important with juice fasting as it is with water fasting: It is vitally important on a juice fast to continually record your glucose and blood pressure numbers all day every day and stay in close contact with your physician. Obviously, insulin and oral meds may need to be significantly reduced or even stopped. Be aware of hypoglycemic signs and symptoms and ensure you feel confident in dealing with any hypoglycemia before beginning any fast. Also, be aware of blood pressure reducing—at times, dramatically. If you feel dizzy or light-headed standing up, your blood pressure may be getting too low. Sometimes this is a reason to end the fast in some people.

Breaking the Fast

A famous fasting adage: "Any idiot can stop eating, but it takes a wise man to break the fast correctly." Of course, I am not saying anyone doing a fast is an idiot—absolutely not! If it is a safe procedure for you to do, you would be very smart to fast even a few days at least once per year for a great detoxification process, but how your fast is broken is extremely important. It has to be broken safely and healthily.

Breaking a fast can be the hardest part of the process. You can get used to not eating, but when your mind and stomach decide it is time to eat again and yet you cannot do so fully for a few days, that can test your discipline.

As I've mentioned, when you fast, your intestinal movements slow considerably and so when you start to eat again, at first food cannot be digested well, as your sleeping digestive tract has to turn back on and get back up to normal speed. This digestive process takes time, and the longer you've fasted, the longer it takes. It is not healthy to eat when the gut cannot move; after all, when a patient has intestinal surgery,

KEY TREATMENT NOTE

Environmental toxins are associated with being a strong etiological factor for insulin resistance and autoimmune disease, and an integrative physician can help guide diabetic patients into living a less toxic life, and can decide if any detox protocol is safe, responsible, and effective. Do not do any detox protocol or any fast without your physician's knowledge, approval, and guidance.

the patient is not allowed to put anything into their intestines after they wake up until their gut shows movement, and that can take a few days. Putting food into a poorly functional gut is a bad idea! This is why it is very important to introduce food slowly into the gut and make sure the initial food is full of fiber, to kick in the natural peristalsis action.

The most important rules in breaking a fast are to slowly introduce foods and especially to not overeat. Eat slowly and chew your food extremely well. Watch your glucose numbers very closely with food reintroduction.

DAY BY DAY DIABETIC FOOD REINTRODUCTION

Day one. Vegetables for breakfast, lunch, and supper, either cooked or raw. Vegetable soups are good. You may add in a nut flour "grain" product at meals.

Day two. Vegetables for breakfast, lunch, and supper and nut flour "grains." Can add in smoothies with protein powder, unsweetened alternative milk, with vegetables, avocados, healthy oil, and acceptable sweetener.

Day three. Vegetables for breakfast, lunch, and supper; smoothies, nuts, seed and nut butter, and organic soy. Can add in animal protein such as fish, poultry, meat, and eggs at two meals.

Day four. You can eat normally on your low-carb diet.

Detoxification Summary

I do not prescribe detoxification protocols with all patients. Detoxification is very effective with prediabetic patients, as it can significantly curb their sugar cravings, reduce their high blood pressure, make them less insulin resistant, increase their energy, reduce their toxic burden, and initiate weight loss. For patients with diabetes, it can be a valuable addition to a protocol, especially if the patient presents with clear signs and symptoms that the toxic world is truly having an immediate effect on their diabetes or concurrent problems such as hypertension.

Even if we do not do a fast or more serious detoxification regimen, "tidying up" our lives is valuable to every single one of us. The fewer toxins we are exposed to, expecially those that we have control over avoiding, the better it is for us, our families, and the world.

— CHAPTER TEN —

The Seventh Essential: Diabetes Supplementation

I want to first start off this chapter by stating that supplements are *not* miracle cures! They are vital but not a panacea. They have a decided place in managing diabetes but, in and of themselves, do not reverse diabetes or cure it.

We call them supplements because they are designed to *supplement a comprehensive protocol* and are just one element of care. If your diet is high in carbs, you are sleeping poorly, or you do not exercise, supplements will be significantly less helpful than if they are added to a regimen that is comprehensively designed by itself to help control glucose levels.

Medications have stronger effects than supplements on the body. If you are on insulin and eating a high-carb diet and you switch to a low-carb diet, you will need to immediately reduce your insulin dosing. Adding in supplements to your protocol does not have a drastic effect on glucose levels or insulin needs. It should be safe to add supplements to anyone's protocol, including adults, children with T1DM, and seniors with T2DM. However, you should not add supplements into your protocol without the clear and helpful direction of an integrative physician who understands you, your health, the medicines you are on, and the reactions you might suffer from. You should work with someone who ensures you get the exact supplements at the correct dosages, in a safe, responsible way.

The categories of the supplements I will be discussing include vitamins and minerals (the essential nutrients in foods your body needs to ingest daily to have it work in good order); essential dietary fats; botanicals, that is, herbs from many different countries; and, nutraceuticals, which are other supplements that don't fit in the previous categories, such as amino acids and antioxidants.

Many conventionally treated patients with diabetes are not on supplements. Why is that? I think it is because conventional medicine does not recommend the use of supplements in patients with diabetes outside of treating actual nutrient deficiencies. The ADA has a very odd view of supplements. The ADA sponsors a highly respected peer-reviewed diabetes journal called *Diabetes Care*, and this journal regularly publishes studies on the benefits of supplements, vitamins, minerals, nutraceuticals, and botanicals. Yet, here is a direct quote from the ADA describing their position on using supplements: "There is no clear evidence of benefit from vitamin or mineral supplements for people with diabetes who do not have underlying vitamin or mineral deficiencies. Nor is there evidence to support the use of cinnamon or other herbs or supplements for the treatment of diabetes."

The fallacy of the ADA's opinion on supplements is that many, many studies have shown the positive benefits of diabetic patients taking supplements. An integrative physician such as I am feels very comfortable recommending supplements to all diabetic patients, as science is supportive, and so is my clinical experience.

The following list describes why a patient should take supplements as part of an effective diabetes protocol:

Antioxidants. Many supplements are antioxidants. Damage to a diabetic body from years of high glucose levels can cause the development of diabetic complications due to pro-oxidative biochemical pathways. As you have learned, an A1C over 5.5 percent means damage of some sort may likely be occurring in diabetic cells. Taking antioxidant supplementation can help your body stop rampant oxidative damage. In chapter 14 I'll discuss how many natural supplements have been proven medically beneficial to patients with fatty liver, retinopathy, nephropathy, and neuropathy.

Deficiencies. Many people in America, including diabetic patients, are nutrient deficient. High serum glucose can cause the loss of many

KEY TREATMENT NOTE

All integrative physicians recommend appropriate diabetic supplements to their patients. Ensure what you are taking is approved by your physician and is the best quality at the best price.

nutrients—such as zinc, chromium, and magnesium—from the body through the kidneys, and some medications that patients take (for example, metformin and proton pump inhibitors) can cause nutrient deficiencies by reducing absorption in the gut. In addition, the unhealthy diet many T2DM patients have eaten for years may have been deficient in essential fatty acids, vitamin D_3, and other nutrients. Many nutrients are needed to help control glucose regulation. Taking daily nutrients can help ensure all deficiencies are corrected, allowing a body to run more efficiently.

Improved glucose control. Some supplements have good data showing that they can be beneficial in decreasing insulin resistance at the cellular level, enabling glucose to enter into the cells easier, and helping to lower A1Cs over time. Studies have shown that supplements can help lower fasting and after-meal glucose, lower A1C values, and lower cholesterol and triglycerides. Supplements can also help reduce the frequency of hypoglycemic and hyperglycemic events.

Reduced appetite and cravings. Some supplements can be very helpful in reducing cravings for food, especially for carbohydrates.

Improved energy and mood. Nutrients can help elevate energy and mood in several ways. Fluctuating glucose levels all day can cause irritability and other unstable moods, and feeling like a victim to diabetes instead of a victor over it can negatively affect self-esteem. Nutrients such as omega-3 oils and bioavailable folic acid are both associated with helping to reduce depression and anxiety. Nutrients can help increase energy by supplying cells with all they need to work better.

Help with weight loss. This is more of an indirect than a direct effect. If a patient is eating healthier, does not have cravings, has good energy and mood, and has lower glucose levels, the patient will be able to lose weight much more quickly and effectively.

Preventing Type 1 Diabetes

Finland has the highest per capita occurrence of T1DM in the world. As a result researchers in Finland, and in other countries, have done some leading-edge studies focused on which supplements can be used with infants to help reduce the risk of developing T1DM later in their lives. Two main nutrients, fish oils and vitamin D_3, were highlighted in these studies. Probiotics have also been shown to be helpful.

Fish Oils

People taking the highest levels of fish oils were shown to have a 55 percent reduced risk of developing T1DM. Fish oils do many good things in the body, including lower the risk of developing autoimmune diseases. Fish oils are good for pregnant moms because they significantly reduce postpartum depression. Fish oils contain eicosapentanoic acid (EPA), and docosahexanoic acid (DHA). EPA and DHA are strikingly anti-inflammatory.

With newborns, a breastfeeding mom can ingest fish oils and the child will receive the EPA and DHA through the breast milk. Once a child is weaned, it's easy to give tasty fish oil to the child each day, which will also help with brain and cognitive development. There are many flavored fish oil products, although avoid gummies with added refined sugar. Fish oils can be found in capsules or liquids. I suggest dosing around 350 mg EPA and 220 mg DHA for infants; 700 mg EPA and 440 mg DHA in children up to ten years old; and 1,000 mg EPA and 750 mg DHA for older children and adults. However, follow what your physician recommends. Read labels to ensure your fish oil capsule is replete enough in EPA and DHA that only two or three capsules a day are needed. Do not look at the fish oil content, but specifically find the EPA and DHA content. Ensure your fish oil company fully verifies their oil product is free from mercury, dioxins, and other environmental toxins.

Vitamin D_3

In one study, children given vitamin D_3 had a 30 percent lower risk of developing T1DM. Another study explained that vitamin D_3 is needed for insulin synthesis, secretion, and sensitivity, and it showed a deficiency in vitamin D_3 was associated with an increase in developing both T1DM and T2DM. An infant can safely take 1,000 IU vitamin D_3 daily. In fact, the American Academy of Pediatrics recommends that all infants be given some vitamin D_3 to prevent them from developing rickets. For older children and adults it's best to dose vitamin D_3 based on the results of a serum measurement, but at least 1,000–2,000 IU per day is a good, safe, protective dose. Vitamin D_3 should be taken with vitamin A (needed for the vitamin D_3 receptor to effectively work), vitamin K (ensures the calcium absorbed as a result of vitamin D_3 signaling can enter the bones, instead of the body tissues), and calcium and magnesium. It's not a good idea to take large doses of vitamin D_3 by itself.

Probiotics

As discussed in chapter 9, a heathy microbiome reduces systemic autoimmunity reactions. Everyone can benefit from taking a broad probiotic from a reputable company. A good probiotic company has different formulas for infants, children, and adults, for different health conditions, in powder and capsule formulas. About twenty to twenty-five billion is a typical daily dose for adults, with infant dosing around ten billion per day. I think the best-tasting healthy children's chewable is Chewable Probiotic by Protocol.

Taking one or more of the above-mentioned supplements does not, of course, guarantee someone will not develop T1DM, but based on the leading studies, it seems they might indeed reduce risk.

Extending a T1DM Honeymoon

A T1DM honeymoon occurs when a newly diagnosed T1DM patient suddenly sees his glucose become completely under control and the need for insulin drastically decreases or is even eradicated. It seems the pancreas begins to work again, and this honeymoon period can last for weeks, months, or even years.

There are some supplements that have been studied for their potential to extend the T1DM honeymoon period. Of course, they work best when diet and other lifestyle aspects are also closely followed. Niacinamide, for example, alone or with vitamin E, has been shown to extend the honeymoon period. Although we generally recommend niacinamide at 1,500 mg per day, in one study the dose used was 25 mg per kg body weight a day, and vitamin E dosing was 15 mg per kg body weight. So, if a child weighed 60 pounds, and we did the mg/kg body weight dosing, she would take only 680 mg niacinamide and 400 mg vitamin E (560 IU) a day, half the standard dose. Ask your physician what dose is best. Do not use niacin, another form of vitamin B_3. Also, please be aware that taking niacinamide does not prevent T1DM onset but may extend a honeymoon period.

Other supplements considered for extending a honeymoon period have been used safely by integrative physicians but are not necessarily scientifically verified:

Pancreatic glandular. A pancreatic glandular is organic pancreatic tissue from a healthy cow or pig, used to stimulate the functioning of the pancreas when taken as a supplement. Patients who follow kosher or halal dietary laws or who are vegetarian or vegan may not want to take this product, although a medicine can usually be taken for a condition even if it is not kosher/halal.

Moducare. This supplement contains sterols and sterolins and is used with many autoimmune conditions to help the immune system veer from autoimmunity. Dr. Bouic formulated this to help against rheumatoid arthritis, but I've used it with other autoimmune conditions, such as T1DM and Graves' disease.

Anti-inflammatory. An anti-inflammatory supplement might contain *Boswellia*, bromelain, curcumin, or other natural anti-inflammatory products.

Gymnema sylvestre. This botanical is from India, where it is known as "gurmar" (sugar destroyer). *Gymnema* has been shown to help regenerate pancreatic beta cells.

It may be a good idea for newly diagnosed diabetic patients to go on one or more of the above supplements as per the guidance of their integrative physicians.

Diabetic Treatment Supplements

The following list of supplements can be used in any type of diabetic patient to achieve the goals listed above.

Essential Dietary Oils

There are many different types of oils used as supplements. We can supplement omega-9 (O-9), omega-6 (O-6), and omega-3 (O-3) oils, as well as gamma-linolenic acid (GLA). O-9 oils are found in olive oil and are associated with reducing the risk of cardiovascular disease. O-6 oils are found in vegetable oils, and when overeaten feed into pro-inflammatory pathways in the body. GLA is found in three plants—black currant, evening primrose, and borage—and I use them mostly in treating skin conditions and female reproductive disorders (such as problematic periods). O-3 oils are found in leafy greens; walnuts; oily fish; grass-fed and grass-finished organic and game meats; O-3 eggs; dairy from grass-fed pasteurized cows, goats, and sheep; soybeans; and flax and chia seeds. These are the golden oils for everyone, especially patients with diabetes.

O-3 oils are considered the most important essential oil, or fatty acid. Historically, we ate an O-6:O-3 ratio of 3:1 or 4:1. Today, due to the high intake of vegetable oils, the ratio is more like 20:1 or 30:1. This means most patients are deficient in O-3 oils and are overeating those pro-inflammatory O-6 oils. I can test for the levels of O-3 and O-6 in body cells through a specific lab. But an accurate diet diary will allow a competently trained, nutritionally oriented integrative medical practitioner to analyze the diet for O-3 food sources without any extra testing needed.

O-3 oils, with both EPA and DHA, can help diabetic patients by lowering lipid panels (reduce triglycerides and cholesterol); reducing insulin resistance; reducing pain and inflammation so exercise and sleep are easier; reducing the risk of cardiovascular disease by lowering blood pressure; reducing the risk of dementia and Alzheimer's disease; preventing and treating anxiety and depression; and promoting antioxidant actions in the body and brain to help reduce developing diabetic complications.

Eating foods high in O-3 is easy on a low-carb diabetic diet, but it's also good to supplement these oils. I generally do not want patients to supplement

O-9 and O-6 oils, as there are already plenty in most diets. I prescribe O-3 oils to every diabetic patient, due to the benefits these essential fatty acids produce throughout our bodies and brains.

Pure fish oils are the main oils you should use to supplement your diet; they are extracted from oily fish such as sardines, anchovies, and salmon. There are also vegan fish oil products from companies that extract the O-3 oils from algae, although they are very low in O-3 dosage compared to actual fish oil. In general, I find the vast majority of patients are willing to use supplemental O-3 oils. I would dose the same fish oils for children as I noted in the T1DM prevention section, but for adults, 1,000 mg EPA/750 mg DHA is the starting daily dose. Sometimes I dose twice that much to some patients I feel really need a more aggressive dose. Most patients like capsules, but there are good, pure oil products, too.

Flax seed oil has both O-3 and O-6 oils, but in the correct ratio. Chia seeds are also high in O-3. However, the O-3 in these seeds is alpha-linolenic acid. These are acceptable for vegan patients, but these oils are poorly transformed into EPA and DHA—only around 10–15 percent of alpha-linolenic acid becomes EPA/DHA—so I prefer fish oils that directly dose the EPA/DHA I find so beneficial to patients. However, using flax or chia seeds is still great! Many patients grind up flax seeds (one to four tablespoons per day) and add them to their drink, smoothie, or food. Chia seeds (one to four tablespoons per day) are also high in O-3 oils. Another option is to take one to two tablespoons of an unrefined organic flax seed liquid. I prefer ground flax seeds because they provide the fiber needed for strengthening the microbiome. It is not helpful to take flax seed capsules because, on average, one tablespoon of flax oils equals many large flax capsules. Remember not to cook flax oils! They are only to be used raw. They can be added to smoothies, poured on cooked veggies, or used to make a very tasty salad dressing with some apple cider or rice vinegar.

Multiple Vitamin with Minerals

It's common for patients to come to me having purchased their own supplements from various stores or from an online company. Many of those supplements are inferior in quality, containing minerals in forms our bodies absorb poorly, synthetic vitamin E, and forms of vitamins that should be

Table 10.1. High- and Low-Quality Forms of Nutrients

Nutrient	High Quality	Low Quality
Vitamin B_6	Pyridoxine-5-phosphate	Pyrodoxine This is an acceptable form but is not bioactive.
Vitamin B_{12}	Methylcobalamin, adenosylcobalamin	Cyanocobalamin This contains a cyanide molecule and is less active in the body.
Carotenoids	Mixed carotenoids	Beta-carotene only Mixed carotenoids are better and safer than beta-carotene by itself.
Vitamin D_3	Cholecalciferol	Ergocalciferol This is a very poor form of vitamin D_3, not well used by the body. It is found in prescription forms of vitamin D_3 and vegetarian vitamin D_3. There are, however, vegetarian cholecalciferol products.
Vitamin E	Mixed tocopherols	DL-alpha tocopherol "DL" means it is synthetic and only half as active as the label states. Mixed tocopherols contain all the different forms of vitamin E the body uses; most vitamins contain only D-alpha tocopherol, which is not bad but not ideal.
Folic Acid	5-methyltetrahydro-folate	Folic acid, folate These are not bioactive forms and may cause problems for bodies with genetic folic acid mutations.
Riboflavin	Riboflavin-5-phosphate	Riboflavin This is an acceptable form but is not bioactive, meaning it is not ready to work immediately in the body.
Minerals	Substrates: citrate, malate, glycinate, bisglycinate, aspartate, picolinate, taurinate	Substrates: oxide, gluconate, carbonate, sulfate These are very poorly absorbed by the gut.

Nutrient	High Quality	Low Quality
Selenium	Selenomethionine, selenium glycinate complex	Sodium selenite This is an inferior type of selenium.

Note: Biotin, vitamin C, thiamine, pantothenic acid, boron, and potassium have no real specific good or bad forms.

avoided or containing extra ingredients called excipients that are unhealthy and should be avoided. Minerals are attached to a substrate for absorption through our intestinal walls. Ideal minerals are chelated or in a bound complex substrate; that means they are attached to a substrate like glycinate, bisglycinate, malate, aspartate, or citrate. Minerals should be avoided if they are attached to a salt substrate; that means they are attached to an oxide, gluconate, or carbonate. Actually, carbonates can be well absorbed by a person if they have good stomach acid, but if not, the absorption is not good, so generally stay with the chelated or bound complex substrates.

With supplements, it's important to beware of what we call "window dressing," which is when a product is advertised as containing some awesome ingredient but upon closer inspection one sees that the dosage is far below clinical activity. Just like prescription drugs have therapeutic doses, so do nutrients, oils, nutraceuticals, and botanicals. The well-known One-A-Day multivitamin, for example, advertises that it contains lycopene, a carotenoid that is a good antioxidant, especially protective of a prostate. There are 300 micrograms of lycopene in the product per serving, but the therapeutic dose is 6–10 *milligrams*. There is no helpful amount of lycopene in that product! A typical person would see lycopene on the front and think they are getting a decent amount of this antioxidant, but, in reality, they are being misled.

I ask all of my patients to bring in their supplement bottles so I can take time educating them about quality of ingredients: which supplements are fine to continue using, what dosage should be used, and which supplements are really inferior, as well as what should be taken instead. People can spend hundreds and hundreds of dollars a month on poor quality supplements.

A good integrative practitioner can guide a patient toward excellent quality products dosed exactly how that individual needs.

There are many different ways nutrients may be listed on an ingredient label. It is very important to work with a physician who can analyze labels correctly to ensure you are paying money for a high-quality multiple. See table 10.1 for help with what to look for. There are many inferior brands out there to watch out for!

A good multiple vitamin and mineral product (or "multiple," for short) is a great way to start supporting nutrient intake in all diabetic patients. This ensures every day that the body receives all the key nutrients it needs so that all its biochemical, hormonal, nutritional, detoxifying, healing, rebuilding, protecting, and strengthening processes can be performed easily and smoothly. The body runs on enzymes, as enzymes speed up reactions to make the body function more efficiently; all enzymes require nutrient cofactors to enable them to effectively engage the action they are designed to do. A good multiple ensures all those cofactors are available every minute, every day.

There are some who believe that "food based" supplements are better than those containing chemically pure vitamins. I do not agree; I think they can both be valuable supplements, depending on the company and the quality. The vast majority of "food based" supplements are made in a huge vat of soy, in which sits a bacteria called *Saccromyces cerevisiae*. Companies usually add into the vat the lowest quality vitamins and minerals that contain preservative and other excipients I do not wish patients to ingest. The companies advertise that the *Saccromyces cerevisiae* turn these poor quality nutrients into excellent supplements. I know that if I put the same poor quality nutrients into my intestine, filled with beneficial bacteria, it would not magically turn into the highest quality forms! Each of those products may contain 1–2 mg of soy, and I do not know if the soy vats contain GMO-free soy or not.

My choice for whole-food vitamins, if a patient wishes to use that type of product, is Whole Earth and Sea (www.wholeearthsea.com) because they use totally organic, non-GMO, sustainably farmed foods, with some high-quality nutrients added in.

The other main type of vitamin is the clean pharmaceutical grade product, and while you might shy away from the word *pharmaceutical*, they are very pure, contain no allergens, can be made into the bioactive forms of the nutrient, have been studied for decades, and are indeed safe for the human body. Of course, eating a high-quality diet will provide you with all the other sources of nutrients the multiple may not. Here are a few recommendations.

First, avoid the One-A-Day brand. All of the well-known One-A-Day products contain poor-quality products at low doses, and are full of unhealthy excipients, fillers, and preservatives. A high-quality multiple will require you to take three to six capsules a day, but will cover all the nutrients your body needs. For children, there are good liquid or powder multiples. Right now, I am using a powder multiple, Vitavescence, from Designs for Health, that turns into a nice berry fizz for pediatric patients and adults who cannot swallow capsules.

Second, all minerals and vitamins should be taken in the most absorbable, bioactive forms. This makes the product a little more expensive, but there is a huge difference in the body's ability to absorb and metabolize different forms of nutrients. I recommend Pure Encapsulations' Polyphenol Nutrients to my patients. It is a very good product, does not cause stomach upset, and even contains some antioxidant botanicals. Remember, all good multiples will turn your urine a bright yellow/green, due to vitamin B_2, riboflavin, a vitamin that colors the urine.

Lastly, patients should take supplements that contain good quantities of the nutrients they advertise and few excipients. Patients should avoid taking products that contain nickel or tin, talc, food colorings, food flavorings, preservatives, allergens such as (usually GMO) soy lecithin, sweeteners, and fillers such as maltodextrin. Look for pure products.

I believe every single patient with diabetes should be on a fish oil supplement and a good multiple vitamin and mineral product. Every single one!

Diabetic-Specific Nutrients

There are many vitamins, minerals, nutraceuticals, and botanicals advertised as being "the answer" to diabetes. I am going to discuss those that have the best research behind them and also those that I have used clinically for twenty-five years with good success in my diabetic patients. I will list the most important ingredients to search for and the typical doses that may help you attain your diabetic goals.

Vitamins and Minerals

Zinc. Zinc is needed to produce, secrete, and activate insulin receptors on the cell. Studies have shown that adding zinc to diabetic patients' diets can be helpful. Hyperglycemia can cause pathological losses of zinc in the urine. It has been shown to lower fasting and after-meal glucose, A1C levels, and lipid panels. Zinc also has an antioxidant effect on cells in diabetic patients. You need to make sure you do not take too much zinc, as it can cause a deficiency in copper, and always take copper with zinc (your multiple probably has copper in it). Taking 15 to 50 mg a day is a good amount.

Chromium. Chromium plays a vital role in binding to and activating the insulin receptor on body cells, reducing insulin resistance. Supplemental chromium has been shown to lower glucose levels, lipids, A1C, and insulin in diabetic patients. It can also help decrease one's appetite, particularly for sweets. A dosage from 200 mcg to 2,000 mcg a day is safe. Higher doses are unnecessary and can cause acute kidney failure.

Vanadium. This mineral has been shown to be an insulin mimetic, to act slightly similar to insulin, reducing insulin resistance. Vanadium has been shown to reduce elevated glucose and lipids. The best absorbed form of vanadium is Bis(maltolato)oxovanadium IV (BMOV) as it is two to three times more potent than vanadyl sulfate or vanadium, typical forms of the mineral. That form also has less toxicity. You do not need much vanadium: 1 to 20 mg a day should be fine.

Magnesium. Magnesium deficiency is common in diabetic patients, as magnesium can be lost in the urine with hyperglycemia. A study in *Diabetes Care* reported that low magnesium status is common in T2DM and showed that when low-magnesium T2DM patients were given an oral dose of magnesium daily for sixteen weeks, the mineral reduced insulin resistance, fasting glucose, and A1C levels. Magnesium is high in green leafy vegetables, nuts, beans, and grains, but we remove most beans and all grains from the diet of diabetic patients. Low intracellular magnesium can cause insulin resistance. Dosing of up to 500 mg a day is fine, but higher than that may result in diarrhea in patients. If you are eating a high-fat, high-animal protein, low-carb diabetic diet, adding in magnesium citrate makes sense.

Potassium. A diet high in potassium has been shown to prevent the onset of T2DM, and when people's serum was made experimentally low in potassium, there was reduced insulin sensitivity and impaired glucose tolerance. Potassium is found in many vegetables and is high in avocados. It's important that patients ensure they are eating a lot of vegetables no matter the type of low-carb diet they are following. Supplements cannot contain a lot of potassium, as it is regulated by the FDA. If you are eating a low-carb, high-fat diet, adding in potassium citrate makes sense to prevent cellular acidosis.

Vitamin D_3. As already mentioned, vitamin D_3 has been shown to help reduce the onset of T1DM. However, once a person has diabetes, vitamin D_3 also helps with glucose regulation. Vitamin D_3 should be measured and should be treated to a level of 40 to 80 nmol/L, a therapeutic reference range based on a serum lab test.

Vitamin C and bioflavinoids. Vitamin C taken as an individual supplement has pros and cons. In general, a person with diabetes should not take more than 1,500 mg a day of vitamin C, as the vitamin C molecule looks very similar to glucose in the body. As a result, taking higher doses could confuse your glucose meter that your blood sugar is higher than it is. Obviously, that can lead to problems! When people get vitamin C IVs, because it is so similar to glucose, sometimes the body produces insulin and the patient can become hypoglycemic during the IV. Nonetheless, vitamin C and bioflavonoids are very useful at decreasing the polyol/aldose reductase pathway in cells. This pathway can cause oxidative damage in a diabetic patient's eyes and nerves. Vitamin C and bioflavinoids help reduce that pathway so oxidative damage is lessened. Taking 250 to 1,000 mg per day of vitamin C is good and safe. Bioflavinoids are safe at any dose and 200 mg and higher are appropriate.

Resveratrol. This bioflavinoid has been shown to protect pancreatic cells, reduce inflammatory cytokines, and increase antioxidants. It may also help improve insulin's actions and lower levels of glucose, A1C, and insulin. It was also shown to help decrease body weight, systolic BP, cholesterol, and triglycerides. It is found in peanuts and red wine. A good dose is around 200 mg a day.

Mixed vitamin E. Vitamin E is an excellent antioxidant and blood thinner. The mixed form, as listed in table 10.1, means that all four forms of tocopherol are included. LDL cholesterol is the "bad" cholesterol, especially when it is oxidized; oxidized LDL is an etiological risk factor for developing atherosclerosis of blood vessels and cardiovascular disease. Vitamin E is effective at reducing LDL oxidation. It is a specific nutrient for preventing further liver damage in fatty liver and nonalcoholic steatohepatitis (see chapter 14). It can reduce formation of advanced glycosylated end products, protein/sugar bonds that also cause diabetic damage throughout the body. A good daily dose is 400 to 2,000 IU.

Biotin. This vitamin was shown to lower blood sugar levels and help improve glucose control. It is needed to increase a liver enzyme, glycokinase, which helps the liver take in glucose and turn it to glycogen. It can be low in patients with diabetes and has been shown, when mixed also with chromium, to be beneficial to diabetic patients. It can help heal dandruff and brittle nails. However, clinically, I have not found it to be a necessary addition to any diabetic protocol, as adding it to protocols did not show any benefits to glucose regulation, so I do not recommend it to patients. A typical dose is 10 to 30 mg a day.

Nutraceuticals

R-alpha-lipoic acid (R-ALA). If I could only prescribe one supplement to a diabetes patient, I would prescribe R-alpha-lipoic acid. Alpha-lipoic acid has numerous benefits to the diabetic patient. It is a water- and fat-soluble antioxidant and has been shown to protect patients with fatty liver from liver disease progression. It can help reduce insulin resistance and has been shown to protect people with diabetes from developing complications in their nerves, eyes, and kidneys. R-ALA can prevent glycosylation of proteins, which reduces the A1C level. It is safe, although very rarely it can cause stomach upset. Alpha-lipoic acid is listed either as ALA or R-ALA. When listed as ALA, this means it contains two forms—the S isomer form and the R isomer form, in a 50:50 ratio. The R isomer form is the only active isomer in the body, and so should be the only form used. If an alpha-lipoic acid product says each capsule contains 300 mg, in actuality, only 150 mg is R-ALA, and will be active. An R-alpha-lipoic acid product that says each capsule contains 300 mg is all active in the body. That is, you can take half the R-ALA dose to equal an ALA dose. The key is to find a product that says it contains "R-ALA" instead of just "ALA." A good daily working dose of R-ALA is 300 to 1,200 mg a day, which is the equivalent of 600 to 2,400 mg a day of regular ALA, if you buy a regular ALA listed product.

Benfotiamine. Also known as allithiamine, this fat-soluble form of thiamine has been shown to be very capable at reducing the formation of advanced glycosylated end products, which are well known to lead to the development of diabetic complications. Benfotiamine is better absorbed than water soluble thiamine. Benfotiamine increases the production of thiamine pyrophosphate, which increases transketolase activity. Transketolase blocks glucose-induced damage by preventing AGE formation. Since AGE formation promotes oxidative damage throughout the body, benfotiamine has been shown to treat and improve retinopathy, nephropathy, and neuropathy. The dosage is 150 mg to 450 mg per day.

N-acetyl cysteine (NAC). NAC is another valuable and inexpensive nutraceutical that has been shown to be a great benefit to diabetic patients. It is also underused in patients with diabetes. It can reduce insulin resistance. It acts as an antioxidant preventing oxidative glucose damage, and can specifically help the pancreas, liver, and eyes, and save kidney and nerve cells from diabetic damage. NAC has been shown to help lower high blood pressure and can help break apart intestinal biofilms, network meshes of dysbiotic bacteria. It is another valuable supplement for patients with fatty liver. The therapeutic dose is 600 to 2,400 mg per day.

Acetyl-l-carnitine. This nutraceutical is very helpful as an aid to fat metabolism, as it takes fat molecules directly into cells to be used for energy production. It can be used to lower LDLs and raise HDLs in T2DM patients. It has been scientifically shown to improve pain, nerve degeneration, and vibratory perception in patients with chronic diabetic neuropathy. I will give acetyl-l-carnitine to every diabetic patient who has any type of neuropathy. The dose is 1,500 to 3,000 mg a day.

Taurine. Taurine is an inexpensive amino acid that is underused as a diabetic supplement. Taurine has been found to be a potent hypoglycemic agent and it can also enhance the effect of insulin. One study showed giving taurine to diabetic patients for a month required a reduction in their insulin dosing, to avoid taurine-induced hypoglycemia. It was also noted that patients had reductions in cholesterol and triglycerides as well. Taurine is found naturally in eye tissue and is the main amino acid in the heart. It prevents glycosylation of proteins and helps the gallbladder work better to digest fats. The dose is around 500 to 1,500 mg per day.

Sulphoraphane. This antioxidant, found in cruciferous vegetables, can reduce blood vessel damage from hyperglycemia. It can substantially reduce oxidative molecules, helping to prevent diabetic complications. It also enhances the formation of enzymes that help the body detoxify. It has been well demonstrated to work against cancer. A dose is 30 to 200 mg a day.

L-carnosine. This product can help reduce glycosylation and may increase beta cell mass. A typical dose is 1,000 mg per day.

Botanical Medicines

There are numerous studies of botanical medicines for patients with diabetes, but not all of them are very good. These studies may have small sample populations or poor methodology. However, there are enough positive studies and patient experiences to inform intelligent, safe, and effective guidance on which botanicals to consider taking regularly. There are a lot of different herbs out there, and I've decided not to discuss every single herb that might be used. Instead, I have listed the most useful herbs with the most documented benefits. A patient does not need to take one hundred bottles a day of everything out on the market, but rather it is important to focus on a few botanicals backed by the most impressive studies and the best clinical evidence. The botanicals listed below are safe and effective.

Gymnema sylvestre. Known as *gurmar*, or "sugar destroyer," in Aryuvedic medicine, *Gymnema* has consistently shown benefits in patients with diabetes. The most active part of *Gymnema* seems to be gymnemic acids, and many products list the percentage each capsule contains. Analyses of the herb have shown it may be helpful in lowering glucose levels. It can delay glucose absorption from the intestine. It was shown to regenerate pancreatic tissues, allowing more insulin to be produced, and help regulate insulin secretion. It also increases the utilization of glucose by the cell, reducing insulin resistance and decreasing appetite, especially for sweets. I usually use it in capsules, or in liquid form in some patients. Due to *Gymnema* having a very similar shape to glucose, it can fit into the taste bud receptors for sugar; it thus has unbelievable power to actually prevent the taste of sweets in the mouth for up to 1.5 hours. When I have a patient who is still struggling to not eat cake and cookies and so forth at parties or celebrations (or just in general), I will give her a tincture of *Gymnema sylvestre*. A tincture is an alcohol-based liquid extract of the herb. It is safe except if someone has a liver condition or is alcoholic. I instruct her to squirt two full droppers of the tincture into her mouth before the celebration, swish it for a minute, and then swallow it. She will usually not be able to taste sweet flavors for at least an hour—when something sweet enters her mouth, it will taste like nothing, an effect that is disgusting to the mouth. As a result, her mouth will oftentimes reject it. This is one of my favorite herbs for diabetic patients. In capsule form doses of 400 to 2,400 mg a day are recommended.

Cinnamon. Cinnamonium cassia and its relative *C. burmanii* are the types of cinnamon that have the best effect on patients. There have been numerous studies on cinnamon and, overall, they have shown cinnamon can slow stomach emptying and lower postprandial glucose levels. It also reduces glucose levels in T2DM patients who have had poor diabetic control. It may also be helpful in lowering insulin levels, blood pressure, and A1C, and reduce AGE formation. This is a safe herb. A good dose is 1 to 2 g a day or 200 mg or more of a concentrated extract.

Berberine HCL. A leading study on humans showed that berberine HCL equaled the effects of metformin on diabetic patients. In the pilot study, the A1C, fasting and postprandial glucose, plasma triglycerides, total and LDL cholesterol, and measures of insulin resistance were reduced, as well as body weight. Berberine is also a liver protectant and activates AMP protein kinase. Cellular AMP protein kinase promotes GLUT 4 translocation and GLUT 4 is what signals the cell to absorb glucose. Berberine increases the activity of insulin receptors, increases insulin sensitivity of the cell, and helps lower glucose numbers. It can also increase GLP-1 incretin secretion. Beyond all the medical jargon, what this means is that berberine promotes cellular uptake of glucose from the blood, lowers blood glucose, and reduces insulin resistance. It is an antioxidant, and may help strengthen pancreatic beta cells. It helps prevent the liver from overproducing glucose. All these actions are very significant and berberine is an important component in diabetic supplements, due to its efficacy and its safety profile. Dosage can be problematic, as higher doses can upset the small intestine. I recommend patients slowly increase their dosage of any product containing berberine. Also, it's important to take the pill right after a meal, when food is already in the stomach. A therapeutic dose is 1,000 to 1,500 mg per day.

Bilberry extract. Bilberry extract is rich in anthocyanoside bioflavinoids and has a specific affinity for the eyes. Bilberry has been studied in T2DM patients with retinopathy and was found to induce a clear improvement in that condition, with marked reduction or disappearance of retinal hemorrhages. It may also be beneficial in improving microcirculation and lowering glucose levels. As retinopathy is a leading complication in diabetic patients, and diabetes is the main cause of adult blindness, this study is remarkably important. A recommended dose is 100 to 350 mg a day.

Green tea leaf extract. Green tea contains the bioflavinoid epigallocatechin gallate (EGCG), which has been shown to be a safe and effective antioxidant. In a study in Japan, green tea was shown to reduce the risk for T2DM onset. It has been shown to improve glucose tolerance in patients, and decrease hepatic glucose production and over-secretion in T2DM patients. Green tea has also been shown to have an effective anti-angiogenesis factor, that is, it reduces problematic overgrowth of blood vessels, which may have a significant effect on preventing diabetic retinopathy. It has also been shown to promote fat oxidation and thermogenesis. Last, green tea can provide antioxidant protection for the pancreas and the fatty liver. A good dose is 200 to 400 mg a day. It's also beneficial to drink organic green tea.

Curcumin extract. Curcumin is a bright yellow chemical produced by the spice turmeric, among other plants. Curcumin seems to have multiple benefits in diabetes. It has been shown to be a marked inhibitor of reactive oxygen species that promote oxidation damage in cells. Curcumin lowers inflammatory chemicals like tumor necrosis factor-alpha, and that's good because TNF-a causes insulin resistance and irritates fatty livers. Curcumin can reduce another pro-inflammatory chemical called NF-KB. The above-mentioned actions provide a benefit in diabetes protection and reduce the risk of developing diabetic complications. Curcumin has also been shown to enhance pancreatic beta cell functioning and reduce fatty liver deposition. It reduces glucose, A1C, and insulin resistance. It was also shown to reduce the onset of Alzheimer's disease, and that is a higher risk in diabetic patients than in nondiabetic patients. What is the best form of curcumin to use? Certainly it is found in Indian cuisine, and that is a tasty way to ingest curcumin. It is difficult to absorb, so mixing in black pepper can aid absorption, and most products with curcumin in them have added pepper. There are many products on the market that have attached the curcumin to a fatty layer or some other substance to enhance absorption. A knowledgeable integrative medical practitioner can guide you on a good product selection. A good dose is 200 to 3,000 mg a day.

Gingko biloba. This plant has been associated with reducing the risk of dementia and cognitive decline, but it has also been shown to reduce blood clotting and to improve retinal and kidney function in T2DM patients with retinopathy. This botanical is a valuable addition to a diabetic supplement protocol, but it should not be taken by patients on blood-thinning medications or patients with the rare condition of hemophilia. A good dose is 160 to 240 mg a day.

Garlic. A tasty plant whose bulb is used commonly in recipes, garlic has been shown to reduce dyslipidemia in patients with T2DM. In one study it lowered total and LDL cholesterol and increased HDL cholesterol. In another study 150 mg of garlic powder was shown to lower fasting glucose, fructosamine, and triglyceride levels. I encourage patients to regularly include garlic powder and cloves in their cooking.

Fiber. Fiber is very helpful; as discussed in the microbiome section last chapter, it is that part of food that is not broken down and absorbed by digestion in the gastrointestinal tract. Removing grains from the diets of diabetic patients means that fiber intake is likely reduced. As we now know, fiber feeds beneficial bacteria that produce SCFAs, reduces glucose levels after meals, and reduces the appetite. For children, the fiber guideline is their age plus 5 g a day. For adults, at least 25 g per day. The greater amount of fiber one eats, the better! Fiber intake may cause increased gas and bloating, and is contraindicated in diabetic patients with gastroparesis and in people having an acute flare of inflammatory bowel disease. There are three kinds of fiber: water soluble, water insoluble, and resistant starch. I've noted earlier that I do not recommend daily intake of resistant starch, so I'll just clarify the other two types of fiber. Water-soluble fiber means that the fiber is absorbed in water and turns into a viscous gel. It includes fibers such as chia seeds, flax seeds, and psyllium. It binds with fatty acids, thus lowering cholesterol. Water-soluble fiber also prolongs stomach emptying, making people feel fuller sooner and longer. It lowers glucose levels by slowing the absorption of glucose from the gut. Water-insoluble fiber is not absorbed in water, and does not form a gel, but instead adds bulk to the stool and helps decrease transient time of stool in the gut, removing toxins. This is made up of many different types of brans and psyllium. Many fiber products have a mixture of these two types of fiber.

Another source of diabetic-related fiber is defatted fenugreek seed. This has been shown to reduce fasting blood sugar levels, triglycerides, LDL cholesterol, and A1C levels. It also improved glucose tolerance. Studies used doses of 100 g once a day and 50 g twice a day. Most patients do not choose to take that much fenugreek! Also, fenugreek and hemp seeds have calories, another reason T2DM patients needing to lose weight should not choose to add them as a daily supplement. Most of my diabetic patients use ground up flax seeds, chia seeds, or a mixed fiber product I recommend. Fiber supplements can be added to smoothies or mixed into yogurt, mixed with water and swallowed, sprinkled on cooked vegetables, and included in nut grain recipes. If using ground flax or chia seeds, one to four tablespoons a day is good. I do not suggest patients buy already ground up flax or chia seeds, as these can oxidize and go bad quickly. I suggest patients buy a little coffee bean grinder and flax or chia seeds, and grind up their daily dosage each day, or at most, grind up three days at a time, and store the extra in the refrigerator. A total daily dose of adding 3–10 g of fiber is recommended.

American and Asian ginseng. Ginseng has been shown in studies to reduce fasting blood glucose, reduce body weight, improve A1C, and improve mood. It is also a good adrenal support to help against fatigue. A good dose is 200 mg a day. Some people over time might have hormonal side effects to taking ginseng, so if something changes in your body in this way, alert your integrative physician.

Recommended Antioxidants

For patients with A1Cs over 5.5 percent, but especially over 6.0 percent, extra antioxidant protection is vital, to prevent damage to the body. Taking one (or more!) of the below makes good sense:

- R-alpha-lipoic acid
- N-acetylcysteine
- Curcumin
- Green tea leaf extract
- Berberine HCL
- Benfotiamine

Momordica charantia *(bitter melon)*. You can find this melon at Asian markets, and yes, it is bitter. It has a reputation for helping patients with diabetes by improving glucose tolerance and lowering A1C levels. It is best taken as the liquid or as an extract. A dose of the extract, if you wish to bypass drinking the unpleasant juice, is 200 to 800 mg a day.

Holy basil. This herb has been shown to reduce fasting and after-eating glucose levels. 200 mg a day is a good dose.

For further discussion of supplements for individual complications, see chapter 14.

Diamend

All diabetic patients should be on a supplement protocol: multiple vitamin and mineral, EPA/DHA, and a diabetic comprehensive supplement. The need for a super high-quality diabetes specialty supplement is why I created my own product called Diamend. Diamend contains numerous leading-edge supplements at therapeutic dosing; no "window dressing" here.

Diamend is a diabetes specialty product manufactured by Priority One Supplements, a high-quality company. It is only sold to physicians in order for them to properly prescribe it to patients.

Here are the ingredients in a bottle of Diamend (seven capsules):

Zinc bisglycinate chelate: 25 mg
Chromium picolinate: 801 mcg

Berberine HCL: 1,000 mg
R-ALA: 600 mg
Gymnema sylvestre (75 percent gymnemic acid): 1,000 mg
Benfotiamine: 450 mg
Bilberry fruit 4:1 extract: 200 mg
N-acetyl cysteine: 600 mg
Green tea extract (70 percent EGCG, 90 percent catechins): 200 mg
Tumeric extract (Meriva): 500 mg
Vanadium (BMOV): 5 mg

As you can see the ingredients are excellent, and in good quantities. The daily maximum dose of Diamend is seven capsules a day, in divided daily doses. Your medical practitioner can prescribe how many capsules and how to divide them. My patients love that they only need to open up one bottle to get an immense amount of scientifically verified benefits, instead of the seventeen bottles they walk into my office with, and they do notice the difference this product makes. If you are thinking of getting what I believe is the best and most comprehensive product on the market for people with glucose imbalances, at therapeutic dosing, please (1) get approval from your physician, and (2) take it right after meals, due to the berberine content in it, as the food will buffer most if not all if the possible stomach upset.

What about helping to reverse diabetic complications? If you have any diabetic complications, chapter 14 will help you and your integrative physician learn what additional supplements may need to be added to specifically help heal and reverse them. Supplements are the seventh essential of a comprehensive diabetes protocol. Using the right ones at the right doses can maximize your ability to really feel great while getting your diabetes under control.

— CHAPTER ELEVEN —

Diabetes and Pregnancy

A woman who is a diabetic patient, either T1DM or T2DM, who becomes pregnant is called a diabetic pregnant woman. Whether the woman is T1DM or T2DM, the key with pregnancy is ensuring excellent glucose control before pregnancy and striving to maintain that during the pregnancy. It is best if the diabetic woman has a great A1C before the pregnancy occurs, ideally lower than 6.0 percent, even lower than 5.8 percent (and of course best if not that low due to frequent hypoglycemic reactions).

A woman who is not diabetic before pregnancy and becomes a T2DM patient during pregnancy is said to have gestational diabetes. Gestational diabetes (GDM) generally occurs at the end of the second trimester or during the third. GDM occurs in 7 percent of all pregnancies. Usually, the woman is either obese before becoming pregnant or gains excess weight during pregnancy through overeating and lack of exercise. Women with Latino, Pacific Islander, and Native American heritage have the highest risks of developing GDM. Other risk factors include family history of gestational diabetes; previous delivery of a large infant; strong family history of T2DM; past history of a baby being stillborn or having a birth defect; and history of polycystic ovarian syndrome, a genetic hormonal condition due to insulin resistance.

What drives the development of GDM? Every woman naturally becomes insulin resistant during pregnancy, and in fact, her microbiome bacteria change to promote systemic insulin resistance; this allows the woman to gain the weight she needs for her fetus's natural growth and development.

While GDM is dangerous for the developing fetus, it can bode poorly for the mom, too. Fifty percent of GDM patients become full-blown T2DM patients within a decade after delivery. One of the earliest ways to assess for GDM in pregnancy is measuring sex hormone binding globulin (SHBG); if levels are low in the first trimester, it is a warning sign of developing diabetes, because insulin suppresses the formation of SHBG. Thus, if insulin is increasing too much, showing early insulin resistance, SHBG can be found to be too low. The earlier the detection, the more effectively GDM can be avoided, or at least properly identified and treated.

Since GDM is mostly related to excessive weight gain during pregnancy, eating correctly during one's pregnancy, getting exercise, taking supplements safe for pregnancy, getting good sleep, and working on stress management can prevent GDM even in a woman whose family is rife with T2DM and even though she is naturally insulin resistant. GDM is entirely preventable. Losing weight before pregnancy, establishing a regular exercise routine, getting dietary counseling, taking natural supplementation, and metformin, if necessary, can be quite helpful.

My patient Lori, for example, is a thin, attractive woman whose father was an uncontrolled T2DM diabetic. He eventually died of his disease after experiencing amputation of his lower legs and then having a fatal heart attack. In her first pregnancy, Lori ate everything she had always held herself back from eating. She gained sixty pounds during the pregnancy and developed GDM. Her baby ballooned to ten pounds, and she had to have a C-section to deliver him. Realizing that had not been a good idea, Lori controlled herself in her second and third pregnancies and did not develop GDM. She became an aerobics instructor and decades later still has never developed T2DM. So, we see quite clearly that diabetes is not a destiny a person cannot escape. Lori did everything right when she realized she was heading down the same path as her father, and she has lived a healthy life free of diabetes. She is a great inspiration to other pregnant women with a family history of diabetes!

Gestational Diabetes Screening

The ADA states that all nondiabetic women should be screened for T2DM at the first prenatal visit if they have any of the aforementioned risk factors and especially if their BMI is equal to or greater than 30 and the woman has a strong family history of diabetes. Unfortunately, more than half the pregnant population in the United States meets the criteria. All women with or without risk factors should have a formal GDM screen between twenty-four and thirty weeks of gestation. If a woman's test is positive, she should have the test repeated six to twelve weeks postpartum to ensure her diabetes went away, which it often does after delivery. Moreover, the ADA adds that if a woman has ever had GDM, she should have a screening for T2DM every one or two years.

It's okay not to screen those women who have the lowest risk of developing GDM: women less than twenty-five years old; women who have a normal pregestational weight; women who belong to a low prevalence ethnic group; women who have no family or personal history of insulin resistance or glucose intolerance; women who have no personal history of poor obstetrical outcomes; and women with no known diabetes in first-degree relatives.

Serum glucose should be very tight in pregnant women.

The glucose targets for pregnant women without preexisting T1DM or T2DM:

Preprandial: ≤ 95 mg/dL
One hour postmeal: ≤ 140 mg/dL
Two hours postmeal: ≤ 120 mg/dL
A1C: 6.0–6.5 percent

The glucose targets for women with preexisting T1DM or T2DM who become pregnant:

Premeal, bedtime, and overnight glucose: 60–99 mg/dL
Peak postprandial glucose: 100–129 mg/dL
A1C: lower than 6.0 percent

How does the oral glucose tolerance test (OGTT) work? There are two ways to diagnose GDM using an OGTT (see table 11.1).

In the one-step method the woman fasts at least eight hours and then drinks 75 grams of glucose. Her glucose is then retested one and two hours after the drink. In the diagnosis column you can see when numbers indicate the test is positive.

The American College of Obstetricians and Gynecologists (ACOG) believes in a two-step approach—fasting glucose, then administer 50 grams

Table 11.1. One- and Two-Step Methodologies for Diagnosing Gestational Diabetes

Step Method	Glucose	Time	Hours	Diagnosis
One-step diagnosis	75 g OGTT	Test after fasting ≥ 8 hours at 24–28 weeks	Fasting One hour after Two hours after	Fasting: > 92 mg/dL One hour after: > 180 mg/dL Two hours after: > 153 mg/dL
One → two-step diagnosis				
Step 1: If (+) move to step 2	50 g OGTT	Nonfasting screen at 24–28 weeks	One hour after	Glucose ≥ 140 mg/dL
Step 2:	100 g OGTT	Test after fasting ≥ 8 hours	Fasting One hour after Two hours after Three hours after	Fasting: > 95 or 105 mg/dL One hour after: > 180 or 190 mg/dL Two hours after: > 155 or 165 mg/dL Three hours after: 140 or 145 mg/dL

Note: The American College of Obstetricians and Gynecologists (ACOG) recommends the two-step method; the ADA recommends either the one-step or two-step method.

of a glucose solution followed by a one-hour glucose check. If the glucose is equal to or higher than 135–140 mg/dL, the test is considered positive. The woman would proceed to a 100-gram glucose solution OGTT, where she has her glucose tested fasting and then one, two, and three hours after the drink. This more complicated and involved protocol is confusing, time-consuming, and causes maternal stress. The one-step guidelines are the ones most established now for GDM analysis.

What is so important about GDM, and why do we take it so seriously? Because when the pregnant woman's glucose is elevated, it goes through the placenta and is high in the fetus. High glucose in the fetus is dangerous; GDM can be devastating to the developing fetus. It can cause birth defects and spontaneous miscarriage in the first trimester. Later in the pregnancy, it can cause premature delivery and delayed growth and development. Elevated glucose can promote large fetal birth weight (macrosomia) causing birthing difficulties and increasing the risk of neonatal morbidity, neonatal damage, maternal injuries, and C-section. Macrosomia is estimated to occur in up to 20 percent of GDM pregnancies. Newborns delivered from mothers who had high glucose throughout much of their development are at risk for suffering from severe hypoglycemia postdelivery. In the womb, the fetus produced high insulin and the newborn continues to do so postbirth even though it is no longer surrounded by elevated glucose levels. Newborns might have seizures, respiratory distress syndrome, enlarged hearts, low calcium levels, jaundice, and polycythemia (a blood problem).

One of the biggest problems with a fetus developing in a GDM womb is that the newborn child has a strikingly high risk of developing T2DM themselves during their life.

Treatment of Gestational Diabetes

Keeping regular diet diaries and glucose graphs will ensure you and your integrative physician continue to control your glucose while your OB/GYN physician organizes the specifics about your prenatal care.

As we have discussed, the ADA's diet for diabetes is very high in carbohydrates: 50–60 percent of calories from carbs, 10–20 percent from protein, and 25–30 percent from fat. ACOG and the Endocrine Society recommend 33–40 percent of calories from carbohydrates in GDM. Lois Jovanovic, MD, a clinical professor of medicine at UCLA Medical Center is a leading international expert in the treatment of GDM and is an advocate of a low-carb diet in GDM. She states that a high-carb diet leads to significant weight gain and hyperglycemia, requiring the addition of insulin. While the ADA recommends a pregnant woman eat 2,000–2,500 calories per day, Dr. Jovanic recommends a lower calorie intake for pregnant woman: 30 calories per kilogram of body weight for normal-sized women; 24 calories per kilogram of body weight for overweight women; and 12 calories per kilogram of body weight for obese women. Dr. Jovanic summarizes that women with GDM have a choice: If a woman chooses to eat low carb, she likely won't need insulin; if a woman choose to eat high carb—that is, she refuses to give up her rice, bread, and tortillas—she will wind up on insulin, because one way or the other, glucose must be controlled during pregnancy. My recommendation is usually for a GDM woman to choose the omnivore low-carb diet, the easiest one for most patients to do, and the one that allows the widest variety of food.

I believe that GDM women, and T2DM/T1DM pregnant women, should follow essentially the same protocol as diabetic patients who are not pregnant. They should measure their glucose several times a day, and, if they are prescribed medicine, take it as dosed by their physician. They should eat a low-carb diet, and only take supplements that were approved for saftey for women with diabetes by their integrative physician. Some excellent diabetic supplements, like berberine, for example, are contraindicated in pregnant women with diabetes. This is how I manage my pregnant patients and it works quite well for them.

Typical diabetic medications that are not approved for pregnant women and should be not taken include incretins, meglitinides, DPP-4, SGLT-2 inhibitors, and TZDs. These nondiabetic medications typically used in diabetic patients are also contraindicated in pregnancy: statin drugs, ACE-inhibitors and angiotensin receptor blockers for hypertension, and many anxiety and antidepressant medications.

No oral hypoglycemic medication is approved for use in GDM by the ADA. The only OHAs considered for use are metformin and glyburide. Metformin has been shown to be safe to use for both mother and fetus during pregnancy, even though the drug crosses the placenta. Metformin is not considered teratogenic, that is, it is not a risk factor for inducing birth defects. It is also considered safe to take during breastfeeding. Glyburide does not cross the placenta, though it can increase the risk of hypoglycemia in pregnant women. It also does not seem to be teratogenic. A study showing that glyburide does not enter into breast milk was conducted with very few women, but it seems it is safe to take during breastfeeding.

OHAs can be used as monotherapy or as an adjuvant to insulin therapy in severe hyperglycemia cases requiring high dosing of insulin, but they are not the drug of choice in GDM. In fact, Dr. Jovanovic clearly states women should not use oral hypoglycemic agents at all with GDM and reaffirms that only insulin should be used.

Insulin is, in fact, the "gold standard" of GDM treatment in conventional care, although it carries with it the risk of hypoglycemia. The ADA recommends stopping oral hypoglycemic agents and transitioning to insulin before pregnancy to achieve better glucose control, but as you can imagine, most women and physicians do not wish to do that. Certainly, when a woman has a positive OGTT, the general rule is to recommend insulin. Insulin is safe to use in GDM because although glucose transfers through the placenta, insulin does not; it has no effect on the developing fetus. It also can be used during breastfeeding. Insulin is thus considered the best drug to use, even with the complications of using insulin responsibly and matching it to carb and protein intake. Historically, NPH and regular insulin were used in GDM patients but, now, using long-acting basal and rapid-acting bolus insulin is allowed. Levemir is rated better than Lantus in diabetic studies in pregnant women. Both Humalog and Novolog are rated the same. They would be dosed as discussed in the insulin chapters, but the dosing is complicated due to worsening insulin resistance as a pregnancy continues.

Of course, insulin is still injected with any T1DM woman already on insulin when she becomes pregnant. However, insulin resistance will significantly increase needs, as noted in the insulin chapter. I discuss that phenomenon in a case study of a T1DM pregnant patient at the end of the book.

Women may need 0.7–1.0 units of insulin per kilogram of body weight a day. Most GDM women do not need insulin after delivery, as their GDM quickly dissipates. It is vital to ensure that a pregnant woman with T1DM, T2DM, or GDM never develops diabetic ketoacidosis, as if she does, there is a 95 percent risk the fetus could die. GDM patients need to keep themselves well hydrated and monitor their glucose regularly. If her glucose goes very high (higher than 160 mg/dL) a diabetic pregnant woman should immediately check her ketones and contact her physician.

A GDM woman may not need to start on any medications if she immediately and fully commits to a radical change in her diet, in exercising, and elsewhere in her lifestyle, as needed; she also might need to lose weight during her pregnancy. Her glucose levels have to come down for her safety and especially for the safety of the developing child. She would need to take the supplements recommended by her integrative medical practitioner. A significantly lowered glucose level would need to be seen within two weeks to ensure a drug-free protocol was a safe and responsible protocol.

Supplement Safety in Pregnant Women with Diabetes

It is good to know which supplements are safe to use with a pregnant woman. A good prenatal multiple vitamin and mineral is required. Fish oil should also be taken, as pregnant women on fish oils have a significantly reduced risk of suffering from postpartum depression. All these additional supplements are safe for a pregnant woman: benfotiamine; cinnamon; vitamin D_3; *Gingko biloba*; N-acetyl cysteine; taurine; green tea; turmeric; and garlic. That's a good mixture of support!

While other supplements have not been shown to be potentially dangerous to a pregnant woman (except berberine), they have also not been shown to be safe.

What about during labor and delivery? There are many muscle groups working during labor and delivery. GDM patients can stop their insulin (and so can most T1DMs) and allow the contractions to use up the serum glucose quite effectively. I strongly urge GDM and T1DM patients to create a hospital plan detailing exactly how they wish to use their medications, check their glucose, deal with highs and lows and other nuances of labor, childbirth, and postdelivery. I help patients develop a plan if they are not comfortable creating one on their own. Women usually are receptive to their physician helping them create a safe, logical methodology for insulin or medication use for their labor and delivery. After childbirth, a woman can usually switch to metformin or sulphonylurea—as I said, safe for breastfeeding—or even be medication free, usually within six weeks postpartum. Close monitoring of glucose and medications will quickly discern changes to be made.

The key, of course, is always to *monitor*, *monitor*, *monitor* glucose, diet, and exercise and work in a team with your OB/GYN and an integrative physician who has expertise in all types of diabetes and working with pregnant women.

— CHAPTER TWELVE —

Pediatric Diabetes

Diagnosis of T1DM means a huge transition for a child, their parents, their friends, and their relatives. But although life indeed changes with regard to consciously having to control blood sugar, it's important to realize and understand that children can live long, healthy, happy, fulfilled lives, and do whatever they want, even with diabetes. Adults with T1DM are professional football quarterbacks and other athletes, supreme court judges, politicians, models, actors and actresses. It's vitally important for children diagnosed with diabetes to not develop low self-esteem or believe they are broken in some way. Everyone involved in their care needs to support them in having a happy childhood and to validate that their dreams are all attainable.

From 2001 to 2009 there was a significant increase in the occurrence of both T1DM and T2DM. In the United States, around 15,000 children a year are diagnosed with T1DM, and about 151,000 people younger than twenty years old have T1DM. We are never quite sure why a child "comes down" with T1DM; there are many etiological risk factors, as discussed in earlier chapters, but how they all come together in any specific child is currently unknown. Around 3,700 children a year between the ages of ten and nineteen are diagnosed with T2DM. The ADA recommends T2DM screening for all children who are overweight and have two or more of the following factors: a family history of T2DM in a first- or second-degree relative; Native American, African American, Latino, Asian American, or Pacific Islander heritage—these ethnicities are at the greatest risk for developing T2DM; signs of insulin resistance or conditions associated with insulin resistance; and maternal history of diabetes or gestational diabetes during that child's gestation.

Screening and After-Diagnosis Testing of Pediatric Patients

Screening for children who meet the ADA's guidelines consists of measuring the child's A1C beginning at age ten or onset of puberty. I suggest also measuring fasting or postprandial glucose and insulin, as well. I like to get both of those readings for an accurate diagnosis and to investigate insulin resistance, as described in chapter 4.

If a child is diagnosed with T2DM, the child should have a dilated eye exam. Blood pressure, fasting lipids, and urine micro albuminuria should also be measured, and should be regularly evaluated at future office visits. The child should then engage in a comprehensive diabetic protocol, consisting of diet changes, good daily exercise, stress management, good sleep, supplementation, and gentle support of their microbiome. I would not detoxify a child, and I strive to avoid using medications. Often, compliance with diet and exercise can be enough to reverse this course of events. While not possible for T1DM, integrative medicine can reverse T2DM entirely in both children and adults.

Five years after a child or teen is diagnosed with T1DM, we begin annual screening of micro albuminuria and creatinine with eGFR based on age and race, and watch their kidney health. After the child has been diagnosed with T1DM for three to five years, and is at least ten years old or at puberty, she should also receive an annual dilated eye exam. The child with T1DM should have a yearly test for thyroid antibodies and a thyroid panel of TSH, free T3, and free T4. The ADA suggests a T1DM pediatric patient should be tested for celiac disease only if there is a family history of celiac or if the child fails to grow or gain weight, has diarrhea, flatulence, or abdominal pain. Those are signs of classic celiac disease and malabsorption. Another sign of malabsorption is repeated hypoglycemia of unknown cause.

However, most patients with celiac disease do not present in the classic presentation. A person may be overweight and constipated and have celiac disease. Thus, I feel all toddlers should be tested for celiac disease to catch it before it might lead to the development of T1DM, and I feel all T1DM patients should be immediately tested for celiac genes and antibodies upon diagnosis. If a child hasn't been tested and comes to me already on a grain-free diet, they would have to eat daily gluten for at least a month before being tested for celiac, and that is contraindicated; I would not recommend it. We can always test for the most common celiac genes to give us an idea of the potential for celiac disease. A positive celiac test or positive gene can be excellent motivation to remain gluten free, and also suggests the rest of the family should be tested, as this is a genetic disease and other family members may also be positive.

KEY TREATMENT NOTE

If you feel gluten is bothering you or a family member, be tested for celiac disease before stopping gluten intake.

There are many other alternative diagnostic tests that can be performed on children with T1DM, to help uncover possible reasons the child developed the disease. These include food sensitivity testing, stool testing, intestinal permeability testing, environmental toxicity testing, genetic testing, comprehensive (and expensive) nutritional evaluations, and so forth. Unfortunately, some parents of kids with T1DM hope that if a result of these tests is abnormal and treated, the child will no longer have T1DM. I have seen this over and over throughout my career. The child is put through numerous tests, and at the end the child maintains their T1DM status. A sense of failure and a stigmatization of the condition can occur.

My view of doing the above-mentioned tests is based on two thoughts. If a child with T1DM also has asthma, psoriasis, migraines, or another treatable condition on top of T1DM, I usually recommend a food sensitivity test to help remove a food trigger if the diabetic diet does not clear up the condition. It also doesn't hurt to do the other tests and see if there are any imbalances and help heal them, perhaps to maximize the functioning of the body system or prevent further autoimmunity. However, at the outset, it should be made clear that the child's T1DM will remain. I do not feel it is right for physicians or others to suggest a "cure" or "reversal" of the child's T1DM in order to put the child through endless integrative tests.

Have I ever seen a child with T1DM be cured of their diabetes? I have not seen it among my patients. A cure would mean the child could eat anything, including whole-grain bread, baked potatoes, and rice, and still have completely normal glucose values, and even have positive diabetes antibodies return to negative status. I have seen *very* long honeymoon periods, where the glucose and A1C are outstandingly normal, as I mentioned, but as puberty kicks in, insulin usually becomes necessary, and once insulin is started, the patients usually cannot be removed from it. I think it is better for a parent to face the difficult reality that their child has T1DM and instead of believing they are losing the child to the disease, allow the child to be accepted as a child with T1DM, be supported, and still have fun and play.

I am hoping that stem-cell or other research may one day lead to a cure for T1DM. To do that, researchers need to figure out how to fully regenerate beta cells and stop an overactive autoimmune system from attacking them. However, until then, I think parents should work hard to keep a child on a good diet and in good control, and at some point accept the condition as permanent. I wish I could say integrative medicine cures T1DM diabetes, but it cannot. It can, however, control it! The best way to help control T1DM in a child is by putting them on the vegan low-glycemic diet.

Guidelines for Control of Pediatric Diabetes

The ADA currently suggests that all children should have an A1C lower than or equal to 7.5 percent, although lower than 7.0 percent is ideal if it can be achieved without frequent, significant hypoglycemia. This represents a change from previous ADA recommendations that depended on the age of the child. The ADA also recommends glucose before meals to be in the range of 90–130 mg/dL (5.0–7.2 mmol/L) and glucose at bedtime and overnight to be in the range of 90–150 mg/dL (5.0–8.3 mmol/L). Unfortunately, having an A1C of lower than or equal to 7.5 percent is still too high, although a child can grow and develop normally if their A1C is lower than 9.0 percent.

I believe the reason the ADA pediatric A1C recommendation is higher than I feel it should be is due to fear of children having hypoglycemia, especially at night when they are sleeping. And it also may be connected to the main axiom of conventional treatment given to T1DM kids, which is "eat what you want, and cover it with insulin." As you can imagine, I find this recommendation dangerous and irresponsible. Diabetic children do not need bread and pasta for energy, or to enable growth; they can do fine without it, especially with lower glucose levels as a result! With gentle education and constant parental love and support, pediatric patients can learn the low-carb diet they need to eat to control their glucose throughout their lives. They will have plenty of energy to play sports, do well academically, and thrive.

However, on the other hand, it can be more difficult to get children with T1DM under good glycemic control due to the following factors:

- Eating irregularly and eating snacks means one has to "stack" insulin for coverage and risk loss, or not covering and risking highs. For kids with T2DM, regular snacking may mean eating too many calories.
- With children under ten years old, a parent is not always sure their child will eat everything on the plate. Thus, it is standard for a parent to inject insulin after the meal, based on the food the child ate. After ten years old, the child will generally eat what is served, and it is safe to transition to injecting before meals, but we need to assess that for each child. Another way to inject is half before the meal and half after, or, if using a pump, set the pump for a dual-wave injection where the pump does the same type of dosing.
- Children grow, and growth spurts require more insulin and can raise glucose numbers.
- Children are active; figuring out how to eat and use insulin with their activities can take some time.
- Children, and teens in particular, experience peer pressure and may eat what their friends eat even when they know they shouldn't.
- It's also natural for teenagers to rebel and act out, which can make it difficult for parents to keep them following the diet, checking their glucose numbers, and injecting insulin. I work with teens and parents to set up positive methods for the teen to care for their diabetes while being rewarded with things important to them, such as computer time, or use of the car, a higher allowance, and so forth.
- Sex hormones cause insulin resistance, and during puberty, before monthly periods, and during pregnancies, humans are naturally insulin resistant. During puberty, sex hormone levels are high, and that is when we mainly see T2DM being diagnosed and when kids

with T1DM will need to increase their insulin doses. It may be harder for kids with either T2DM or T1DM to keep glucose levels under good control during those adolescent years.

Children with T2DM diabetes may or may not need oral hypoglycemic medications and insulin. If they are on insulin, they have the same difficulties as their T1DM peers. If they are not on insulin, T2DM kids still share some of their struggles. Role modeling is very important, including getting the entire family to give up junk food and eat healthier. Exercise—getting the child to initiate a fun, positive, and active exercise regimen—is also vital. It doesn't hurt for the entire family to work out or be active together, either. Lastly, body image is a concern. Children who are overweight or obese may or may not have a body image issue. If they do, counseling may be helpful. While the goal is to establish good control of a child's diabetes, I would encourage protocols that ensure the child feels positive about themselves and who they can become. We want to empower, motivate, and support, not criticize and judge.

Diabetes Supplies

Parents of pediatric T1DM patients, especially those under ten years old and on insulin, generally test their child's glucose typically around ten times a day. The child's physician has to write a prescription script for around three hundred glucose test strips a month, to ensure insurance will cover them.

The child on insulin, whether T1DM or T2DM, must have a medical ID on at all times and must also carry glucose tabs and gels in case of a hypoglycemic event. Be creative with the ID and allow the child to choose if it is a necklace, bracelet, or attached to shoelaces; however they wish to wear the ID is fine.

For children needing insulin, it is now standard to use the same long-acting basal and rapid-acting bolus insulin that we recommend for adults. Children are extremely sensitive to insulin—if a pediatric T1DM patient weighs 40 pounds, one unit of rapid insulin will lower his glucose 210 mg/dL. One unit of basal insulin will lower his glucose 280 mg/dL. If a T1DM child weighs 70 pounds, one unit of rapid insulin will lower her glucose 120 mg/dL and one unit of basal insulin will lower her glucose 160 mg/dL. If children are using syringe and vial, ensure the child uses a BD 3/10 half-unit marked syringe, as half-unit markings will be helpful for better insulin dosing. It is possible to dilute insulin, if necessary, for very young children who require a syringe for their insulin, but it is not commonly done; instead a pediatric patient will ideally be put on a pump.

If using rapid pens, make sure to get a NovoPen Echo or HumaPen Luxura HD, as these are the only rapid pens with half-unit markings. The vast majority of pediatric patients I see come to me on typical rapid pens without the half-unit dosing capabilities, so they can only dose one-unit intervals, which sets a child up for a high risk of hypoglycemic events. Most pharmacies do not carry pens with half-unit markings; they usually have to be special-ordered.

Children typically just need one shot of basal for twenty-four hours if they are on syringe or pen, and it's common to inject that in the morning when they are very young. Once they reach puberty, they likely will need to be on both an evening and a morning dose, adding the second dose to control their background glucose.

A pump should be seriously considered for pediatric patients on full basal/bolus dosing to be able to dose the precise, small doses of insulin many children require. Using the pump gives increased accuracy to basal dosing, which can ensure parents sleep better through the night, with their child at less risk for hypoglycemic reactions. Pumps are recommended in standard care for pediatric patients, although a child can be just as poorly controlled on a pump as on a syringe and vial if diet, exercise, sleep, and supplements are not in good order.

Although conventionally oriented—it does not promote low-carb diets—the website Children with Diabetes (www.childrenwithdiabetes.org) is very informative and has a weekly newsletter.

Diabetic Diet for Pediatric Patients

Diets for children with diabetes are similar to what we recommend for adults, and should ideally be grain free and low carb. It's a common mistake to believe that diabetic children need grains to grow and have energy. They do not; they need low glucose levels. Children can easily thrive on a grain-free low-carb diet.

It is good to have all children with diabetes help do the food shopping and a little cooking with their parents, so they can help choose what they will eat, which will help them feel more in control and more willing to eat the new foods and recipes. Adding in nut, coconut, or cauliflower flour muffins, cookies, tortillas, granolas, pizza crusts, lasagna, and cookies—all foods that all kids like to eat and that can easily be adapted to a low-carb option—can make the diet really successful, tasty, and fun.

Of course, it's not helpful if the entire family eats all the restricted foods in front of the child with diabetes. The entire household needs to outwardly conform to the child's diet; if a sibling or parent needs to eat some bread or a bag of pretzels, they should do so out of the child's sight, unless the child is older, understands, and is okay with family members eating what he or she cannot.

For newly diagnosed T2DM and T1DM pediatric patients it's good to keep a diet diary of a typical day's food intake, both the good and the bad, both at the beginning of their treatment (their typical diet) and as it changes, including entering it into the USDA's SuperTracker website to determine calorie content, fat, carbs, protein, salt, and so forth.

Neither T1DM nor T2DM pediatric patients should eat or drink refined sugar, junk food, fast food, poor quality processed foods, or grains.

With T1DM children we need to ensure they have enough calories and protein intake. If the child is eating a vegan diet, monitor their growth every three months, and if the child is not clearly growing, it's a sign of protein malnourishment and animal food must be added back into the diet. Also, if eating vegan, supplementation should occur but nonetheless check for iron and vitamin B_{12} serum levels at least once a year.

In T2DM pediatric patients, conventional care starts with diet, exercise, lifestyle modifications, and metformin, and encourages either weight loss or weight maintenance, allowing growth to help the child become more lean. The diet the American Academy of Pediatrics advises consists of regular meals and snacks; reduced portion sizes (use smaller plates); calorie-free beverages except for milk; juice limited to one 8 ounce cup a day; increased fruits and vegetables; three to four servings of low-fat dairy products; limited high-fat foods; and reduced calories eaten in fast-food meals. There are some good aspects to those diet recommendations, certainly, but I think they need to be a great deal tighter.

Low-calorie diets are at times suggested for for T2DM pediatric patients. In general, these are normal calorie intakes for pediatric patients:

Four to eight years old: 1,200 kcal per day female and 1,400 kcal per day male
Nine to thirteen years old: 1,600 kcal per day female and 1,800 kcal per day male
Fourteen to eighteen years old: 1,800 kcal per day female and 2,000 kcal per day male

In general, in T2DM kids, instead of reducing calories, just removing the worst offenders—soda pop, candy, cake, chips, and French fries—can have amazing benefits in glucose control and weight loss. Of course, this reduces calories, but the key is to add in foods that the child finds equally delicious, and get them exercising, so it doesn't feel like a "diet." In lean T1DM patients, adding calories may be important to ensure lack of weight loss from removing the calories from sugar and grains, through using nut products and adding oils or adding high calorie smoothies.

The T2DM pediatric dose for metformin is 500 mg once per day, slowly titrating up over one to two weeks to the maximum dose of 2,000 mg per day, which is actually the same dosing as for adults. Adding in basal or bolus insulin is considered an acceptable next step, if necessary—if diet, exercise, and metformin are not lowering glucose, reducing insulin resistance, and allowing weight loss.

For both T1DM or T2DM pediatric patients on bolus insulin dosing, meal and correction, I always use the same insulin dosing for meals and corrections as discussed in chapter 6 of this book. If you have an Android phone, you can use my CarbProtein Insulin Calculator app for children, too.

Pediatric Diabetes Supplementation

Whether I am working with a newly diagnosed T1DM pediatric patient, a T1DM pediatric patient who has been diagnosed for a while, or a T2DM pediatric patient, the supplement list in table 12.1 can be used for any of them.

If a newly diagnosed T1DM pediatric patient has a "honeymoon" period, the supplements are designed to help protect the pancreas and safely strive to reduce the autoimmune reaction.

For established T1DM and T2DM pediatric patients, supplements are also beneficial to increase energy, help learn and have good focus, protect the body from high-glucose damage, reduce insulin resistance, and give all nutrients needed for the cells of the body to maximize functioning. Please do not put any child on any supplemental protocol without first having the guidance and approval of the child's physician.

Table 12.1. Recommended Daily Dosages of Supplements (One or More), by Patient Type

Supplement	Dosage per day	Patient Type[a]
Alpha-lipoic acid	300–1,200 mg	ND, T1DM, T2DM
Chromium drops	200–800 mcg	ND, T1DM, T2DM
Cinnamon capsules	200–1,000 mg	ND, T1DM, T2DM
Curcumin	200–1,000 mg	T1DM, T2DM
Vitamin D_3, if deficient	Dosed per need via labs	ND, T1DM, T2DM
Diamend	1–7 capsules	ND, T1DM, T2DM
Extra zinc	5–25 mg	ND, T1DM, T2DM
Fish oils	250–1,000 mg EPA / 250–750 mg DHA	ND, T1DM, T2DM
Gymnema sylvestre	400 mg or more	ND, T1DM, T2DM
Mixed vitamin E	400–800 IU	ND
Moducare	1–2 capsules	ND
Multiple vitamin/mineral	3–6 capsules	ND, T1DM, T2DM
Niacinamide	1,000–1,500 mg	ND
Pacreatic glandular	1–3 capsules	ND

[a]ND stands for newly diagnosed T1DM; T1DM and T2DM: established diagnosis

A good supplement regimen would consist of one or more of the supplements listed in table 12.1. If dairy is removed from the diet, then a calcium and magnesium supplement also needs to be added in.

Of course, children should not take all those supplements. Diamend is a good option for children who can swallow capsules; they may take fewer than the full seven capsules a day. For children who cannot swallow capsules, getting supplements in powder or liquid form is necessary. Many, but not all, capsules can be opened up and added to food or smoothies; R-ALA is too acidic for that and needs to be swallowed in the capsule, or it comes in a safe liquid form, as well. From this extensive list, I choose the best protocol for each child.

Diabulimia

In teenage T1DM or insulin dependent T2DM patients, we have to watch for diabulimia, a terribly serious condition with grave consequences for the child's health. It tends to occur between the ages of fifteen and thirty. Diabulimia is considered a disordered eating behavior and occurs when an insulin dependent teen stops or underdoses required insulin to lose weight and stay thin. It is mostly seen in diabetic female teens who realize they can eat whatever they want if they are not using insulin, as it will not enter their cells, and they will urinate out their calories. However, these teens will have strikingly high glucose levels, put themselves at high risk for diabetic ketoacidosis (DKA), and cause devastating damage to their bodies. It is important for parents to monitor their child's insulin use, glucose levels, weight, diet, and so forth, to ensure that DKA is discovered as soon as possible. If it is, the child can then receive counseling and get their glucose and insulin dosing back on track.

Parents should test their child's A1Cs every three months. If any of the following are occurring, parents need to immediately have a discussion with their child and seek care with her physician and psychological practitioners:

- There is a lack of finger sticks, and no need to get more glucose test sticks.
- The child is not running out of insulin.

- The recorded glucose numbers on a glucose graph do not match the A1C and Glycomark labs.
- The child has significantly elevated glucose levels (over 400 mg/dL) for no reason, such as illness.
- The child has a DKA event, or has weight loss, excessive appetite or urination, indigestion, increased thirst, weakness, fatigue, lack of concentration, or elevated ketones in urine or blood.

Diabulimia is massively damaging to the teen's body and may even be fatal due to DKA. Teens who stop or underdose insulin can end up in kidney failure or blind, have severe neuropathy, cardiovascular disease, or osteoporosis even in their twenties. While this condition is not common, all family members should keep alert for any signs of diabulimia, a fully treatable condition.

For anyone reading this book who either has diabulimia or knows a friend or family member who does, there is a crisis hotline available online at diabulimiahelpline.org. Please contact it!

Schools and Camps

No matter where my T1DM pediatric patients live, all the schools they've attended have been excellent to work with: helpful, accommodating, understanding, and willing to work with the protocol created by the parents for their diabetic child. There is a 504 Plan for diabetes as well as an individualized education program (IEP), since diabetes has been listed by our government as a "disability." These forms allow parents, with their physician, to create a formal plan for how their child should be treated at school regarding their diabetes: when the child needs to check glucose levels, and inject insulin; when and how to treat a hypoglycemic episode; and so forth. I always suggest parents meet with the principal, teachers, and nurses, and alert them that their child is an insulin dependent diabetic. It is common for the school to ask for supplies for the child, such as insulin, syringes, pens, glucose meter, glucagon, glucose tabs, and so forth. Working in a positive way with school officials enhances the child's school experience. Don't worry—in my experience, schools tend to be great working with children who have T1DM.

Having things worked out at school can be a huge relief for parents, the child, and the school.

As for camps, I am sure we can all imagine that it would be great fun for a child with T1DM insulin dependent diabetes to go to a camp where she is surrounded by other insulin dependent kids. Being accepted for having what everyone else has, knows about, and understands is valuable to all children. There are many camps specific to T1DM kids all around the country.

In an article in *Diabetes Care*, the ADA recommended the following:

- Daily record of camper's process should be made—all glucose and insulin doses should be recorded, and multiple glucose checks should occur each day.
- Follow the home insulin dosing level, although usually the child needs 10–20 percent less insulin due to activities.
- Meals should be monitored for carbohydrate counts (of course, I hope parents would press for a low-carb diet menu!).
- There should be a formal relationship between the camp and a nearby medical facility.
- Universal hygienic procedures should be followed by camp personnel, such as wearing gloves when taking glucose checks and disposing of sharps in a responsible manner.
- The camp should have personnel on staff who are experts in treating diabetic pediatric patients and are confident in treating hypoglycemia, ketoacidosis, and other diabetic concerns (e.g., switching to syringe and needle if the pump breaks). Clear treatment guidelines should be established with personnel trained in applying them as necessary.
- The camp should have a "Camp Management Plan" reviewable for all to read. It should contain sections on all aspects of working with and managing diabetes, treatment of problems, handling of diabetic supplies, emergency protocols, and so forth.

I suggest all parents read the article on the ADA's website before sending their child to camp, to give them the ability to analyze the camp setup and ensure they feel it is well run.

Children going to camp should take with them a written medical management plan that contains their medical history, immunization record, and clearly written diabetes regimen. Their insulin dosages and blood glucose monitoring and ketone testing schedule should be explicit and clear. Also, it would be good for parents to include data on any hypoglycemic and hyperglycemic/ketoacidosis tendencies/times the child has experienced, their recent A1C levels, any medications or supplements they are on, any dietary restrictions the child has, any medical conditions the child has in addition to their diabetes, and if they suffer from any psychological issues. It also needs to be clear when the camp should contact parents/guardians, a primary care practitioner, and a diabetes care provider.

In this way, the child can have a wonderful time playing, enjoying nature, doing new activities and learning new skills, making friends, and being well cared for by personnel who are competent in working with insulin dependent children.

It is very rewarding to work with children with diabetes, helping them deal with a condition that needs to be dealt with twenty-four hours a day, seven days a week. Setting up comprehensive protocols for kids and seeing them thrive and develop is one of the best parts of being a physician who specializes in diabetes. When parents are stressed, it is rewarding to help them relax and accept the situation, ensuring their child still enjoys life and feels positive about who they are and what they can become, which is anything they want to become! Using integrative medicine to help reverse T2DM in children, and educating on diet and insulin (when needed) with kids who have T1DM means creating a win-win scenario for everyone involved.

— CHAPTER THIRTEEN —

Diabetic Challenges

In this chapter, I will cover how to correctly address several diabetic challenges: diabetic ketoacidosis, hypoglycemia, an ill diabetic patient, and safe diabetic travel.

Diabetic Ketoacidosis and Hyperglycemic Hyperosmolar State

The definition of diabetic ketoacidosis (DKA) is an absolute or relative insulin deficiency causing hyperglycemia, dehydration, and metabolic acidosis. About 3 percent of the T1DM population will have an episode of DKA, and if it is caught early and treated, there is, luckily, only a 2 percent fatality rate. However, we never want any diabetic patient to die from DKA! DKA is more prevalent in pediatric patients—and, in fact, many children with new onset T1DM are in DKA upon diagnosis—but it can occur at any age. DKA tends to develop quite quickly and is considered to be a medical emergency. For safety's sake, all patients in DKA should be immediately sent to the emergency room.

When the body burns fat for energy, the breakdown of the fat creates ketone bodies and fatty acids. There are three physiologic ketone bodies: acetoacetic acid, acetone, and B-hydroxyl-butyric acid. Ketone bodies go to the brain, which uses them for energy instead of glucose. A higher amount of ketones in the blood is called "ketosis." As discussed earlier, ketosis is a safe biochemical phenomenon, and is often seen when patients are eating a strict low-carb diet or when they are eating fewer calories on a weight loss program and their body is burning fat. A diet containing fewer than 40 or so grams of carbs will often initiate a ketone-producing or ketogenic reaction.

Many, if not most, overweight T2DM patients who are not on insulin but are losing weight on a low-carb diet can be in daily ketosis. Other people using a ketogenic diet for other reasons will be in a safe state of daily ketosis, as well. DKA is *not* ketosis, and this is an important differentiation that every parent, child, and medical practitioner should know.

Ketoacidosis is a more complicated and dangerous biochemical event than ketosis. It starts with a lack of insulin in an insulin dependent diabetic. As the blood glucose increases and cannot be absorbed into body cells to nourish and feed them, the body secretes glucagon, growth hormone, and catecholamine, substances that direct the body to break down triglycerides to fatty acids and ketones. Ketone bodies are acidic, and they can rapidly deplete extracellular and intracellular acid buffers, so the serum becomes more acidic. Meanwhile, the liver and kidneys begin gluconeogenesis, breaking down starches into glucose, and raising the serum glucose even more. This causes the person to urinate more, which causes sodium, potassium, phosphates, and water depletion through the kidneys. It is the multifactorial situation of decreased or no insulin, high glucose, ketone bodies, acidic serum, and dehydration that collectively defines DKA and causes the body to start failing.

When should you check for ketones?

- Glucose is higher than 250 mg/dL for more than a few hours.
- The patient is feverish, has an infection, is vomiting, or has diarrhea.
- The patient does not feel "well," and has some symptoms of DKA.
- The patient is a pregnant woman with T1DM whose glucose numbers are not strictly controlled and are not being regularly checked.

Common presentations of DKA include:

- Fruity breath (exhaled ketone bodies have a sweet smell)
- Abdominal tenderness ("stomachache")

- Nausea, vomiting, diarrhea
- Polyuria (urinating a lot), polydipsia (drinking a lot)
- Signs of dehydration: thirst, weakness, dry skin and mucous membranes, skin tenting, lack of urination
- Tiredness, fatigue
- Disorientation, confusion
- Coma
- Hyperventilation (breathing more frequently than normal)
- Signs of infection such as fever and chills

DKA is highly associated with infection in insulin dependent diabetics; in fact, 40 percent of patients had a urinary tract infection, gastroenteritis, or flu precede DKA onset. Newly diagnosed T1DM patients account for another 15 percent of patients with DKA. Moreover, a deliberate or accidental omission of insulin injection accounts for 25 percent of patients. The last category of DKA onset includes miscellaneous events: trauma, heart attack, stroke, stress, cocaine, surgery, and dental abscess.

Testing for Ketones

The diagnosis of DKA is well established via labs: elevated blood sugars, elevated ketones, low potassium, arterial pH lower than 7.2 (the blood is acidic), and plasma bicarbonate lower than 15 mEq/L (the blood is low in buffers). The last two readings show that the body is in an "acidosis" state.

Checking for elevated ketone bodies, a sign of the first stage of developing DKA, can easily be done at home. Ketones can be measured in the blood: Precision Xtra and Nova Max Plus are both combination meters that measure blood glucose and blood ketones. The ketone measured is B-hydroxy-butyric acid, and 80 percent of ketones in the blood are B-hydroxy-butyric. Blood ketones are helpful, as they measure in the moment what is occurring in the body regarding ketones; however, the test strips are very sensitive and expensive.

Ketones can also be measured in the urine on Ketostix test strips, which anyone can buy at a pharmacy. These strips measure for acetoacete ketone bodies. The strips are inexpensive, but a urine analysis can reflect what was happening in the body two to four hours ago. So, if a T1DM patient has had any DKA events outside of initial diagnosis of his diabetes, then having a glucose meter that measures ketones in the blood, which is an immediate reading, is very helpful. Otherwise, the Ketostix are fine to measure ketones to prevent the chance of DKA during a future illness. In general, ketone urine test strips are typically used due to convenience and cost.

You can have a false negative (it shows negative, but it is wrong) urine ketone test if the patient has very acidic urine from ingesting high doses of vitamin C, from aspirin intake, or if the test strips were exposed to air for quite a while. You can have a false positive (it shows positive, but it is wrong) urine ketone test if the patient is taking certain drugs or is fasting or the test is performed on a pregnant woman with hyperemesis gravidum—severe nausea and vomiting.

We also need to ensure we know what type of ketones we are dealing with. We've mentioned benign *dietary ketones*, which will occur with normal glucose levels and normal insulin dosing on a low-carb diet. *Starvation ketones* are ketones that are elevated with low glucose levels. This is due to hypoglycemia from having too little glucose in the serum, so the body turns to burning fats. The treatment for this is simply to eat glucose tabs and then food, injecting the proper amount of insulin to allow the glucose to rise in the serum, but also to enter the cells. *DKA ketones* are the ones we are most concerned about.

Table 13.1 is helpful for knowing how serious the urine or blood ketone test results are (but, of course, always call your physician!):

Table 13.1. Ketone Test Results and Their Seriousness

Seriousness	Urine Ketone Level: mg/100 mg	Blood Ketone Level: mmol/L
Negative	White, light pink	0–0.5
Small	Mid-pink	0.6–1.0
Moderate	Magenta	1.1–1.5
Large	Dark purple/black	1.5–3.0

A person should immediately be referred to a hospital emergency department if the ketone level is severe, over 3.0 via the blood, or if the urine test is very dark and the patient is still suffering symptomatically.

Table 13.2, adapted from the book *Type 1 Diabetes*, by Ragnar Hanas, MD, helps clarify the different types of ketosis and how to monitor and treat them.

There are four scenarios that can occur when waking up in the night:

1. Blood glucose is slightly high, around 150 mg/dL, urine glucose is slightly present, and ketones are negative. ANALYSIS—Glucose

Table 13.2. Types of Ketosis and How to Treat Them, Based on Glucose Levels

Ketones	Glucose: < 180 mg/dL	Glucose: 180–250 mg/dL	Glucose: 250–400 mg/dL	Glucose: > 400 mg/dL
Blood: < 0.5 Urine: Negative	Normal	Normal	Check in 1–2 hours	Check in 1–2 hours
Blood: 0.6–1.0 Urine: Small	Check in 1–2 hours	Consider insulin, if active	Inject 0.25 units/10 lb	Inject 0.5 units/10 lb
Blood: 1.1–1.5 Urine: Moderate	Starvation ketones: eat and give fluids	Eat, give fluids, and inject 0.25 units/10 lb	Give fluids and inject 0.5 units/10 lb	Give fluids and inject 0.5 units/10 lb
Blood: 1.5–3.0 Urine: Large	Starvation ketones: eat and take insulin after glucose has elevated	Eat and inject 0.5 units/ 10lb, stop vomiting and give fluids	Inject 0.5 units/10 lb, check glucose in 2–3 hours and inject again if necessary, stop vomiting and give fluids	Inject 0.5 units/10 lb, check glucose in 2–3 hours and inject again if necessary, stop vomiting and give fluids
Blood: > 3.0 Urine: Severe	ER	ER	ER	ER

Source: Adapted from *Type 1 Diabetes*, by Ragnar Hanas, MD.

was higher during sleep, high enough to go into the urine, but not enough to cause ketosis. Don't worry; don't eat; and don't inject.

2. Blood glucose is around 60 mg/dL, urine glucose is negative, and ketones are positive. *Analysis*—Starvation ketones. Eat.
3. Blood glucose is very high, around 270 mg/dL, urine glucose is high, and ketones are elevated. *Analysis*—Hyperglycemia during the night due to lack of insulin. Inject insulin; drink fluid.
4. Blood glucose is very high, around 270 mg/dL, urine glucose is high, and ketones are elevated. *Second analysis*—Somogyi phenomenon, where a hypoglycemic event caused reactive hyperglycemia. Not everyone agrees this phenomenon occurs, but some patients feel they have experienced it. Inject insulin; drink fluid.

Of course, always call your physician as soon as possible if you notice ketones that are not due to dietary ketosis. Unless you have been well trained by your physician, please *do not* follow the aforementioned guidelines on your own!

When someone with T1DM is ill, is exercising outside on a hot day, or is otherwise at risk for DKA scenarios, keeping the person hydrated is very important. Dehydration is a key aspect of developing DKA. Pushing fluids is always safe for a person with diabetes of any type and at any time. Many patients who are poorly controlled (glucose over 200 mg/dL, and especially over 250 mg/dL) will be able to find high ketones in blood or urine. This is not a crisis, yet. By correcting the high glucose and keeping hydrated, these elevated ketone situations can be easily treated, and no one needs to panic. It's good to have a way of contacting your physician to get an immediate response to any ketone question. Once a patient or a parent is well trained and understands ketones and DKA extremely well, it's easy for a calm, cool, and collected demeanor to get ketones down and glucose back into cells, and avoid any dangerous situation.

I do find that children with T1DM on a low-carb diet tend to have higher ketones even though they are thriving, have good energy, and are growing well. This can be nerve-wracking for parents, of course! But as long as the patient is fine overall, their glucose is under control, and they are drinking a lot, I do not see the ketones in the urine or blood as much of a problem. I think pediatric patients, with their high metabolisms, burn fat more readily. It's important for these children to eat enough calories each day; we do not want them to lose weight. The USDA's SuperTracker website to measure calorie intake can be used to record a daily intake of all food—it will automatically list out calorie, carb, fat, and protein intake (this website also can list micronutrient intake). But, please note: early on in a low-carb diet, some kids with T1DM can be spilling ketones regularly into their urine and this can be fine.

Hyperosmolar Hyperglycemic State (HHS)

This crisis mainly occurs in senior T2DM patients, and the average time of onset is in the seventh decade of life. Unlike diabetic ketoacidosis, which can occur very quickly, within hours, HHS has a very slow onset and, in general, takes days to a week to develop. There is no significant ketoacidosis with HHS. It is less common than DKA but has a higher mortality rate, mostly due to the fact that the patients experiencing it are older and often have co-morbidities—several serious medical conditions they are dealing with, such as cardiovascular disease, renal disease, or congestive heart failure.

These patients can still make some insulin, so it prevents ketone formation, but their insulin level is not high enough to lower glucose levels. Adding in dehydration, they can have a serious collapse.

HHS is diagnosed by these lab values:

Glucose. Higher than 600 mg/dL
Profound dehydration. Often up to 9L deficient in fluid. (Tachycardia [rapid heartbeat], hypotension [low blood pressure], and skin turgor [tenting] are signs of dehydration.)
Low ketones in the urine, and no or very low ketones in the blood
Serum osmolality. Equal to or higher than 320 mOsm/kg
Serum pH. Higher than 7.30
Bicarbonate concentration. Higher than 15 mEq/L

The serum pH and bicarbonate concentration values indicate that patients are not in DKA.

There is also often some alteration in consciousness, such as the patient being drowsy or lethargic. The patient can have visual changes or disturbances, sensory deficits, hemiparesis (one-sided paralysis), or seizures, or may fall into a coma. The patient may have a high temperature.

These older T2DM patients might be on medications, such as diuretics, beta-blockers, or antipsychotics. They might be abusing alcohol or illegal drugs. They might be noncompliant with taking their oral diabetic medicines or injecting their insulin. Sadly, they might also be victims of elder abuse or neglect in that their caregivers are not giving them enough fluids, and are thus leading them to slowly developing dehydration.

HHS is a very urgent medical emergency and, unlike in DKA, it is very important that no one gives the patient any insulin. In HHS, rapid lowering of glucose without vigorous fluid replacement can result in devastating complications, including an increased risk of shock. A person with HHS must be referred to an emergency room immediately for detailed and precise treatment under close medical care, so simply call 911.

After the crisis is over, it is important to prevent HHS from ever happening again. The person will have to be counseled on taking their oral diabetic medicines or injecting their insulin as prescribed. Their living situation will need to be evaluated to ensure the patient can administer appropriate self-care or that the family member or assisted living situation is not neglectful. The patient will need to be educated on how to better control their glucose numbers (including going on a low-carb diet!). Moreover, it will need to be firmly established that the patient has access to half their body weight in water a day (in ounces), which is the amount people should drink to stay well hydrated.

Hypoglycemia

Hypoglycemia, by medical definition, is when a person's glucose sinks below 70 mg/dL. While the brain can still function until the glucose falls below 30 mg/dL, most people feel awful the lower the glucose goes. It's important to learn how to prevent hypoglycemic events, and, once one occurs, how to quickly and effectively treat it.

Hypoglycemia is a common phenomenon in patients with diabetes, especially those injecting insulin or those taking a sulphonylurea. On average, a diabetic patient has two or three hypoglycemic events every week and one hypoglycemic event so severe it initiates loss of consciousness or a seizure one or two times a year. Patients obviously and understandably dislike hypoglycemia, and avoiding severe lows is a huge benefit to them in a well-rounded treatment regimen.

How does hypoglycemia occur? When a nondiabetic person's serum glucose lowers inbetween meals or during prolonged exercise, they secrete glucagon from their pancreatic alpha cells, epinephrine and cortisol from the adrenal gland, and growth hormone from their pituitary; these hormones signal the liver to create glucose and secrete it into the bloodstream. Also, insulin secretion is inhibited. Thus, glucose levels naturally increase and can stay within normal limits.

A person with insulin dependent diabetes might have a deficiency of glucagon production, might have a blunted adrenal response (especially if she has repeatedly had hypoglycemic events), and might have normal or elevated levels of insulin still active in her system. Thus, instead of glucose naturally elevating due to appropriate physiological responses to hypoglycemia, it does not rise and might also continue to decrease.

Hypoglycemia in diabetes can be due to:

Excessive insulin injection. Overinjecting basal, meal, or correction insulin, or receiving too aggressive a dose of oral medication, in combination with food and exercise, can easily cause a hypoglycemic reaction. Also, injection mistakes can cause hypoglycemia. More than once, I've had patients call me at 11 p.m. and report that instead of injecting Lantus, their nightly basal dose, by mistake they injected Humalog, a rapid insulin. Just like checking twice before sawing in carpentry, a patient with diabetes should check the insulin type twice before injecting. It's also good to put different color bands on each type of insulin bottle, such as a blue band for basal and a red band for rapid.

Decreased or delayed food ingestion. A patient may have injected correctly before their meal but got distracted and forgot to eat on time or ate less food than the insulin was designed to cover.

Use of alcohol or drugs that interfere with liver production of glucose. Alcohol breaks down not into glucose but into acetaldehydes, which do not raise the glucose, and on top of that, alcohol interferes with gluconeogenesis, a pathway the liver uses to break down proteins into glucose to raise the sugar levels. Because of this, alcohol tends to lower glucose levels. Thus, drinking alcohol, injecting insulin or taking oral medications, and eating a low-carb diet can cause hypoglycemia if it is not all balanced and appropriately handled.

Increased exercise from usual regimen or *did not reduce insulin appropriately post-exercise.* Doing unplanned extensive exercise, doing a notably longer or more intense exercise session, by mistake having injected insulin into a muscle instead of subcutaneous fat, or adding insulin back in too strongly after exercise can lead to significantly low glucose during or after exercise.

Medications, particularly beta-blockers and SSRIs. As discussed earlier, beta-blockers mask early signs of low glucose so that patients cannot feel the slower onset of hypoglycemia, and fall victim to it once it is quite advanced. Beta-blockers are contraindicated in all insulin dependent diabetic patients, unless absolutely necessary for some serious medical reason. Serotonin selective reuptake inhibitors (SSRIs) are antidepressants that can also stop symptoms of hypoglycemia in some patients. Caffeine, on the other hand, can help the adrenals detect hypoglycemia, even when the glucose levels are higher, so it can be beneficial to deterring hypoglycemia.

Hypoglycemia Signs and Symptoms

What does hypoglycemia feel like? Both adrenal and neurological systems can create signs and symptoms in a patient experiencing hypoglycemia.

The brain physiology of glucose changes as it lowers. When the body's serum glucose is 82.8–540 mg/dL, the brain glucose level is similar to that of the blood; in fact, a nifty study showed that even as low as 54 mg/dL, the brain and blood glucose levels may be similar. Things get murky in the brain as the blood glucose lowers but one study showed that the brain glucose level approaches zero when plasma glucose is approximately 21.6 mg/dL. Zero is not a good glucose number for the brain!

Hypoglycemia reactions basically fall into two categories: an adrenal autonomic reaction, caused by the adrenals secreting a lot of epinephrine as a result of low blood sugar, or a neuroglycopenic reaction, caused by the brain changes from low blood sugar. When the glucose goes below 65–70 mg/dL, hunger is the first sign. Due to the adrenal autonomic reaction, a person may become irritable or experience trembling, anxiety, and heart palpitations. They may be pale and have a cold sweat.

When the glucose goes below 50–55 mg/dL, the neuroglycopenic symptoms start occurring due to the brain getting low in glucose: blurred vision, weakness, dizziness, headache, fatigue, poor memory, slurred speech, and unsteady walking or loss of coordination. The diabetic person may begin having abnormal behavior or confusion, and can have poor judgment of situations, for example, feeling they will be good drivers when, under 70 mg/dL, diabetics are not supposed to drive, as they often are cognitively impaired. If the glucose continues to lower below 50 mg/dL, the patient may fall unconscious and have a seizure.

Hypoglycemia unawareness (HU) is a term used when a patient does not experience any notable signs or symptoms when going low. HU is usually due to frequent hypoglycemic events that "burn out" the adrenal glands' capacity to respond, so the body skips the early adrenal autonomic symptoms and moves into the neuroglycopenic ones. Children, in general, tend to have fewer hypoglycemic symptoms innately, or may not be able to express them to parents, so they are more susceptible to hypoglycemic unawareness. HU is easily treated by simply not having hypoglycemic episodes. Having no episodes for even two weeks can reset the adrenals, strengthen them again, and allow the body to experience early symptoms if another hypoglycemic event occurs.

Patients doing a low-carb comprehensive program with an integrative medical practitioner have extremely low risks of having serious hypoglycemic events and developing hypoglycemic unawareness.

Hypoglycemia Treatment

Hypoglycemia can be mild, moderate, or severe. If the hypoglycemia is mild, mild symptoms are noticed, and the diabetic patient can treat it himself. If it is moderate, adrenal symptoms usually occur and the diabetic patient will feel worse, but can still self-correct. When hypoglycemia is severe, the

Feeling Hypoglycemic When You Are Not

It is common that when a diabetic patient with fairly poor control (an A1C higher than 7 percent and glucose numbers regularly over 200 mg/dL) comes to an integrative physician and begins his new diet and comprehensive protocol, serum glucose numbers can lower dramatically even within the first week. I've had patients see me with glucose numbers regularly over 300 mg/dL and, within a week, their glucose numbers are down to 90–110 mg/dL. These patients very often will experience significant low blood sugar feelings, even though their glucose is not medically defined as hypoglycemic.

This feeling of hypoglycemia is because the body has a kind of "glucostat" that keeps track of where, on average, the blood glucose levels are, in the same way a thermostat in your house measures the temperature. If the glucose is around 300 mg/dL all the time, the glucostat of the body believes that is the normal glucose level. Having the glucose suddenly descend to 100 mg/dL will be temporarily interpreted by the body as a notable hypoglycemic event. Although the patient cannot fall unconscious or have a seizure at those lowered numbers, which are still

patient will need help from another individual to recover, and will perhaps need a glucagon shot.

How is hypoglycemia treated? First, if you feel hypoglycemic, test your glucose on your fingertips (no alternate site testing). Remember that fingertip testing gives us our glucose level right now, while in the less painful alternate sites, results show where it was ten to fifteen minutes ago. When hypoglycemia is occurring, we need immediate data, and can only use fingertip testing. If you are below 70 mg/dL, do not drive, operate machinery, or exercise until the glucose is back up to a healthy normal. Physicians and parents should not leave patients alone during or immediately after a hypoglycemic event, especially if the patient is a child. Most importantly, the hypoglycemic event needs to be fully analyzed to uncover the reason the low occurred, in order to prevent a similar event in the future.

clearly above 70 mg/dL, the patient can feel awful, as if their glucose is around 40 mg/dL. They can often have blurry vision, a common symptom, and other symptoms, as listed above.

There are ways to deal with this situation. First, a physician should warn patients this might happen. Having a patient be aware that this type of scenario might occur is much better than having it occur out of the blue, surprising and upsetting them. Second, a physician can slowly introduce the dietary restrictions over a week or two, so that the glucose lowers very gradually, instead of in one big drop. A slow, gradual decrease may decrease the development of symptoms. Last, body glucostats are very competent at resetting themselves, so a patient may feel low for seven to ten days before the glucostat resets itself to the newer, lower number, and the symptoms fade away.

If, however, there has been a great deal of blurry vision or even vision change with the lowering of the glucose, it is a good idea for the patient to revisit an ophthalmologist and get a dilated eye exam to ensure that no serious damaged occurred to the eyes as a result. Patients may even need changes to their eyeglass prescriptions. I've never had that happen, but it might, and being safe is always best.

Glucose Tablets and Gels

I am a huge advocate of using glucose tabs and gels to raise glucose levels. I am always a bit confounded by a patient's desire not to use glucose and instead use fruit, fruit juice, or other food, as that is "healthier." It is not healthier to do that! We do not call the sugar in our serum *glucose* for no reason. We call it that because it is a straight monosaccharide called glucose. When someone is iron anemic, we give iron; when deficient in vitamin B_{12}, we dose vitamin B_{12}. When glucose is low, what your body and brain need right away is glucose.

Fruit sugar is fructose, dairy sugar is lactose, white sugar is sucrose—all of these forms of sugar have to be enzymatically changed by the body into glucose before they can raise glucose levels. This takes time and is a reason that when a diabetic patient experiences a significant low, and he uses food to try to reverse it, his symptoms are not alleviated quickly and so it is easy for him to start overeating, because the brain is screaming for glucose. I've had patients report in first office visits with me that they eat entire packages of cookies and entire quarts of ice cream during their hypoglycemic events. That's because those foods did not quickly raise the glucose levels, the brain was still "hungry," and it sent out signals for more and more food. Once patients begin using straight glucose to raise their glucose levels, their hypoglycemia, their symptoms, and their increased appetites are very quickly resolved.

I am adamant that my patients need to correct low glucose with straight glucose—they will feel better almost immediately. Glucose comes in tablets, such as Dextrotabs, and glucose tablets are almost always regulated to contain 4 grams of glucose per tab. By the way, glucose and dextrose both describe the same sugar. Glucose gel packs are gels a person does not have to chew. They can be squirted directly into the mouth without fear of choking and so are useful for patients entering severe hypoglycemia who need more glucose and may not be fully aware. Gel packs tend to contain 15 grams of glucose, equivalent to almost four glucose tabs.

I prefer my patients go online and buy GlucoLift glucose tabs, which are healthier than typical brands. This company makes glucose tabs with only natural flavorings in them. However, if that is not feasible, then using any old glucose tab is fine, and every pharmacy carries them in many different flavors. All the ones I have seen in drugstores state that they are gluten-free, but it's good to check, especially for any person with T1DM who also has celiac disease.

For a person who weighs 120 pounds, one gram of glucose tends to raise the blood sugar 5 mg/dL, so a 4 gram tablet might raise a person's glucose around 20 mg/dL. If you weigh less, one tablet might raise your glucose much more, and if you weigh more, one tablet will probably raise your glucose less (see table 13.3 for glucose elevation according to weight).

However, general guidelines do not always relate exactly to a particular patient. Thus, I have all patients do a test in the morning to see how much one glucose tablet raises their individual glucose. Here is how to do this test:

1. Wake up in the morning and check your glucose; if it is less than 150 mg/dL, then you can do the test. (If it is over 150 mg/dL, there

Table 13.3. Glucose Elevation according to Weight

Weight (pounds)	Glucose Elevation from 1 Gram of Carbs	Glucose Elevation from 4-Gram Glucose Tab
50	8	32
75	7	28
90	6	24
120	5	20
160	4	16
200	3	12

may be some insulin resistance that may negatively affect how your body reacts to the glucose tab and not give an accurate result.)

2. Eat one glucose tab (for children under ten, use half a tablet).
3. Wait fifteen minutes and then retest your glucose level. The difference between fasting and post-glucose-tab test is how much one glucose tab increases your glucose level.

For example, if you wake at 91 mg/dL, eat a glucose tablet, and in fifteen minutes your glucose is at 116 mg/dL, then we know one glucose tab can raise your glucose 25 mg/dL. This is very helpful, as then if you ever wind up at 65 mg/dL and our correction goal for you is 100 mg/dL, you know that eating 1.5 glucose tabs should get you right to that glucose level, in a stable, steady, yet immediate way.

What is so valuable about knowing this information is that one can correct a low without shooting into the glucose stratosphere afterward. Using fruit juice, fruit, ice cream, or candy will certainly raise the glucose, but invariably the glucose then winds up high, in the 200s or 300s. Then it has to be corrected with insulin, and one begins the "brittle" battle all day long—hypoglycemia, overeating, hyperglycemia, injecting insulin, repeat! Breaking this cycle is vital, and by correcting glucose in an exacting manner, raising the glucose specifically to a safe correction number without going very high is pragmatic, safe, and efficient. Once I explain that all to patients, and they see how helpful the tabs are, they are convinced this is the best way to go, which it is!

In conventional medicine, hypoglycemia is treated via the 15-15 Rule: when a person is hypoglycemic, he eats 15 grams of carbohydrates, waits fifteen minutes, and then rechecks glucose. If the glucose reading is still lower than 80 mg/dL, the process is repeated: eat 15 grams of carbohydrates, wait fifteen minutes, recheck glucose.

STANDARD MEDICAL LIST OF FOODS WITH 15 GRAMS OF CARBOHYDRATES

- 3.5 glucose tabs
- 4 dextrose tabs
- 1 glucose gel/drink pack
- 4 ounces fruit juice
- 5–6 ounces regular pop
- 3–4 teaspoons sugar in water
- 4 Gummi Savers
- 6 Sweet Tarts (3 pieces per pack)
- 9 Sweet Tarts Classic
- 14 Giant Smarties (a little more than half the roll)
- 7 pixie sticks
- 4 Starbursts
- 7–8 jelly beans
- 1 tablespoon honey or maple syrup
- ½ ounce cake icing

In table 13.4, the last two foods raise the glucose slowest because they are mixed up with protein and fats, which slow down digestion and absorption of nutrients, even of sugar.

My problem with the 15-15 Rule is that many people do not always need that much elevation, and they end up at a risk for a high that will need to be corrected. Also, obese T2DM patients may need more glucose, due to insulin resistance, which means we end up wasting fifteen minutes, after which they are still very low. That is why it makes sense to test people individually for how dextrose affects their own glucose levels.

Please do not use anything but a glucose or dextrose tab or gel for a hypoglycemia reaction, unless you do not have either of those on hand, and you have to make do otherwise. With a glucose gel, be aware that you do not have to ingest the entire packet at one time; you can dose just the percentage of it you know you need. If in fifteen minutes the glucose levels are not elevated significantly, taking more glucose is necessary. We'll discuss that in the next section.

Table 13.4. How Foods Raise Glucose, from Quickest to Slowest

Quickest
Glucose drink (like Glucola)
Glucose tabs
Glucose gels
Honey
Lemonade
Fruit syrup
Milk
Ice cream
Chocolate bar
Slowest

Teaching people to have a protocol that initiates very tight control, eradicating the vast majority if not all of their glucose highs and lows, and instructing them to use gentle glucose tabs for instant corrections helps glucose regulation, elevates moods, boosts energy, gives patients confidence, and is indeed a great empowering tool.

Severe Hypoglycemia

Severe hypoglycemia is medically defined as a glucose level lower than 55 mg/dL, whereby the diabetic needs treatment help from another individual. Like mild hypoglycemia, it is caused by very similar factors: injecting the wrong type or amount of insulin; missing a meal when insulin had been injected for it; increasing exercise intensity or length; combining exercise with alcohol ingestion; being on a medication that blocks symptoms of hypoglycemia; injecting too high a basal dose; and so forth. With the glucose level so low, the hypoglycemia reaction is much more serious. This possibility is why I require patients to have diabetic IDs on them at all time, and also to get a glucagon emergency kit.

A person is at serious risk of seizing due to low blood sugar when their glucose fingertip value is lower than 20 mg/dL. Seizures occur mostly in children, who have more delicate nervous systems that are still developing. If a child has repeated hypoglycemic seizures, it may negatively impact his or her intellectual development.

Treatment of Severe Hypoglycemia

The first key is always being attentive and trying to catch the hypoglycemia in a mild or moderate state, and also calling a caregiver or physician if an

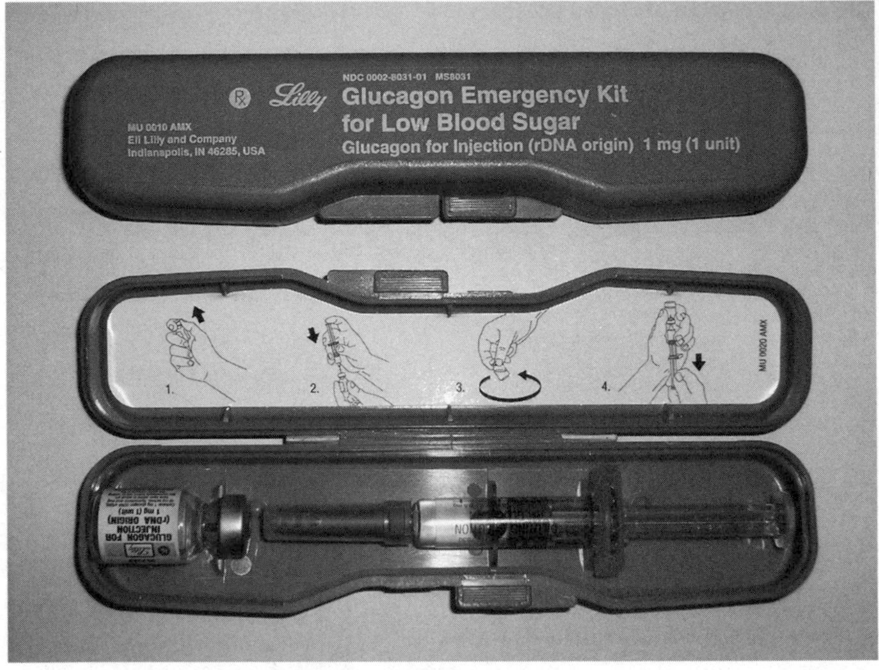

Figure 13.1. Glucagon kit.

insulin injection mistake has occurred. If you are alone, your glucose is going low, and you are starting to experience concerning symptoms and signs, immediately call 911.

Here is the basic methodology of handling a serious hypoglycemic event. First check glucose through the fingertip. If the patient is still awake and can chew, give glucose tabs or gels. If they are awake but getting fuzzy-headed, skip the tablets and squeeze a glucose gel pack into their mouth. Repeat the glucose test in fifteen minutes and give more tabs or another glucose gel if numbers have not substantially risen higher than 70 mg/dL.

If the patient is passed out and seizing, call 911 immediately. Then inject glucagon, and if the patient is not conscious within fifteen minutes, inject glucagon a second time. Glucagon is the hormone from the pancreatic alpha cells that immediately signals the liver to produce as much glucose as it can, by breaking down stored starches and proteins. Glucagon comes in a red kit, but may be out in a pen form in the future, which will make it much easier for people to feel comfortable using it. Right now, a glucagon kit comes with a syringe full of a clear fluid and a little vial with glucagon powder in it.

DIRECTIONS FOR USING A GLUCAGON KIT

1. Take off the silver lining that covers the vial top.
2. Inject all the fluid in the syringe into the vial.
3. Mix the vial up a little with the syringe still in the vial—roll it back and forth in your palms to get the powder dissolved evenly in the fluid, or keep turning it upside down.
4. Pull back on the syringe to get the dose loaded: 0.5 mg for pediatric patients (weighing less than 44 pounds) and 1.0 mg for heavier children and adult patients.
5. Inject glucagon nearly anywhere: arms, legs, upper outer hip, and abdomen are fine, but do not inject in the neck, face, or groin.
6. You cannot overdose on glucagon so don't worry about that. The website www.lillyglucagon.com has information, a tutorial, and videos showing how to use a glucagon kit.

Glucagon can make a person nauseous, so if you inject it into someone, turn the peron on his side so that if he vomits, he will not swallow or inhale the vomit. Once he wakes up, give him some glucose gel, and then once he is feeling better, it is best also to give him food. If he goes a little high that is fine at this point; he can correct it at the next meal. We don't like going high with mild or moderate hypoglycemia, but with significant hypoglycemia if we get the person up and away from the low and go a little high, okay, we'll deal with that. Don't leave the person alone for at least an hour to make sure his glucose is stable at a good level.

Once the glucagon syringe has been used it must be discarded, and a physician will need to write a new prescription. Keep unopened glucagon kits at around 68–77° F ideally. Glucagon kits expire after a year, so ensure you are aware of the expiration date on yours, and change the kit to ensure effectiveness each year.

The last thing to do after a severe hypoglycemia event is to figure out what variables were involved that caused it to happen. Analyze food eaten, insulin injected, illness, exercise, and medications, and uncover why such a serious low occurred. That way, you can be assured it never happens again!

Nocturnal Hypoglycemia

Nocturnal hypoglycemia is a fairly common problem, especially among children with T1DM who are following the conventional treatment axiom of eating what they wish and covering it with insulin, leading to endless poor control. Hypoglycemic events can occur as easily during the long hours of sleep as during the waking hours.

Nocturnal hypoglycemia signs and symptoms include waking with nighttime perspiration or with a headache, bed-wetting (which hyperglycemia also can cause), waking from a nightmare, and waking up in the morning very tired, with no energy.

Nocturnal hypoglycemia can be due to basal insulin injection at night being too high; undereating at night in relation to injected bolus insulin; doing late night strenuous exercise or having done lengthy exercise during the day without lowering later insulin dosages; or, ingestion of alcohol. And, of course, the most frustrating thing is when hypoglycemia occurs without any discernable reason.

Long-acting basal insulin tends to peak around five hours after injection, so right then is a good time to check for hypoglycemia. If someone injects and goes to bed around 10 p.m., checking glucose at 3 a.m. is a good time. For kids injecting and going to bed at 8 p.m., checking their glucose at 1 a.m. is best.

Historically, for people who had hypoglycemia during the night, particularly children, it was suggested they use resistant starch bars—time-released glucose bars containing some protein and uncooked cornstarch—to slow production of glucose throughout the night, because the bars are slowly broken down and produce a subtle glucose effect for a long time. Extend Bars contain resistant starch but are not that healthy otherwise. Resistant starch can also be bought as powders such as Bob's Red Mill potato starch or Hi-Maize non-GMO resistant corn starch.

Alternatively, 2 tablespoons of corn flour mixed with 100 ml (about a half cup) of cold water will produce some resistant carbs throughout the night.

Young kids, those less than three years old, may also require a chewable digestive enzyme to help digest the starch. But resistant starch is not now commonly used today in any form.

Obviously, if someone is having consistent hypoglycemia during the night, reducing the evening basal insulin dose would be something to consider. I also at times have people eat a little food before bed, like some turkey breast; protein will slowly turn to glucose over time. Some patients eat a cheese stick or a couple of tablespoons of nut butter, instead, to achieve the same results.

The absolute worst consequence of a very low hypoglycemic event, especially in pediatric patients, is Dead in Bed syndrome. A curtly named horror, this is seen only in T1DM patients using insulin and occurs in general in patients between five and forty years old. Dead in Bed can account for 5–6 percent of the mortality rate of T1DM patients.

In this syndrome, the T1DM person goes to bed looking fine, and they die without any apparent symptoms of illness, low or high blood sugars. The theory is that low blood sugar, in these tragedies, initiates a severe cardiac arrhythmia that the heart cannot recover from and that silently kills the person as he sleeps. Without getting too technical, research shows that hypoglycemia can induce prolonged QTs and ventricular arrhythmia, EKG heart rhythm abnormalities that can be fatal.

So, it is very important to ensure that all patients, both T1DM and T2DM, can sleep smoothly without having to worry about hypoglycemia plaguing them. This is why a continuous glucose monitor system (CGMS) can be such a valuable tool for patients, caregivers, and medical practitioners. For any diabetic patient experiencing lows, especially during the night, learning where the glucose is throughout the entire night can be incredibly helpful in order to change insulin dosing and eating habits. For any child or adult with a regular history of low glucose events, it is important to have your physician guide you to companies that make CGMSs. Insurances do cover CGMS machines when lows and highs are a common part of problematic glucose control. CGMS units come with hypoglycemia warning alerts, although people sometimes unfortunately sleep through them. Even if a patient is not on a pump, a CGMS can still be obtained if glucose is not tightly regulated. Having a CGMS is much easier than having a parent get up to check her child's glucose levels several times a night!

There is a certain phenomenon to know about regarding a CGMS, however, especially when it is attached to a pump with an inappropriate automatic shut-off based on the CGMS numbers. It's called pressure induced sensor attenuation (PISA). PISA occurs when a patient has a CGMS, and recordings show dips in glucose levels for a brief amount of time and then the glucose record elevates back to normal. This is caused when a person rolls directly onto the inserted sensor during sleep, which may push the needle into the muscle tissue, changing the accuracy of the glucose reading. When the person naturally rolls off the sensor, it goes back into the subcutaneous fat and picks up again with appropriate glucose readings. Unfortunately, sometimes that may trigger a rapid hypoglycemia alarm, and prevent insulin from being delivered from the pump.

If you have questions about CGMS readings during the night because someone is having lows lasting fifteen to twenty minutes before then getting back to healthy levels, it may indeed be a PISA event. A good analysis of a CGMS report can help uncover PISA.

Hypoglycemia Summary

In summary, it is vital for a diabetic patient to check glucose levels regularly. Act immediately if hypoglycemia is noted via symptoms or a glucose meter. Always carry a medical ID, so if you do wind up with a significant low glucose situation in public, and are confused or unable to care for yourself, emergency medical technicians and others can quickly identify you as diabetic and proceed with effective treatment right away.

Always have some glucose replacement with you and always have a glucagon kit prescribed to you and ensure that someone in your household, work, and school knows how to use it and that is it not expired. Alert school, parents, family, teachers, and others who care for your child, or someone who is around you if you if are an adult, if frequent low-glucose struggles are occurring and how to treat them. Keep good records of food intake, glucose levels, insulin injections, and exercise habits. Be careful increasing exercise, especially new intensities, new lengths, and new activities. Don't panic if you feel yourself getting low. These episodes are easy to treat and it is much easier to do so if you are calm, cool, and collected. Last, if you are having frequent hypoglycemic events, it's best to find an integrative medical practitioner who might put you on a comprehensive protocol designed to stabilize glucose levels day and night.

Patient Case #1: Lean Forty-Two-Year-Old Woman with LADA

I put this lean, petite forty-two-year-old female LADA patient on 2 units of Lantus at night and her morning glucose was around 130 mg/dL for several days. I increased her bedtime Lantus to 3 units. She called the next morning at 8 a.m. and her glucose was at 60 mg/dL, and she didn't feel good; she was having hypoglycemic symptoms.

I should have just raised her dose to 2.5 units, not by a full unit. Petite LADA patients need to have slight increases in insulin. She was using a syringe and vial, so a half unit was feasible.

I told her only to use her fingertips to check her glucose levels and to check her glucose every fifteen minutes the first hour. She had no glucose tabs or glucose gels, even though I had asked her to get some. So, we were left with fruit juice. She drank 6 ounces of orange juice; her glucose rose temporarily but fell again by the end of the hour. I directed her to drink 6 ounces of orange juice each hour, and by noon, four hours later, she was fine, her glucose was stable at 101 mg/dL, and she stopped the juice. She did perfectly on 2.5 units of insulin at night thereafter.

Patient Case #2: Lean Twenty-Eight-Year-Old Woman with T1DM

This patient mistakenly injected 14 units of Humalog at bedtime instead of 14 units of Lantus. She called me at home on my cell phone around 11 p.m.

First, I told her to stay calm and that I would walk her through this. Moreover, I told her not to inject her Lantus that night.

Having done the morning glucose test, we knew that one Dex4 tab raised her glucose 20 mg/dL; I told her to eat eight of her Dex4 tabs, to raise her glucose 160 mg/dL. We did this preventively to try to stave off any sudden drop. With a serious insulin error like this, if she got a little hyperglycemic, I did not care; we could correct it at her morning breakfast Humalog dose. She checked her glucose every fifteen minutes and kept calling me up to report. In another hour, we started to see a little glucose dip, so I instructed her to take six more Dex4 tabs, which would raise her another 120 mg/dL. After another hour, three hours total, her glucose stabilized; remember, rapid-acting insulins only last three to four hours total in the system. So, after three hours, she felt fine, her glucose was in good numbers, and she went to bed. She woke a little high, because she hadn't injected her Lantus, and she corrected at breakfast. She then injected her morning Lantus and did fine after that.

When there is a huge risk of a serious low, like with mistaken insulin injection in a young child, I am less concerned that the child will get a significant high than I am that the child not have a serious low. We can always correct the glucose later, and in general, since this happens very frequently at bedtime, the whole next day may not be as well controlled as normal and may be hyperglycemic, especially if there is not a second basal shot injected in the morning. However, being high the next day after an evening injection error is not a huge worry.

As you can see, hypoglycemia, while unfortunately a reality for almost all diabetic patients at some time, is something that can be caught early and treated effectively, preventing problematic consequences. With a comprehensive alternative protocol, patients get off the constant lows and highs of typical diabetes management.

Diabetes and Sickness

I want to start out this section by discussing the naturopathic philosophy of sickness, particularly of colds and flus. Everyone tends to get sick one or two times a year, and that is normal. To a naturopathic physician, a sickness is considered a cleansing of the body, when toxins from food, drink, too little sleep, and other negative impacts on the body accumulate, particularly in the intestines. A microorganism that stimulates a fever, runny nose, coughing up mucous, diarrhea, and so on, is a great way to expel toxins and reset the body to a cleaner state. This is one reason it is so common to get a fall cold.

In the summer, it is very easy for mammalian bodies to live; the weather is warmer and so keeping ourselves at regular body temperature, 98.6° F or so (it is a myth that human temperature should be 98.6° F twenty-four hours a day), is easier. If we eat hot dogs, ice cream, and soda pop all summer long, along with other unhealthy foods, we can accumulate toxins in our body, but we also put up with them because the body does not have to work that hard to maintain a normal core temperature and metabolism. However, once the summer heat dissipates and the fall cold in comes in, it is very common for people to get sick.

Why? Because when the temperature sinks substantially, the body needs to be cleaner to keep up the steady mammalian temperature humans require, activating our metabolism and our energy processes effectively. So, the body joins with a microorganism to stimulate a sickness purge of accumulated toxins. If a person goes through their illness under the care of an integrative physician, and doesn't use over-the-counter suppressive medications, such as cough suppressants, decongestants, or NSAIDs to artificially lower their fever, and doesn't use unnecessary antibiotics, the sickness usually lasts between three and seven days. After that the person is ready to face the winter cold with a healthier body.

People who stop a fever or who use over-the-counter suppressive medicines disallow the body to cleanse fully as it needs to. I often get patients who have been sick for three to six weeks, because the body needs to detoxify and the medications they have taken are slowing down or preventing the body from doing so.

The problem with antibiotics is that many illnesses are from viruses, and antibiotics do not kill viruses; they only work against bacteria. Many times patients with an obvious virus are still given an antibiotic "to prevent a secondary infection" or because the patient expects to get some medicine from their physician; antibiotics are handed out all too often in medical clinics. Antibiotics negatively affect our microbiome, and it's unfortunately fairly common in my practice to see patients who have had the most antibiotics now on cycles of frequent sickness. A normal, healthy microbiome, devoid of multiple antibiotic doses, keeps our systemic immune system strong, and fighting off an illness with the natural immune system can strengthen the system. A healthy microbiome can also reduce the risk of autoimmune disease, help reduce insulin resistance, and protect us from getting many systemic body and mind disorders.

Thus, the more we take antibiotics—especially if they are taken without a probiotic during the prescription and for two to four weeks afterward—the more our beneficial bacteria are killed, the weaker our immune system becomes, and the more we get sick. It is a catch-22. Taking a probiotic to help protect the gut microbiome is beneficial, though we do not have a supplement that fixes all the bacteria that are destroyed, so we can only replace a few. Even still, that is very helpful. Patients have come to me with concerns about taking a probiotic while taking an antibiotic; I will say here: yes, it is safe, and yes, it makes sense. Take the probiotic at a meal, as probiotics should always be taken at meals, and as far away from an antibiotic dose as possible.

In many instances, I do not have to use antibiotics to treat typical infections such as ear infections, sinus infections, strep throat, and bronchitis. There are amazingly effective natural medicines that stimulate a body's immune system so it can fight off those bacteria and viruses on its own. I prove this all the time in practice.

If a diabetic patient is ill but does not have vomiting or diarrhea and just has a typical upper respiratory infection (URI), such as a sore throat, strep throat, sinus infection, runny nose, ear infection, chest cold, or bronchitis, it is relatively easy to treat. When I see a diabetic with one of the above infections, this is typically what I recommend:

Notify your physician. All diabetic patients should alert their physicians when they are sick. An office visit may or may not be necessary, but certainly patients should inform their doctors, even about URIs.

Do not eat. Fasting is best when ill. The gut does not need food when we are sick. The less we eat, the fewer toxins we continue to produce, and our bodies can instead focus on increasing the action of our white blood cells to fight the infection. Most of us are not hungry when we are ill, but some people force themselves to eat or just continue to eat as normal. This will make the patient sicker for longer. Especially do not eat refined sugar, refined grains, dairy, and gluten, and do not overeat when you are sick. If you do have an appetite, then only eat cooked veggies, veggie soup, veggie smoothies, nut "grain" products, and some easy to digest protein, like white fish or plain white meat chicken.

Inject basal insulin. You will still inject basal insulin if not eating but will not need to inject rapid insulin unless a correction dose is necessary. Fever can raise glucose levels.

Drink fluids. It is important to keep hydrated when ill. Water, herbal tea, veggie soup, and vegetable drinks are all good options. Electrolyte formulations are not necessary unless vomiting and diarrhea are continual.

Rest. Our immune systems are most active at rest and during sleep. In fact, when we start getting sick, we get achy in our bones because our white blood cells are made in our bones, and when they are revving up white blood cell production, they ache. This is designed to signal us to go to bed and rest. Many people take NSAIDs, instead, such as ibuprofen, to fight the achiness, which lowers the fever and gives us temporary intestinal permeability in our gut, the worst scenario for quickly overcoming the infection. I have patients stay home from work for at least a day, and I write a note to their bosses, if necessary, explaining the medical reason they could not go to work. I also ask them to stop their Zumba class, stop vacuuming, and hold off on doing the laundry. Just rest!

Let the fever go. When you feel the urge to urinate, you do not take a pill to stop feeling that urge. When you feel the need to defecate, you do not take a pill to stop feeling that symptom. We all know that our bodies send us precise information about how they are naturally working, and we respect those signals and almost always follow their directions. We urinate when our bladders inform us they are full; we defecate when our rectums feel full; we eat when our stomachs say they are empty; we sleep when we feel tired; we drink when we feel thirsty. But, unhelpfully, when it comes to having a fever, we screw it up most of the time. Fever is a natural sign of illness, as thirst is a natural sign of dehydration. Fever does everything we want our bodies to do when we get sick: helps kill the microbes; increases our metabolism so we make more white blood cells and our immune system is more active; and signals us we are sick so we will rest and allow the immune system to maximize action against the microbes. Taking an NSAID due to fear of the fever is the absolute worst thing a person can do when sick. Fever is one of the best answers to illness and is by no means unsafe. Fever from 100–105° F is completely safe. In fact, I've seen infants who had temperatures of 105° F from simple ear infections or when they were teething. Infants are full of vitality, so small irregularities can cause high fevers; as we age, we tend to have much lower fevers, and our senior patients may have serious infections without any fevers at all. In general, a fever of 101–103° F is typical for most children and adults getting ill. It is completely benign. Brains do not boil at a fever of 103° F! You should always contact your physician when you are sick and have a fever, but please do not reach for an NSAID. The fever is your friend! The only time to stop a fever is if a person has febrile seizures, that is, has seizures when their temperature starts suddenly increasing. In that case, keeping the fever below 101° F is best.

Hydrotherapy. Hydrotherapy is the use of water to help your body heal. There are numerous home treatments of hydrotherapy patients can do, which stimulate the immune system particularly in a specific area of the body. I regularly instruct patients on doing a heating compress to the throat for throat infections, pharyngitis, and laryngitis; hot foot baths for sinus infections; warming socks for chest and sinus infections; heating compress to the chest for bronchitis; garlic feet for chest infections; and so forth. These are remarkably beneficial, and they are something people can easily do when traveling. You can find a copy of my hydrotherapy handouts on my website, but please do them only with the approval and guidance of your physician.

Supplements. Supplements do not kill the microbes in your body, but they can indeed stimulate your immune system to do so. I use a product that contains as many incredibly effective immune stimulators as a super strong natural antibiotic, and usually combine that with an herbal tincture (an alcohol preparation of herbs) or glycerin preparation specific to the area of the body that is most effective—throat, sinuses, chest, and so on. For diabetic patients, I often will add in vitamin D_3 by body weight in thousands of IU, which is to the immune system what a massive tidal wave is to a drop of water. That means if you weigh 125 pounds, I will prescribe 125,000 IU of vitamin D_3 for four days. This is an extremely effective immune system add-on. It is contraindicated in some conditions, so check with your physician before using such high doses. Liposomal vitamin C, which is vitamin C attached to a fatty molecule that makes it incredibly more absorbent, is also an extremely effective way of boosting the immune system.

Daily check-ins. When a diabetic patient is very sick, I have my office call patients daily to ensure they are getting better. Keeping in touch with patients ensures they feel well cared for, and by doing so I can verify the treatment is effective.

Antibiotics. Okay, I know I just wrote about the negative effects of antibiotics, and they are real. But to play devil's advocate, if a diabetic patient with elevated glucose is both sick and in general has not been under good control, and has an elevated A1C, her innate immune system may be seriously malfunctioning and antibiotics may be necessary. Hyperglycemia can significantly decrease the functioning of our body's immune system, which is a huge concern if the patient is very ill. Since responsible patient care is always more important than medical philosophy, although I have effective natural protocols for ill diabetic patients, now and then I may need to recommend an antibiotic. When I do, I prescribe high dose probiotics during and for at least a month after. It is better to use antibiotics now and then than to have a patient require hospitalization if the infection continues to progress.

Emergency room. If DKA seems to be occurring, the T1DM patient should be taken to the emergency room.

When a patient with diabetes is sick, and their glucose is raised over 170 mg/dL (having a fever can push glucose levels higher), it initiates insulin resistance, increased urination, and ketone formation. Patients will need to drink a lot and, if on insulin, will no doubt need to use more insulin to lower their glucose in correction doses. For diabetic patients who are not on insulin, glucose will likely be higher during days of fever. Measuring glucose and ketones regularly is important, and remember that high doses of vitamin C can cause glucose meters to register inaccurately higher glucose levels. Keeping in touch with your physician is important. Taking medicines as directed is important. The above will work exceedingly well for patients with URIs, sore throats, bronchitis, and viral pneumonia, the majority of cold and flu season illnesses.

For T2DM patients, keep taking your prescribed medications during illness. Integrative immune support as listed above is safe to combine with the vast majority of prescription medications. Avoid eating or eat very little; while this helps the immune system, it can also help keep the glucose levels lower, and lower glucose means a more active immune system. I have found that T2DM patients who are not using insulin can have a harder time with infections than T1DM patients, due to the fact that it is hard to lower glucose with a fever without insulin. Plus, abdominal weight is pro-inflammatory and that can feed into an inflammatory infective process.

For T1DM and T2DM insulin dependent patients, I typically ask them to measure their glucose at least every five hours. If there is significant hyperglycemia (and it's not from excess vitamin C), it's good to inject a corrective rapid acting insulin dose via their correction math to reach their correction goal. They can inject subcutaneously or intramuscularly, with an intramuscular injection lowering glucose quicker than a subcutaneous one.

Once you work with an integrative physician and see how effectively your immune system can be stimulated, it's quite a positive experience. It's good to learn that even with diabetes, you have an effective immune system that, when given support, can overcome illnesses often without the need for antibiotics or over-the-counter medications.

Vomiting and Diarrhea

As we know, dehydration can be a serious part of illness for diabetic patients, especially in T1DM patients. If vomiting or diarrhea is occurring, fluid loss is occurring; if there is a fever, as the glucose rises, hyperglycemia can also cause urination and more fluid loss. We have to watch fluid loss and dehydration in all types of diabetic patients, with additional concerns of DKA in T1DM patients.

There are many reasons people vomit. A few of the most common reasons for acute vomiting include food poisoning; poisoning or overdosage from supplements, medications, household cleaners, and so on; pregnancy; migraines; and viral or bacterial gastroenteritis (stomach flu). We are mainly interested in food poisoning and viral gastroenteritis as sicknesses that commonly lead to vomiting.

There are also many reasons people develop diarrhea. The most common reasons for acute diarrhea include food poisoning; poisoning or overdosage from supplements, medications, household cleaners, and so on (vitamin C, magnesium, metformin); and viral or bacterial gastroenteritis. Use of laxatives, *C. difficile*, or other dysbiotic conditions after antibiotics, eating too much fruit or diabetic food with sorbitol and mannitol in it, and gastrointestinal disorders such as irritable or inflammatory bowel in a flare, can also produce diarrhea, and I've seen those occur with many patients. We are mainly interested in diarrhea caused by food poisoning, viral or bacterial gastroenteritis, and postantibiotic diarrhea.

Regarding vomiting or diarrhea in a diabetic patient, a patient's physician should be immediately contacted if:

- There is any sign of blood in the stools.
- There are more than two episodes of diarrhea a day (that's not a lot, but I want to catch things as early as possible; some physicians recommend calling after six bowel movements a day).
- Diarrhea begins within two months of having taken an antibiotic.
- Severe cramps, urgency, abdominal pain, or joint pain occur with diarrhea.
- There are signs of dehydration—skin tenting on wrist or abdomen, lethargy, lack of urination, or dry lips.
- Glucose is consistently over 200 mg/dL.
- Ketones are occurring above mild in blood or urine.
- Vomiting or diarrhea is not cleared up after one day.

Use of Insulin

If a patient has vomiting and diarrhea, it's best to temporarily stop eating. A patient should call his physician and follow her advice. He should continue his long-acting insulin, but stop his bolus insulin, unless a correction dose is needed, and should check glucose levels every hour, as well as ketones if a T1DM patient and glucose is over 200 mg/dL.

Treatment

If a patient has vomiting and diarrhea that is lasting all day or for a few days, electrolyte replacement is suggested. Do not drink an electrolyte replacement formula if there is no vomiting or diarrhea.

For electrolyte fluid replacement at home, this is what I recommend:

1. Start with 1 liter or quart of water, iced tea, herbal iced tea, club soda, carbohydrate free bullion, or veggie soup.

2. Add electrolytes. Ideally *do not* use coconut water, Gatorade, or Pedialyte. Gatorade and coconut water are not full electrolyte replacements, and neither is Pedialyte. If Pedialyte is used for nourishment, it contains 25 grams of carbs in each liter of fluid, 1,035 mg of sodium and 780 mg of potassium. That may increase the glucose levels, especially with a fever, depending on the liters ingested.

   This is a good homemade formula: Mix 1 level teaspoon salt (approximately 2,000 mg), ½ teaspoon potassium chloride salt substitute (approximately 500 mg), and, optionally, 1 level teaspoon sodium bicarbonate. An easy way to go is to get LoSalt (original with no iodine), which is sold at grocery stores. 1 teaspoon of LoSalt contains 1,800 mg of potassium chloride and 680 mg of sodium chloride. It is not exactly the ratio found in Pedialyte, but it provides potassium, sodium, and chloride, and those are the main electrolytes we need to replace in cases of vomiting and diarrhea. It is very inexpensive. If your physician directs you to, you can add in a little more straight salt to increase the sodium. Add lemon juice or stevia, if desired, to taste.
3. Do not add anything with carbs, such as honey or fruit juices, into your drinks.

Using glucose tabs, gels, or drinks for sugar is helpful to elevate glucose if necessary, but the first thing to do is to keep electrolytes and fluid up. A patient should drink at least 8 ounces of fluid an hour, getting in at least half their body weight in ounces a day, especially when fever accompanies the vomiting and diarrhea. That means if a patient weighs 150 pounds, he should drink *at least* 75 ounces a day, or a little over 2 liters. It's best to drink a little more to ensure good fluid content in body cells.

If dehydration is nonetheless happening due to a patient not being able to keep anything down, watery diarrhea is frequently occurring, and the patient has a fever, a trip to the emergency room at a hospital for an IV saline drip might be indicated. Intravenous saline is safe, but it's best to avoid IV dextrose and Lactated Ringer's solutions, as they both will likely increase glucose levels. You may have to make a bit of a fuss to ensure the emergency room doctors are not using dextrose fluid replacement, but most understand that in a sick diabetic with high glucose who is suffering from dehydration, adding more glucose in solution is completely medically contraindicated.

Other reasons to go to the hospital include elevated glucose levels, elevated ketone levels, lethargy, and signs of dehydration; in other words, if the patient cannot reduce risk factors for DKA.

VOMITING

There are natural medicines for vomiting, such as ginger tea or capsules, peppermint tea, slippery elm gruel, the indicated homeopathic remedy, or acupuncture. If none of those are significantly helpful, a patient's physician should prescribe Phenergan rectal suppositories. This is an antiemetic medication, which the patient would get from a drug store and which can be inserted every three hours into the rectum to reduce nausea or vomiting. Also, another stronger drug, such as Zofran/ondansetron tabs, can be tried.

DIARRHEA

Diarrhea from food poisoning or a stomach virus can often be treated with high-dose probiotics mixed with natural antimicrobials specific for gastrointestinal microorganisms. Some natural antidiarrheal antimicrobials include garlic, berberine, uva ursi (an herb), lactoferrin, neem, caprylic acid, and oregano oil. Activated charcoal can bind with gut toxins to help eliminate them; the capsules turn stool black, though! Your physician should decide which natural medicine, at what dose, is best and safest for you. I do not recommend patients use antidiarrheal agents, as in general diarrhea occurs when the gut is attempting to detoxify, and allowing diarrhea to occur can help expedite healing.

If the ill insulin dependent diabetic patient is sleeping, a loved one or friend can continue to check her glucose while she sleeps and wake her only if a correction dose is needed. If the ill insulin dependent diabetic patient is alone, she should set an alarm to help wake and check her glucose every few hours. If the patient is very ill and is alone and is sleeping through alarms, then it might be best for her to take a tepid bath, or if absolutely necessary, an NSAID can artificially lower the fever to reduce the elevation of glucose. One thing to recall—aspirin can cause false positive ketones on the urine dipstick. Tylenol does not do that. Watch Tylenol intake, though, and do not overdose, as it is harmful to the liver. NSAIDs, if overdosed, negatively affect the kidneys, and those organs may be suffering a little if dehydration is occurring to any degree. And, again, NSAIDs should only be taken if absolutely necessary.

Treatment Summary

When a diabetic patient becomes ill, he needs to call his physician, and probably should go in for an office visit or have a phone consultation, if possible. Depending on the presentation, natural treatment or antibiotics may be prescribed. Dehydration is important to avoid. Monitoring glucose and ketones must be done. Continuing basal insulin and correcting elevated glucose are key treatment guidelines.

For T2DM patients on oral hypoglycemic medications, we are not concerned with DKA, and continuing their diabetic medications is fine. For those on GLP-1 inhibitors, if nausea caused by them is aggravated during the stomach illness and is causing more vomiting or diarrhea, it may be helpful to reduce or stop the GLP-1 meds temporarily. Your physician can direct you along those lines.

Traveling and Diabetes

There is no need for a patient with diabetes to feel nervous about traveling. Smart preparation can easily ensure that a diabetic patient enjoys vacations and work travel without having any problem with maintaining good glucose control. I have had many diabetic patients travel without any problems at all.

The patient preparation list:

- Check with your physician to make sure you are cleared to travel.
- Have letters from your physician stating your diagnosis of diabetes and that you need to carry insulin, oral hypoglycemic agents, or non-insulin injectables (if you are on any of those medications); syringes and needles; glucose meter, test strips, and lancets; glucagon kit; glucose tabs; ketone dipstick and ketone strips, and so on—all the required tools you need. Carry copies of prescriptions for all of the above pertinent to you.
- Patients on pumps should carry a backup vacation loaner pump, infusion sets and cartridges, sensors (if you use a CGMS), extra

batteries for your meter/pump, extra battery cap and cartridge cap for pump, extra pump clip or pump case, a current list of pump settings, and skin preparation dressings or adhesive.

- Carry contact information in case you need hospitalization overseas.
- Check your medical insurance to see if you are covered outside the United States.
- Always carry your medical ID if you require one.
- If flying, don't pack diabetic supplies in checked bags, which have a higher rate of getting lost, but carry all your supplies with you onto a plane.
- Carry food in case there are delays when you are on the tarmac longer than expected or you wind up in other situations where you need to eat to maintain your glucose and activity levels and healthy food is not available.
- Wear comfortable shoes, such as sneakers, Rockports, or your diabetic approved footwear.
- If you use syringes, definitely carry the BD Safe-Clip to cut off your needles and allow you to safely and respectfully throw out needleless syringes without putting anyone at risk.
- Carry your pump company's contact phone number, in case anything happens to your pump overseas.
- Do not order diabetic meals on planes (if they are still serving food!); instead order seafood or kosher meals. As you might expect, a diabetic meal will probably be high in carbohydrates and low in fat.
- Carry antidiarrheals and antiemetics unless you are going to a country where typical drug stores abound and you can buy them there, if needed.
- Take probiotics for two weeks before your trip and throughout it; studies show that doing so significantly reduces the risk of getting gastroenteritis on the trip. Ask your integrative physician for natural antibiotics in case you get sick, and for homeopathic remedies for diarrhea. If nothing else, a good strong garlic product is a good idea to take while traveling too, to help reduce the risk of illness and food poisoning.

- Notify the TSA official at the airport that you have diabetes and have your supplies with you. All diabetic supplies are allowed through the checkpoint after the screening. Pumps and CGMS should *not* go through the x-ray or millimeter wave scanner; you can disconnect it to go through those; it will only take a minute or so being disconnected. You may have a TSA agent pat down the pump, and your hands may be tested for explosive chemicals.
- Monitor, monitor, monitor! Check glucose frequently, maybe more than you typically do, to ensure any highs or lows are caught as soon as possible.

All patients on insulin should carry a backup vial and syringes, no matter if they use pens or are on a pump. If you are on a cartridge pen, then the cartridge can be used as a vial, as you can easily remove insulin with your syringe from an insulin cartridge. This ensures that if you lose your pen or your pump malfunctions, you will have backup insulin to protect your health.

In fact, it is important to have a backup of pretty much everything: glucose meter, pens, pen needles, and medications. You never know when your luggage will be lost or stolen. There are little backup glucose meters like the Sidekick Testing System, where you get a disposable glucose meter with fifty test strips. You would need lancets for the device, however. This is a small and easy-to-carry backup glucose meter. Insulin pump companies will also allow you to use a free vacation loaner pump. Give the company at least two weeks notice to get that set up.

Depending on where you are traveling, you might need a cooling or heating pack, like a FRIO kit, such as if you are traveling to a place where the temperature will be over 86° F or under 34° F, and you will be outside for considerable time.

Insulin Types

As mentioned previously, in North America insulin is U-100; that is, one milliliter of insulin contains 100 units. Most other countries also use U-100;

however, in some countries U-40 or U-80 is used, although all insulin pens are U-100. This is why it is important to carry backup U-100 insulin, as it may not be found in a country you visit.

If you must use U-40 insulin, you must use it with a U-40 syringe. It is very confusing to mix U-40 insulin with a U-100 syringe or U-100 insulin with a U-40 syringe. Here is how the math works:

20 units of U-100 insulin with a U-100 syringe is: 20 units
20 units of U-40 insulin with a U-40 syringe is: 20 units
20 units of U-40 insulin with a U-100 syringe is: 20 units × 2.5 = 50 units (confusing!)
20 units of U-100 insulin with a U-40 syringe: 20 units ÷ 2.5 = 8 units (confusing!)

So, either stick with U-100 insulin with a U-100 syringe, or, if necessary, use U-40 insulin *only* with a U-40 syringe at the same dosage of your U-100 insulin.

United States Embassies and Organizations

If you have serious health trouble abroad, call a US embassy in the country you are visiting, and ask about which hospitals have physicians who speak English. The embassy personnel may also be able to track down a diabetic specialist for you.

There are helpful travel organizations to know about, as well, including Overseas Citizens Services, International SOS, and the International Association for Medical Assistance to Travellers. Through these organizations, you can find English-speaking physicians, get emergency medical assistance, and learn where all US consulate offices are located.

Ensure your family knows your itinerary day by day, where you are going and where you are staying, with contact numbers.

Insulin Use and Time Changes

If you are traveling and are just on OHA or a non-insulin injectable, you can continue to take them as you have been. There is no concern about taking those medicines when traveling.

Insulin is another thing, however! It can get a little confusing figuring out how to maintain a p.m./a.m. insulin schedule when one is traveling through multiple time zones. I'll give you some basic guidelines that might be helpful, but make sure you check with your physician on how to use your insulin when traveling.

If the time change is less than three hours, you should continue to inject normally in the new time zone.

If your travels take you through more than three time zones going *west*, the day will be longer and so extra insulin later in the day may be necessary. If you are on one shot of basal a day, you can take the same amount or increase it by 20 percent to cover the extra hours; or, sometimes it is better to give a little morning boost (if you only take a shot at night—or a night boost if you inject your basal only in the morning). Alternatively, on this travel day, instead of doing just one basal dose, split it in half and dose 50 percent in the evening and 50 percent in the morning of the day you are traveling. Or, you may inject your normal pretravel basal but then inject a little more, around 10 percent more the evening after your travel is ended. As you can see, there are several methodologies, and your physician should help you choose which is best for you. If you are already injecting basal twice a day, keep doing it at the usual times you inject. If you are on bolus insulin, too, just continue to inject that normally before meals and for correction doses. Nothing changes with bolus dosing (and correction dosing) on a trip. When you arrive, reset your insulin as normal to your new location time. That may mean you have a day when you are a little higher or a little lower than normal, so checking glucose levels frequently is absolutely necessary for the first day or two.

If your travels take you through more than three time zones going *east*, the day will be shorter. One shot a day of basal can be taken as normally, or you may need to decrease it by 10–20 percent. Alternatively, like going west, you may wish to split the dose in half and inject half in the evening and half in the morning. If you already inject twice a day, continue to do so but watch glucose levels to see if a decrease in dosing is required. Again, ask your physician for advice on how to best adjust this. Bolus dosing before meals and for corrections is the same. Then, start your basal insulin on the new time zone's local time. Again, you may be a little high or low the first day or two; monitor glucose levels closely.

Going either west or east, if you are unsure what to do, underdose your basal, and if your glucose elevates, you can correct it at meals. This is not ideal, but it is better than having a low when traveling.

For those using a pump while traveling through time zones, it is important to keep updating the day and time on your pump and your glucose meter. This is done when your basal rates vary significantly throughout the day, you have a noticeable dawn phenomenon, you have a risk for low blood glucose during the night, and, as stated above, when you are traveling through multiple time zones.

Maintaining the typical basal rates throughout the day and changing the time regularly is one way to manage traveling. Changes to the bolus dose at meals can correct for highs, and if you are low, lowering the bolus dose, skipping it, or increasing glucose with a glucose tab before a meal and then injecting the normal bolus dose are all options.

Another method is setting an average daily steady rate, and injecting for meal and corrections as needed. An average daily steady rate would be one set level throughout all the hours, instead of differing values. Then once you reach your destination, reset typical basal times based on the new location's time. You might not have the typically great control you are used to, but you should do okay for just one day of travel.

If the pump breaks down during travel, add up your total daily basal dosing with some basic math, and then use your backup insulin and syringes either in one shot or split in half in the evening and morning.

How do you add up your daily total basal insulin? Let's say this is your basal rate during the day:

10 p.m. to 2 a.m. 0.75 units per hour—0.75 × 4 hours = 3.0 units
2 a.m. to 6 a.m. 0.85 units per hour—0.85 × 4 hours = 3.4 units
6 a.m. to 9 a.m. 1.05 units per hour—1.05 units × 3 hours = 3.15 units
9 a.m. to 10 p.m. 0.8 units an hour—0.8 units × 11 hours = 8.8 units

Total daily dose: 18.35 units

With a BD 3/10 half-unit syringe, you are able to inject 18 or 18.50 units; either would probably suffice. Inject all of it in the evening or inject 9.5 units at night and 9 units in the evening the day of traveling.

Traveling Summary

Travel can be fun, exciting, and safe if you work with a knowledgeable physician and are comfortable with your diabetes. You must make the effort to be prepared. Many of my patients have traveled throughout the continent and abroad and have done just fine. Diabetes never has to interfere with you seeing the world and having wonderful experiences in new places, meeting new people, enjoying new (low-carb) food, and enriching your mind with new cultures, architecture, activities, and scenery. You might lose control of your glucose a little during travel, which is understandable, and we prefer highs to lows. Being a little flexible and realizing good control can be reinstituted upon arrival at your travel destination can help you enjoy the trip and not excessively worry about your glucose levels.

— CHAPTER FOURTEEN —

Diabetic Complications

No matter the diagnosis, all types of diabetes can cause the same complications if uncontrolled. Well-controlled diabetes should never cause complications.

The complications of uncontrolled diabetes mellitus are fundamentally due to the elevated glucose levels in the person's body. No diabetic patients ever have to have any complications if their glucose numbers are normal enough that they are not initiating damage to body cells.

There are two types of diabetic complications: macrovascular and microvascular. Macrovascular complications relate to the blood vessels and are associated with an increased risk of myocardial infarction (heart attack) and cerebral vascular accident (stroke). It is a sad fact that most patients with diabetes do die of a heart attack or stroke. Microvascular complications are associated with smaller blood vessels and affect the eyes, kidneys, and nerves.

Way back in the early 1990s, two keynote studies were done that are still discussed and referenced. The United Kingdom Prospective Diabetes Study (UKPDS) studied two groups of T2DM patients—one group was given conventional treatment and one group was given "intensive" treatment. In the end, the conventional group had an A1C of 7.9 percent, but the intensive group had lowered their A1C to 7.0 percent. Of course, 7.0 percent is not a very good A1C, but it is better than 7.9 percent. They followed these patients for over ten years and found out that those in the lower A1C group had a 12 percent decreased risk of cardiovascular disease; 25 percent decreased risk of microvascular disease; 21 percent decreased risk of developing retinopathy; and 33 percent less chance of developing early kidney disease.

Around the same time, a second similar study, the Diabetes Control and Complications Trial (DCCT), was done with T1DM patients. In this study, the conventionally treated T1DM patients had an A1C of 9.0 percent, while the intensively treated T1DM patients lowered their A1C to 7.2 percent. The results were similar to the UKPDS—the intensively treated patients had a 50 percent decreased risk of developing kidney disease; a 60 percent decreased risk of developing nerve disease; and a 76 percent decreased risk of developing diabetic eye disease.

So, we know that having better glucose control significantly reduces the risks of developing diabetic complications. Other studies have shown that even lower A1Cs give more protection. Using the A1C score as an indication of when damage starts occurring in the body is supported by other studies. An A1C greater than 5.5 percent (average glucose at around 113 mg/dL) increases one's risk for endothelial (blood vessel) lining damage and retinopathy; an A1C over 6.0 percent (average glucose at around 126 mg/dL) significantly increases the risk of developing chronic diabetic kidney disease. Unfortunately, most Americans with diabetes have A1Cs greater than 5.5 percent, and few are on appropriate supplementation to help stave off the damage.

Aside from the personal aspect of developing diabetic complications, the economic burden of diabetes on our country is substantial. In 2012, the cost of diabetes in the United States was $245 billion dollars. And the cost is climbing each year. Much of that cost consists of hospital stays for diabetic complications and is highest in our over-sixty-five-years-old population, which is growing each year as baby boomers become seniors. Controlling hypertension is a big help toward reducing complications, as well. Reduction of just 10 mm systolic (the first number) and 5 mm diastolic (the second number) reduced the onset of microvascular complications by 37 percent in the UKPDS blood pressure study. Unfortunately, costwise, T2DM patients require on average 2.5 medications, and nearly half require 3 or more medications to get their high-carb-diet-induced high blood pressure under control. Moreover, on top of all that, less than 30 percent of patients obtain the blood pressure goal of lower than 130/80 mmHg. So, we know lowering blood pressure is helpful, but if you are doing conventional care and following a standard high-carb, low-fat diet, you need many medicines, which insurances have to pay for. In those patients it's likely poor control will also lead to the development of diabetic complications.

Diabetic complications create some scary statistics:

- 28.5 percent of diabetics over forty years old have diabetic retinopathy.
- 13 percent of patients have diabetic macular edema.
- 33.4 percent of diabetics have nephropathy.
- 60–70 percent of diabetics have neuropathy.

Diabetes is the number one cause of blindness in the United States for adults over thirty. It is the number one reason in the United States that a patient develops kidney failure. It is the number one reason in the United States—outside of trauma—that a person has a part of their body amputated. Those are categories none of us want to belong to, and no diabetic patient should have to belong to!

The big question is, why do diabetic complications occur? Moreover, why do they occur in the cells of blood vessels, eyes, kidneys, and nerves?

Most cells in the body—adipose, liver, muscle cells—can become insulin resistant, so when the glucose level in serum is elevated, the cells can block the uptake of glucose (remember that even in T1DM patients, if glucose is elevated above 150 or 170 mg/dL, insulin resistance also occurs). Often in T2DM patients those adipose, liver, and muscle cells become insulin resistant when they are full of fat and do not want to absorb glucose and form even more fat.

However, there are four types of cells in the human body that do not become insulin resistant: blood vessels, eyes, kidneys, and nerve cells. These cells are so vital for life, they are made to absorb glucose easily and without resistance. Thus, whatever the glucose in the serum, those cells absorb that much glucose into them. If your glucose level is 240 mg/dL, that's what is in those cells. Those high levels of glucose inside the cells wreak havoc. Moreover, if glucose levels are elevated for extensive periods of time, those four types of cells are damaged the most, and that is why cardiovascular disease, diabetic retinopathy (eyes), nephropathy (kidneys), and neuropathy (nerves) are the main complications of people with uncontrolled diabetes.

Biochemically, there are several ways in which having high levels of serum blood sugar and insulin cause imbalances in a person with diabetes.

The key to understanding all the problems, however, is to know that hyperglycemia significantly increases reactive oxygen species (ROS), also known as free radicals. ROS are chemically reactive molecules that contain oxygen, such as superoxide anion radicals, hydroxyl radicals, peroxynitrite radicals, and lipid peroxidation. ROS production is a normal part of metabolism, but when the body is under stress, for example from high glucose in uncontrolled diabetes, the formation of ROS can increase significantly, and this is called oxidative stress.

The amount of oxidative damage occurring in a diabetic who is uncontrolled is excessive and life-threatening over time. When the ROS are very high, that notably reduces the amount of antioxidants in the cells, such as glutathione and catalase, and so the body math is pretty simple: high oxidative products plus low antioxidants equals cellular damage. Hyperglycemia also causes a pro-inflammatory state via the production of chemicals that promote inflammation. That leads to other troublesome concerns, such as increased risk of blood clots, liver inflammation, deterioration of pancreatic beta cells, and increased risk of cancer and Alzheimer's disease.

There are four main hyperglycemia pathways in the body that initiate oxidative damage:

1. *Increased (diacylglycerol) protein kinase c beta activation (DAG).* This pathway increases inflammatory chemicals (cytokines), ROS, and also vascular cell proliferation, which is a key component of developing diabetic retinopathy.
2. *Increased advanced glycosylated end products (AGEs).* When glucose in our serum reacts with proteins, it forms AGEs, but the protein is warped by the sugar and distorts its shape. AGEs are very destructive and pro-inflammatory, and lead to oxidative damage in the cell. They damage proteins, lipids, and DNA. AGEs are factors in causing damage all throughout the diabetic body. RAGEs are *receptors* where AGEs bind, and initiate the production of ROS. So we have AGEs, landing on receptors and becoming RAGEs and those cause ROS that damage body cells.

   AGEs also become proteins the body can no longer recognize as normal—for example, LDL cholesterol proteins that are covered with sugar are no longer recognized by the liver. Thus, high levels of AGE-LDLs do not signal the liver to stop producing more LDLs, so the liver keeps pumping that out, and cholesterol increases. AGE-LDLs oxidize quickly and oxidized LDLs increase the risk of a person developing atherosclerosis.

High cellular glucose can increase the production of triphosphates. Triphosphates can go down two main pathways—one that is not damaging and one that is. The nondamaging pathway is called the ribose-5-phosphate pathway and is promoted by an enzyme called transketolase. Thiamine pyrophosphate increases transketolase so triphosphates are shunted down the nondamaging pathway more. The damaging pathway makes those AGEs. Benfotiamine is a key supplement that increases transketolase enzymes and helps shunt triphosphates into the nondamaging pathway, preventing AGE formation, which is why you'll see benfotiamine in so many studies helping to prevent and treat diabetic complications.

3. *Polyol pathway.* In general, this biochemical pathway is not frequently used by the body, but it occurs with hyperglycemia. When glucose enters cells, in this pathway the enzyme aldose reductase converts the glucose into sorbitol, and then, via the enzyme sorbitol dehydrogenase, the sorbitol is converted into fructose. However, too much glucose in the cells messes up the whole conveyor belt and the process gets stuck in sorbitol buildup. When too much sorbitol is made, it causes oxidative stress in the cells, ROS are made, and antioxidants are reduced. The cell can experience proliferation, death, tissue dysfunction, and damage.
4. *Hexosamine pathway flux.* In this pathway, under normal conditions, glucose is converted to glucose-6-phosphate and used as a substrate for glycolysis (breaking down glycogen) or pentose phosphate metabolism. When there is too much glucose in the cell, this pathway can also be increased, which greatly increases inflammatory chemicals, increases insulin resistance, prevents clot breakdown, and causes scar formation to occur, causing tissue damage. (Luckily, N-acetyl cysteine can prevent this pathway from going aberrant.)

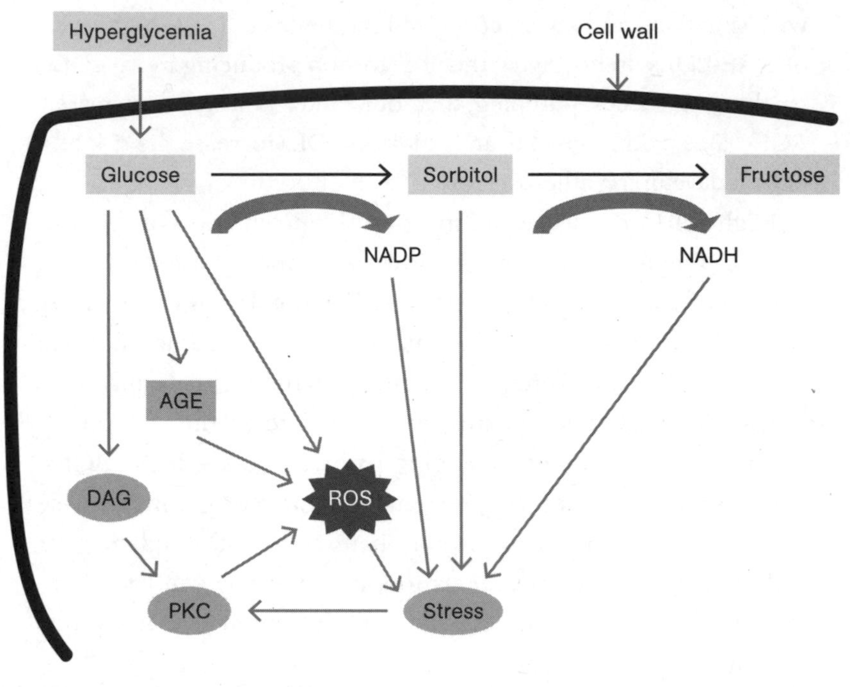

Figure 14.1. DAG and PKC: diacylglycerol and protein kinase c beta activation. NADP and NADH: metabolites can increase ROS. ROS: reactive oxygen species. AGE: advanced glycosylated end products.

Figure 14.1 sums up how hyperglycemia enters into cells and stimulates the pathways discussed above. Note that all the dysfunctional pathways lead to cellular oxidative stress and that means cellular damage.

More things can go wrong in the diabetic body. An overweight or obese T2DM patient's fat cells produce chemicals and hormones that are pro-inflammatory, increase insulin resistance, and can negatively affect glucose regulation. Hyperglycemia also promotes the development of atherosclerosis by interfering with nitric oxide production in the blood vessels. Nitric oxide is a gas that opens up blood vessels, helps lower blood pressure, and promotes good blood flow. Hyperglycemia causes nitric oxide to convert into a free radical itself, reactive nitrogen species, thus promoting vasoconstriction of the arteries, and a pro-clotting, pro-inflammatory state. In other words, high blood sugar is not good! The body falls apart in many ways when it is faced with chronic hyperglycemia.

The Good News about Complications!

In conventional care, diabetes is a relentlessly progressive disease invariably causing complications that worsen over the years and then lead to an early death. However, that is not how it has to be!

If they have not progressed too far, all these degenerations of the body can be reversed. I've seen neuropathy heal and limb numbness return to full feeling; kidneys improve; eyes stabilize, and even improvements in retinopathy; and fatty liver inflammation resolve. Remember, the main principle of naturopathic and integrative medicine is to remove the obstacles to cure: high blood sugars, high insulin levels, nutrient and antioxidant deficiencies, and unhealthy lifestyle choices. Once those are back in balance, the natural wisdom and healing capacity of your body can be active. Of course, a patient may present with complications so advanced, such as late stage kidney disease on dialysis, that it's too late for reversal. But, the goal of the future is to have enough medical practitioners and clinics out there so that millions of diabetic patients can discover and thrive on comprehensive integrative medicine, preventing the development of complications and catching them when they are not too far along.

It must be reemphasized that complications should never occur in the first place. Only people with uncontrolled diabetes develop these problems. If you have one or more of these complications, perhaps the protocol you are following is not as beneficial to you as it could be, and it's time to seek a totally different one.

Elevated insulin can also lead to diabetic complications. Whether a T2DM patient is making too much insulin innately, or any diabetic patient is injecting more than 40 units of insulin a day, it's too much insulin. Here is what high levels of insulin can do in the body:

- Increase production of plasminogen activator inhibitor (PAI). PAI inhibits clot breakdown. That means there are more clots in the body that are not broken down, which can increase the risk of a heart attack or stroke.

- Cause the liver to increase production of triglycerides and LDL cholesterol. Elevated lipids are one risk factor among many that might increase the risk of cardiovascular disease.
- Cause increased levels of angiotensinogen II. Angiotensinogen II stimulates blood vessels to constrict, promotes pro-inflammatory chemicals, and promotes the rupture of atherosclerotic plaques in blood vessels. Those all might increase the risk of cardiovascular medical events.
- Promote vascular endothelium growth factor in the arterial lining, which makes arteries leaky. As a result, the body grows new blood vessels in that area that are fragile and lose blood easily. As discussed in the retinopathy section, this is a main reason diabetic patients can develop serious vision problems.
- Cause the retention of sodium and the loss of potassium and magnesium, which helps raise blood pressure levels.
- Reduce nitric oxide production. Nitric oxide dilates blood vessels, so making less of it can lead to higher blood pressure.
- Cause a loss of magnesium. Among the hundreds of actions magnesium does in the body, it is a vital nutrient involved in lowering the blood pressure, reducing insulin resistance, helping produce anti-inflammatory chemicals and energy, and aiding liver detoxification.

KEY TREATMENT NOTE

No diabetic patient willing to follow a comprehensive integrative treatment protocol ever has to develop complications. And I'm not saying that irresponsibly. The patient needs to commit to following a protocol as directed for life. But, if there is a good team dynamic between doctor and patient, this can occur. As a result, complications can be prevented and, if already in existence, if not too far along, can heal.

Specific Diabetic Complications

I'll discuss the following diabetic complications one at a time: nonalcoholic fatty liver disease and nonalcoholic steatohepatitis, Alzheimer's disease, cardiovascular disease, diabetic eye disease, nephropathy, and neuropathy.

Nonalcoholic Fatty Liver Disease (NAFLD) and Nonalcoholic Steatohepatitis (NASH)

Fatty liver is the most common chronic liver disease in the United States. Although nonalcoholic fatty liver (NAFLD), or just fatty liver, is not listed as one of the classic diabetic complications, it is so common and potentially so dangerous over time, I want to spend some time discussing it.

There are three main disease conditions in which a liver becomes fatty and then may progress further into more severe liver abnormalities: alcoholism, chronic hepatitis C, and NAFLD.

Fatty liver is highly associated with metabolic syndrome, when patients have abdominal obesity (men over 40 inches; women over 35 inches), elevated triglycerides (higher than 150 mg/dL), reduced good HDL cholesterol (lower than 40 mg/dL), hypertension (higher than 130/85 mmHg), and elevated fasting glucose (higher than 99 mg/dL).

The statistics are astounding and frightening. Around 30 percent of the US population, or one hundred million people, have NAFLD, and more than 90 percent of these people have at least one of the metabolic syndrome problems listed above. Statistics show that around 70–80 percent of obese patients (BMI greater than 30) have NAFLD, and up to 100 percent of morbidly obese patients (BMI greater than 40) have NAFLD. Around 36 percent of adults in the United States, around 78 million, are obese, and even worse, around 17 percent of children, 12.5 million, are obese, as well. Fatty liver is seen in both obese adults and obese children. Around 70 percent of T2DM patients have fatty liver, and 5–20 percent of those patients will progress to developing cirrhosis of the liver.

Since misery loves company, it is important to note that the United States is not alone in its obesity status. In 2014, globally, 1.9 billion adults aged eighteen and older were overweight, of which 600 million were obese. That means 39 percent of all adults are overweight and 13 percent of those are obese. Forty-two million children under the age of five were overweight or obese in 2013. Those numbers have doubled since 1980. Of the obese population, depending on the study, 40–90 percent of that population has NAFLD; 240–560 million people. So, this is a worldwide crisis.

What exactly is fatty liver and how does it form? There are two stages to fatty liver. The first stage is the liver becoming, well, excessively fatty. A typical liver contains about 5 percent fat in its tissue, and fatty liver occurs when the fat in the liver is greater than 10 percent. It is the number one medical reason liver enzymes, which show liver inflammation, are elevated. Overall, though, fatty liver is a benign condition of fat accumulating in the cells of the liver, even though there can be so much fat in the liver cell it risks bursting.

There are many reasons why a liver can become fatty. Although NAFLD is the primary reason, this list contains all the medical etiologies and risks for NAFLD:

- Overweight/obesity with insulin resistance and metabolic syndrome
- Severe acute or chronic hepatitis C
- Certain medications: valproic acid, corticosteroids, tamoxifen, estrogens, methotrexate
- Environmental toxins: organic solvents, PCBs, petrochemicals, dimethylformamide
- Genetic abnormalities: galactosemia, glycogen storage disease, homocystinuria, Wilson's disease, hemochromatosis, alpha-1-antitrypsin deficiency
- Metabolic abnormalities: PCOS, obstructive sleep apnea
- Nutritional problems: overnutrition, starvation diet (causing rapid weight loss), total parenteral nutrition, protein-energy malnutrition, celiac disease, vitamin A toxicity
- Autoimmune liver diseases: hyperthyroidism and hypothyroidism, primary biliary cirrhosis, primary sclerosing cholangitis
- Surgery: bariatric surgery—if it causes rapid weight loss
- Age: most patients with NAFLD are between forty and sixty-five years old, but it can occur at any age

- Ethnicity: Latinos, Asians, Caucasians (it seems lower in African Americans)
- Positive family history of NAFLD
- Gut microbiome. According to a fascinating new look at the body, the gut and liver have extensive "cross-talk." The gut determines how ingested calories are processed; it is the caloric gatekeeper and the metabolic control tower. The gut can contribute to the development of fatty liver if it produces bacterial metabolites that promote the deposition of fat in the liver and encourages the fat to become inflamed. The gut microbiome can also increase or decrease the effect of insulin resistance in the systemic body.
- Gut permeability and small intestine bacterial overgrowth. When the gut is unhealthy it can lose the integrity of its cells and become "leaky." When it becomes leaky, it may activate immune system pro-inflammatory responses, and bacteria from the gut may leak through and wind up in the liver with toxic effects.

Remember I said earlier that one reason the liver develops insulin resistance is because the abdominal fat cells dump free fatty acids, triglycerides, into the portal venous system. This is the vein that takes everything from the intestine, including the fat cells around it, to the liver first, before it enters the body as a whole. These free fatty acids wind up being stored in the liver cells, and there they can oxidize, turning into pro-inflammatory substances. White blood cells are drawn to the fatty liver cells and release their own pro-inflammatory chemicals such as tumor necrosis factor-alpha, interleukins, hydrogen peroxide, and superoxide. These can both damage the liver cells and promote systemic insulin resistance. As a result of this situation, the liver cell mitochondria, the source of energy production, can develop dysfunction and not work as efficiently. Liver insulin resistance develops and increases, causing elevated serum glucose, noticeably in the fasting morning glucose, and more abdominal fat deposition, which then releases more fat into the liver at night, promoting this dangerous cycle. Last, patients with fatty liver are often found to be low in antioxidants, such as vitamin A and vitamin E, so more oxidative damage can occur in their liver cells.

In stage two of this condition, when all of the above has been happening, nonalcoholic steatohepatitis (NASH) develops. *Steatosis* means fat, in medicine; *hepatitis* means liver inflammation. In NASH, the smoldering embers of NAFLD become a fire, causing inflammation and damage to liver cells. Liver cells develop ballooning degeneration, swelling in size even to bursting. When they erupt, more white blood cells from the immune system are drawn there, releasing more pro-inflammatory cytokines.

If NASH continues for years and years, then liver cells can develop fibrosis, a kind of scarring. If that continues, then the liver can develop nonfunctioning nodules definitive of cirrhosis, leading to liver failure and either death or a requirement for liver transplantation. The very damaged liver cells may also transform unfavorably into hepatocellular carcinoma, or cancer.

Unfortunately, there are very few symptoms of NAFLD and NASH. The vast majority of patients are asymptomatic. Some minor signs might develop, such as what we see with metabolic syndrome. We might also note on a physical exam that there is hepatomegaly (enlarged liver) or splenomegaly (enlarged spleen), or if the patient presents with an advanced case, there might be some signs of cirrhosis and liver failure. But that is extremely uncommon.

When a person with T2DM diabetes comes to me, I always do the following lab work first to pick up any possibility of NAFLD:

Ferritin. This is usually the first elevated lab value indicating a person has fatty liver. Most, if not all, conventional physicians do not include ferritin in their lab tests, so you may need to request it to be drawn. Ferritin is elevated if you have an uncommon genetic disease called hemochromatosis, whereby you absorb too much iron from your food; if you have a severe bacterial infection in your body; or, most typically, if you have NAFLD, with ferritin showing there is some acute inflammation occurring in your liver. If ferritin comes back elevated, your physician will need to rule out hemochromatosis through another serum lab test. It would be obvious if you had a serious bacterial infection; those don't hide the way fatty liver can!

GGT (gamma-glutamyl transferase). This is another early warning lab value showing fatty liver, but this is found less often than elevated ferritin. This test is also not commonly done by conventional physicians.

Liver enzymes called AST (aspartate aminotransferase) or ALT (alanine aminotransferase). These enzymes are classically the first lab values showing inflammation in the liver cells, but they will be elevated after the ferritin rises. When these are elevated, I am more concerned that the patient has NASH, instead of the more benign NAFLD. With one or both liver enzymes elevated, a good physician will also rule out viral hepatitis, alcoholism, autoimmune liver diseases, medication-induced liver disease, or even supplement-induced liver disease.

Serum fibrosis bloodwork. I am not very impressed with these tests. Labs will check for extracellular matrix proteins (ECM) indicating activation of hepatic stellate cells, activated due to liver inflammation and injury. Production of these ECM cells can promote liver fibrosis. The NASH FibroSure lab checks ten biochemical markers, but none are that unique or diagnostic. The FibroSPECT II from Prometheus Labs checks three biochemical markers (hyaluronic acid), tissue inhibitors of metalloproteinases (TIMP-1), and alpha-2 macroglobulin, which may pick up either no or mild fibrosis or more moderate to severe fibrosis, but it may not clearly diagnose patients in the middle.

Abdominal ultrasound. It is typical that I will schedule a T2DM overweight or obese patient for an abdominal ultrasound if I find elevated ferritin and hemochromatosis is ruled out. An ultrasound, which is not invasive, and is covered by insurances, will diagnose fatty liver when 15–30 percent of fatty content exists in the liver. The more the liver has "increased echogenicity," the more fatty liver exists. However, an ultrasound cannot differentiate between NAFLD and NASH.

FibroScan. This simple, noninvasive machine is exceedingly helpful in diagnosing the extent of fatty liver, fibrosis, and cirrhosis. There is now a lab doing this test in Scottsdale, Arizona, close to my office, so I can refer my NAFLD patients there to see if any significant damage is occurring in their liver as a result of it being fatty. I highly recommend medical practitioners search their cities to find labs doing FibroScan analyses for patient diagnostic referrals.

Liver biopsy. Injecting a thin needle into the liver to take a biopsy is the gold standard of liver analysis, and the most comprehensive way to specifically diagnose NAFLD and NASH. There are some risk factors, such as bleeding or puncturing a lung, but they are not common and the procedure is quick. The liver biopsy will grade inflammation, hepatocellular ballooning, and fibrosis. However, this is a very invasive procedure, and most physicians (including myself) and gastroenterologists do not wish to do a biopsy to diagnose fatty liver, so this is really never done.

Neither a CT scan or an MRI is helpful in diagnosing NAFLD or NASH, so I do not recommend these.

NAFLD is reversible if the liver is not yet cirrhotic. An analysis on NAFLD in the *World Journal of Gastroenterology* noted that patients who lost 5 percent or more of their body weight over nine months saw improvements in insulin resistance and a decrease in their fatty liver. Five percent weight loss is not that much! If a patient weighs 220 pounds, 5 percent is only 11 pounds. That, and much more, is doable for all overweight T2DM patients on a comprehensive integrative protocol.

Conventional Treatment of NAFLD

There are no conventional treatment guidelines specifically for NAFLD or NASH. Here are some key conventional treatment ideas:

Avoiding alcohol. If the liver is unhealthy, alcohol is the absolute worst substance a person can ingest. Even though alcohol lowers the morning glucose if drunk at supper, it is still completely contraindicated for a person with fatty liver. Alcohol promotes further degradation of a NAFLD or NASH liver, and accelerates the rate of damage.

Weight loss. As noted, 5–10 percent weight loss can make a substantially positive impact on the fatty liver. The body is wise, and if you allow it to lose weight, it will naturally remove it from the liver as well as the abdomen. There is one key aspect of weight loss that should be highlighted, from a study of extreme weight loss in forty-one patients. Although biopsies confirmed less fatty tissue in their livers, 24 percent of patients developed liver inflammation or fibrosis. That is, one in four experienced hepatic aggravation from the weight loss. So, even if the liver loses fat, there could be an increase in liver inflammation. The idea is that one's initial weight reduction goal should be to lose 10 percent

KEY TREATMENT NOTE

Weight loss of more than 3.5 pounds per week puts the patient at significant risk of developing liver inflammation and fibrosis. I have seen overweight T2DM patients who went on the extreme human chorionic gonadotropin (HCG) diet suddenly have their liver enzymes elevate substantially. This is why I do not recommend rapid extreme weight loss or starvation diets for patients. Another risk of extreme weight loss is the development of gallstones and a resultant cholecystectomy (removal of the gallbladder). Losing weight slowly, over time, is safe and effective and keeps the liver and gallbladder healthy.

of baseline weight and not exceed 3.5 pounds (1.6 kg) a week. In the first month that a patient begins a low-carb diet, there is often up to 12 pounds of weight loss, due to water and fat loss (exercise helps prevent muscle loss). However, on a comprehensive integrative protocol, that significant weight reduction slows down to a consistent loss that is safer for the liver. Slow but steady is the best way to lose weight, cure NAFLD or NASH, and reverse T2DM.

Exercise. Of course, exercise is a key factor in weight loss, ensuring fat is reduced and maintaining (or building) muscles.

Bariatric surgery. Worldwide diabetes associations, including the ADA, now recommend bariatric surgery for morbidly obese T2DM patients with BMIs equal to or over 40 kg/m^2, and they suggest it can also be considered for T2DM with BMIs between 30 and 34.9 kg/m^2 who are not able to get their glucose or obesity under control with conventional lifestyle interventions and medical therapy. In the United States, around 220,000 people annually have bariatric surgery. Conventional care has done many studies showing bariatric surgery can reduce weight, improve glucose levels, reduce A1Cs, and heal NAFLD and NASH, by removing the fat and reducing liver inflammation. The most common forms of gastric bypass include Roux-en-Y gastric bypass, laparoscopic adjustable lap band, and sleeve gastrectomy. With the Roux-en-Y surgery, most studies reported decreased hepatic steatosis, inflammation, and fibrosis. However, four studies showed worsening fibrosis, and in two studies NASH scores deteriorated. So, the most drastic surgery may or may not be helpful for any individual. With the gastric band, in one study, after weight loss there was significant improvement in the liver tissue. However, in one large study with 381 patients who experienced one of those three types of bariatric surgery, liver biopsies were performed at one and five years after their surgeries. Although there was less steatosis and ballooning, there was no change in inflammation and an increase in fibrosis scores. As we can see, bariatric surgery can be very helpful for some obese patients with NAFLD and NASH, but may not resolve it in many. I would certainly hope patients would try a comprehensive integrative medical protocol before resorting to bariatric surgery.

Liver transplantation. This, of course, is the last chance for a patient whose NASH has progressed to significant cirrhosis of the liver causing liver failure.

Supplementation.

- Conventional medicine has done some studies on vitamin E, showing it reduced liver enzymes and steatosis. Vitamin E, milk thistle, and lecithin were shown to improve liver enzymes, reduce fatty liver content, and reduce inflammation.
- In a study in obese pediatric patients, the children were dosed with *Lactobacillus* GG. The probiotic significantly reduced liver enzymes.

Medications.

- Thiazolidinediones (TZDs): These oral hypoglycemic agents decreased insulin resistance and liver inflammation, reducing AST and ALT levels. However, as discussed in chapter 5, these drugs are essentially off the market, and in my opinion, should be. I would not use them in NAFLD patients.
- GLP-1 agonists: These non-insulin injectables have been shown to reduce insulin resistance, lower appetite, and reduce glucose levels. They have also decreased steatosis, inflammation, and fibrosis in the liver.
- Anti-obesity medications: Medications such as Xenical or Alli (orlistat), Qysmia, or Contrave have been shown to reduce AST and ALT but not help with liver fibrosis. They also have some serious side effects such as liver damage, vision problems, seizures, suicidal thoughts, and so on, so it is best to avoid them!

Overall, conventional medicine has some notable ideas for treatment, but I think integrative medicine has a lot more to offer.

Comprehensive Integrative Treatment of NAFLD and NASH

All the aspects of the comprehensive diabetic regimen help a person with insulin resistant induced fatty liver lose weight, reduce fat in their liver, reduce inflammation, and protect the liver from progressive disease.

DIET

It is much easier for a T2DM patient to lose weight on a low-carbohydrate diet. Losing weight means it's likely you can avoid initiating medications, or can reduce or stop them. There is one other important dietary consideration to add, which involves ferritin. Ferritin is stored iron, and it is elevated in many patients with fatty liver. There are indications that patients with iron overload and NAFLD might have worse insulin resistance, liver inflammation, and more tendency to develop fibrosis. In patients with elevated ferritin, avoiding iron in the diet may be helpful for preserving healthy liver tissue. Two of the biggest sources of dietary iron are red meat and poultry. The dietary recommendations for someone with NAFLD or NASH would be to avoid eating any red meat, such as beef or lamb. It would be best to also avoid poultry, or eat just a little a couple of times a week, focusing instead on other diabetic-friendly protein sources: fish, eggs, nuts, seeds, soy, dairy, and protein powders. Also, avoid cooking in cast iron skillets, drink black or green tea if you do eat meat or poultry as those prevent iron absorption, and ensure any supplements you take are iron free. In this way, putting less iron in the body may help protect a fatty liver.

LIFESTYLE

Ensuring that a patient gets exercise, sleeps well, engages in detoxification, supports the microbiome, and manages their stress are important in reducing NAFLD and NASH.

Exercise has been shown to reduce triglyceride levels in the liver, thus reducing NAFLD, and as we know it is also exceedingly beneficial in helping with weight loss.

Ensure the patient gets great sleep and, if necessary, is successfully treated for obstructive sleep apnea (OSA). OSA is associated with promoting

KEY TREATMENT NOTE

Avoid red meat and alcohol if you have high ferritin and NAFLD or NASH.

insulin resistance and NAFLD and NASH. Doing a sleep study and diagnosing OSA, and then having the patient use a therapeutic fix for the OSA is something all physicians should focus on.

Working with patients to reduce and manage their stress can help them avoid emotional eating and engaging in behaviors that harm the liver, such as drinking alcohol or recreational drug use.

The intestine and the liver are intimately connected. A "leaky gut," where the lining of the gut suffers from permeability, can allow bacterial endotoxins to reach the liver and promote liver inflammation. It is important to ensure that the lining is healthy. If indicated, food-sensitivity testing, small intestine bacterial overgrowth testing, or actually measuring specifically for a leaky gut might be helpful to ensure the gut's health is maximized. Supplements such as L-glutamine, slippery elm, marshmallow, quercitin, and licorice are all regularly used by integrative practitioners to heal a "leaky gut," reducing the delivery of toxic gut bacterial endotoxins to the fatty liver. The microbiome should be supported with a good fiber product that provides 3–8 grams of fiber per day, especially because a low-carb, no-grain diet can harm the intestinal microbiome. Fiber can help prevent that. As for using probiotics, although *Lactobacillus* GG was helpful to overweight pediatric patients with fatty liver, we are not sure exactly what probiotic species to use specifically for fatty liver in adults. *Lactobacillus gasseri* has been shown to aid in reducing waist circumference in adults, so a product containing that, among other bacteria, might be a good start. Avoid NSAIDs and other over-the-counter medications, especially microbiome-destroying antibiotics, as much as possible. Eating fermented foods to help restore beneficial bacteria is a great idea, too.

A gentle detoxification might be required if the patient presents with symptoms or has positive signs or a past history that shows detoxification is necessary, such as a positive toxic burden test result or a history of working around solvents and unhealthy chemicals.

LIVER HEALTH

Helping the liver become cleaner and healthier is important because fatty liver is a condition in and of itself in the liver cells. A person with NAFLD or NASH should especially, even during vacations and holidays, stay on a low-carb diet and avoid soda pop, sugar, and all junk food. It is better to switch from coffee to green tea, which can have the same stimulating effect, but is full of antioxidants scientifically shown to be protective to the liver, and also reduces the absorption of iron.

I recommend an increase in the consumption of "bitters," as bitter is the main flavor that specifically promotes bile production and secretion in the liver and helps the liver detoxify. Bitters include cruciferous vegetables (cabbage, broccoli, cauliflower, radish, kale, Brussels sprouts); chicory in alternative coffee drinks such as Teeccino, Pero, and Cafix; bitter greens such as arugula, radicchio, and dandelion greens; and herbs such as gentian, chamomile, and bitter orange peel. If you are going to drink alcohol (though you should not), I suggest sticking with bitter aperitifs such as Fernet-Branca, Angostura, or Campari.

Another way naturopathic physicians help the liver is through the castor oil pack, a hydrotherapy method that has been used for decades to help decrease inflammation in the liver and abdomen, and promote lymph tissue movement. This technique is anti-inflammatory and helps move the lymph tissue, also promoting a type of detoxification.

Another aspect important to helping detoxify your liver is to control your anger and irritability, the emotions associated with the liver and liver disease. Doing stress management to maintain an even mental and emotional balance is always good for the whole body and mind, including the liver.

It is also good to live and work in a green environment. Remember to not use chemical exterminators in your yard or home, and to use "green" chemicals and hygiene products, refurbish your home with "green" materials, and ingest clean water and the organic foods you can afford. The less work the liver needs to do regarding environmental detoxification, the healthier it can stay, and the quicker it can heal. Environmental toxins have been shown scientifically to promote weight gain and insulin resistance, so being as "green" as possible is the best way for any prediabetic or diabetic patient to live!

How to Do a Castor Oil Pack

A castor oil pack is an old medical tool integrative physicians and patients find very helpful for reducing pain and inflammation in abdominal and pelvic conditions.

1. Purchase some high-quality castor oil, which is available at regular pharmacies and health food stores.
2. Get some flannel or cotton, enough fabric so that it can be folded in half and cover your liver.
3. Pour the castor oil onto the flannel until it is soaked through but not dripping oil all over the place.
4. Place the flannel on your abdomen over your liver.
5. Cover the flannel with some plastic wrap, such as Saran wrap, and then place a heating pad over the pack. The plastic wrap is used to protect the heating pad from getting oily.
6. Turn the heating pack on as high as you comfortably can.
7. You can cover all of this with a towel to keep it in place.
8. Leave on for around forty-five minutes.
9. Do this between one and seven times a week, as directed by your physician.

SUPPLEMENTATION

Supplements are a great addition to a fatty liver protocol. They can be used to reduce insulin resistance and protect liver tissue. They can also help with appetite control and weight loss.

BASIC SUPPLEMENTS

Multiple vitamin/mineral. This is a good start for nutrient repletion.

DHA. In pediatric NAFLD, DHA was shown to reduce liver steatosis, reduce liver enzymes, and decrease insulin resistance. 250–500 mg per day.

Fish oils. Can reduce hepatic steatosis, improve NASH, and reduce inflammation. 1,000–2,000 mg EPA per day.

Probiotics. Aside from VSL #3, there are many different probiotics integrative medical practitioners use in their practices. Taking at least twenty-five billion a day of a quality product is recommended.

NUTRIENTS FOR REDUCING INSULIN RESISTANCE

Chromium picolinate. 200–1,200 mcg per day

Vanadium (bis[maltolato]oxovanadium). 5 mcg–10 mg per day

Zinc citrate/bisglycinate. 15–50 mg per day

Vitamin D_3. Dose to 40–70 ng/mL on labs (2,000–10,000 IU per day in combination with vitamins A and K and calcium and magnesium)

BOTANICALS FOR REDUCING INSULIN RESISTANCE

Berberine HCL. 1,000–1,500 mg per day

Cinnamomun cassia/burmanii. 1–3 grams per day

Fiber. 5–20 grams per day

Gymnema sylvestre. 400–2,400 mg per day

GALLSTONE PREVENTION WITH WEIGHT LOSS

A gallstone is formed when there is too much cholesterol in comparison to bile and lecithin. If someone is overweight or obese, and begins a serious weight loss protocol, cholesterol is released by the fat cells being metabolically burned, and this increases the risk of creating gallstones. If a person has a family history of gallstones and begins to lose weight, working to prevent gallstones is very helpful. These are supplements that can help reduce the risk of developing a gallstone:

Lecithin (also lowers lipids, and helps with concentration). Lecithin comes from soy or sunflower generally. Ensure, if from soy, it is GMO-free: around 3,000 mg per day

Taurine and/or glycine (helps form bile salts). 500–1,500 mg per day

Ox bile digestive enzyme. 1 capsule per meal

Peppermint capsules. 1 capsule one to three times per day (might be contraindicated in gastroesophageal reflux disease)

ANTIOXIDANTS

As discussed above, many NAFLD or NASH patients are low in antioxidants, which no doubt increases the risk for more liver damage. The below supplements can help protect the liver:

Carotenoids. Higher doses of carotenoids might make a person's skin turn an orange hue, as carotenoids are stored in the skin. This is a benign event, and stopping the carotenoid intake will quickly remove that slightly unusual tint from the skin. 10,000–100,000 IU per day.

Mixed vitamin E. A well-studied antioxidant for the liver, ensure it is in the "mixed" form with all four types of tocopherols present. 400–1,200 IU per day.

R-alpha-lipoic acid. 300–900 mg per day orally.

Vitamin C. 500–1,500 mg per day (remember, higher doses of vitamin C in patients with T2DM can throw off glucose meters).

Selenium. 200–600 mcg per day.

N-acetyl cysteine. 600–2,400 mg per day.

BOTANICAL ANTIOXIDANTS/ANTI-INFLAMMATORIES

Licorice. Licorice has been shown to help reduce free fatty acid hepatic toxicity. It can come as licorice tea, extract, jam, tincture, or capsules. The glycyrrhizinic acid component of licorice, in some people over time, can elevate the blood pressure due to its similarity to our adrenal hormone aldosterone, which is used to elevate our blood pressure. Licorice is often sold deglycyrrhizinated, with that component removed, making it safe for all patients, including those with hypertension. Around 200 mg per day.

Green tea. Increased green tea and epigallocatechin-3-gallate (EGCG) flavonoid can reduce the risk of liver disease, decrease inflammatory markers in the liver, and is anticarcinogenic. Green tea can be used as an organic tea or taken in capsules. Around 200 mg per day.

*Milk thistle/*Silybum marianum. This antioxidant prevents lipid oxidation; inhibits fibrosis and inflammation; enhances DNA/RNA/protein synthesis in the liver; helps prevent mitochondrial injury; and helps the liver function better overall. Milk thistle has broad base actions of protection of the liver while helping it heal and proliferate healthy cells. Around 200 mg per day.

Cordyceps sinensis. In a good study, the use of cordyceps reduced damage in livers with NASH. 1 gram three times per day.

Curcumin extract. Curcumin can prevent fibrosis development, decrease the inflammatory process in the liver, and promote bile production and secretion, and thus decrease the risk of developing NASH. 200–3,000 g per day.

Resveratrol. This is a strong antioxidant. 100–200 mg per day.

Those are a lot of supplements. Taking a good multiple vitamin/mineral supplement, fish oils, mixed vitamin E, lecithin, and one or two liver protective supplements is a good start. Ask your integrative medical provider for advice on a supplement regimen. Between eating a healthy, appropriate diet, losing weight, avoiding red meat, doing castor oil packs, and taking the appropriate supplementation, fatty liver can be managed well and even reversed. Your liver can be saved and healed.

Alzheimer's Disease

There are some people who call Alzheimer's disease "Type 3 diabetes." While I don't find it helpful to label conditions associated with diabetes with their own diabetes number—why not then call kidney failure "Type 4 diabetes"?—diabetes that is not well controlled can cause an increased risk of developing Alzheimer's disease (AD).

AD consists of damage in the brain causing a loss of synapses, which connect neuron cells together. Loss of synapses leads to less communication among brain cells, memory loss, disorientation, and cognitive impairments.

In the United States, 5.3 million people currently have AD, and statisticians predict that by 2050 up to 13.8 million will suffer from it. AD has been believed to be a random, nonpreventable condition that strikes people somewhat suddenly without any warning. The good news is that this does not seem to be true. It seems there are many precursor years to the development of AD. In 2014, a small study at UCLA showed reversal of mild to moderate AD using exercise, attaining a normal body mass index, and eating a Mediterranean diet. Another study showed that comprehensive diet changes, brain stimulation, exercise, sleep optimization, vitamins, stress management, and some pharmaceuticals were able to improve cognitive decline in most patients. Here are a few specifics of the many varied protocols. The diet consisted of eliminating all simple carbohydrates, gluten, and processed foods; eating more vegetables, fruits, and nonfarmed fish; as well as intermittent fasting of at least twelve hours between dinner and breakfast, and at least three hours from dinner to bedtime. The supplements included melatonin, methylcobalamin, vitamin D_3, fish oil, and CoQ10. Ensuring good dental care was occurring was important, as well. All this is what I have been discussing regarding treating diabetes, and it is very exciting, considering pharmaceutical treatment of AD has generally been a failure.

There seems to be a very strong correlation between AD and metabolic syndrome, hyperinsulinemia (high serum insulin levels), and insulin resistance. As much as 40 percent of the neurological pathology of AD is attributed to hyperinsulinemia. Higher A1Cs correlate with lower cognitive status. In fact, the brain areas that are most sensitive to insulin and insulin-like growth factor-1 are the same areas most susceptible to AD damage, and are associated with increased production of the amyloid proteins found to gum up the functioning of the brain.

Diabetic type diets have been shown to be helpful in preventing AD. One study, called MIND, was a hybrid Mediterranean and DASH diet. DASH, Dietary Approaches to Stop Hypertension, was developed by the US National Institutes of Health to lower high blood pressure without medication. This diet is very similar to the diet shown to prevent prediabetic patients from becoming diabetic and consists of green leafy vegetables (six servings a week); other vegetables (one serving a day); nuts (five servings a week); berries (two or more servings a week); beans (at least three servings a week); whole grains (three or more servings a day); fish (one serving a week); poultry (two servings a week); olive oil used as the main cooking oil; and wine (one glass a day). Foods minimized in the MIND study include red meat (fewer than four servings a week); butter and margarine (less than one tablespoon a week); cheese (less than one serving a week); pastries and sweets (fewer than five servings a week, though I think it should be even fewer); and fried or fast food (less than one serving a week). Sure, eating grains is not on the diabetic protocol, but these people were not diabetic patients.

The 923 people in the MIND study were followed for 4.5 years. Those who most strictly followed the diet had a 53 percent risk reduction in developing

AD. That's wonderful! Even those who were in the middle on observance of the diet had a 35 percent risk reduction. The diet is very anti-inflammatory and also has a low glycemic aspect; inflammation is associated with being a risk for AD occurrence.

Patients who have a positive APOE4 gene mutation have an increased genetic risk factor of developing T2DM, elevated lipid panels, and cardiovascular disease. In another study analyzing eating excess calories and fat in 980 people for over four years, those with that problematic gene mutation had a 2.3 times increased risk of developing AD. Many medical studies have noted that being overweight or obese in middle age, in and of itself, significantly increases one's risk of developing AD.

The brain likes fat, and burns well on ketones. A low-carb ketogenic diet, providing ketones to a brain that thrives on them, makes sense to help neurons function better. Especially beneficial are medium-chain triglycerides, which increase ketone levels no matter if a person is strictly on a ketogenic diet or not. We discussed a low-carb ketogenic diet in chapter 7, but even adding in two tablespoons of coconut oil a day may be helpful. Dr. Mary Newton, MD, has written quite a bit about a low-carb ketogenic diet and coconut oil as a possible treatment for AD (https://coconutketones.com).

It is also very important to ensure there is no folate or vitamin B_{12} deficiency. A folate deficiency alone can cause two to three times the risk of developing AD.

The following supplements may support the brain:

All nutrients used to help reduce insulin resistance
Multiple vitamin/mineral with bioactive vitamin B_{12}, methylcobalmin, and folic acid in the form of methyltetrahydrofolate
Coconut oil: 1–2 tablespoon per day
Acetyl-l-carnitine: 1,500–3,000 mg per day
Fish oils: at least 1,000 mg EPA/750 mg DHA per day
Gingko biloba: 160–240 mg per day
Curcumin: 200–3,000 mg per day, as an anti-inflammatory agent
R-ALA: 600 mg per day
Phosphatylcholine (lecithin): 3,000–12,000 mg per day
CDP-choline: 250–2,000 mg per day, provides neuroprotection

Uridine: 250–1,000 mg per day
Vinpocetine: 5–60 mg per day
Bacopa monniera: 10–300 mg per day

A study at MIT linked choline (as in phosphatylcholine or CDP-choline), uridine, and fish oils to improvement in patients with AD. All three of those nutrients are precursors to the lipid molecules that, along with certain types of proteins, are integral parts of the neuron cells, and they increased the number of working synapses. The study showed all three nutrients had to be administered together for them to be effective.

It seems that following The Eight Essentials is not only valuable to controlling diabetes but also valuable for reducing the risk of AD. It makes good sense for a diabetic person with a family history of AD to follow The Eight Essentials, including taking one or two of the aforementioned supplements.

Cardiovascular Disease

Cardiovascular disease (CVD) is rampant in our society. In people over sixty-five years old, at least 68 percent die from heart disease, and around 16 percent die from stroke. Adults with diabetes are two to four times more likely to have CVD than adults without diabetes.

Damage to the heart and blood vessels is in general referred to as CVD. Blood vessels consist of arteries carrying blood away from your heart, and veins, which return it. Damage to those is called macrovascular disease. Cardiovascular disorders that can develop include coronary artery disease, stroke, peripheral artery disease, damage to the heart muscle, congestive heart failure, and heart attack. CVD is the leading cause of morbidity and mortality in diabetic patients.

The American Heart Association lists diabetes as one of the seven major controllable risk factors for CVD, along with tobacco smoking, elevated total and LDL cholesterol and triglycerides/low HDL cholesterol, hypertension, lack of exercise, overweight and obesity, eating an unhealthy diet, and high blood sugars.

The statistics are astounding—more than 90 percent of diabetic patients have one or more of those noted risk factors; for example, up to 97 percent of diabetic patients have elevated lipids. Studies show that reducing elevated lipids, gaining good control of blood glucose, and reducing hypertension can prevent adverse cardiovascular outcomes by 30–50 percent. Unfortunately, less than 30 percent of diabetic patients achieve the lipid and blood pressure goals, and less than 50 percent achieve an A1C of less than 7.0 percent.

As noted, some of the medications given to diabetic patients need to be reduced as the eGFR decreases. I listed these in the discussion of oral medications (chapter 5). A knowledgeable physician or nephrologist can guide patients through reducing or stopping them.

Controlling hypertension is invaluable for helping to prevent kidney disease. Systolic and diastolic hypertension markedly further the development of diabetic nephropathy. In general, in T1DM patients, hypertension develops as a result of nephropathy; in T2DM patients, hypertension comes in alignment with metabolic syndrome, and also as a result of nephropathy. Thirty percent of T2DM patients already have hypertension when they are diagnosed with diabetes.

What does "blood pressure" mean? When the heart beats, it pumps blood throughout your body, and the blood pushes against the blood vessels containing it. Blood pressure is the pressure of the blood against the vessels and is closely related to the force and rate of the heartbeat and the diameter and elasticity of the walls of the arteries. Two numbers make up one's blood pressure: systolic and diastolic. The systolic number, the top number in a blood pressure number (which is always higher than the second number) measures the pressure in the arteries when the heart beats, that is, when the heart muscle contracts. The diastolic number, the lower number of the two, measures the pressure in the arteries when the heart is at rest and filling with more blood, inbetween the heartbeats. Hypertension means either the systolic or both the systolic and diastolic numbers are above the recommended value for the patient and their health. (Hypotension means the numbers are lower than recommended. Hypotension is not associated with poorly controlled diabetes.)

Regarding hypertension, normal blood pressure is lower than or equal to 120/80 mmHg. Seventy-one percent of diabetic adults (older than age eighteen) have high blood pressure, that is, a reading higher than 140/90 mmHg. Around 20 percent of T1DM patients and up to 70 percent of T2DM patients have hypertension. Unfortunately, it usually takes two to four prescription medications in conventional care to lower elevated blood pressure in patients with diabetes. And, even with medications, only 27 percent of diabetic patients attain a blood pressure lower than 130/80 mmHg. I once saw a morbidly obese T2DM patient on *seven* medications to control his blood pressure!

Blood pressure goals, historically 120/80 mmHg, have now been changed in diabetic populations. The 2016 ADA guidelines for treating hypertension in patients with diabetes consist of systolic targets, diastolic targets, and treatment.

SYSTOLIC TARGETS

- People with diabetes and hypertension should be treated to a systolic blood pressure goal of lower than 140 mmHg.
- Lower systolic targets, such as 130 mmHg, might be appropriate for certain individuals with diabetes, such as younger patients, those with albuminuria, or those with hypertension and one or more additional atherosclerotic cardiovascular disease risk factors, if they can be achieved without undue treatment burden.

DIASTOLIC TARGETS

- Individuals with diabetes should be treated to a diastolic blood pressure goal of lower than 90 mmHg.
- Lower diastolic targets, such as 80 mmHg, might be appropriate for certain individuals with diabetes, such as younger patients, those with albuminuria, or those with hypertension and one or more additional atherosclerotic cardiovascular disease risk factors, if they can be achieved without undue treatment burden.

TREATMENT

- Patients with blood pressure higher than 120/80 mmHg should be advised on lifestyle changes to reduce blood pressure.
- Patients with confirmed office-based blood pressure higher than 140/90 mmHg should, in addition to lifestyle therapy, have prompt initiation and timely subsequent titration of pharmacological therapy to achieve blood pressure goals.

- In older adults, pharmacological therapy to achieve treatment goals of lower than 130/70 mmHg is not recommended; treating to systolic blood pressure lower than 130 mmHg has not been shown to improve cardiovascular outcomes and treating to diastolic blood pressure lower than 70 mmHg has been associated with higher mortality.
- Lifestyle therapy for elevated blood pressure consists of weight loss, if overweight or obese; a Dietary Approaches to Stop Hypertension (DASH)-style dietary pattern, including reducing sodium and increasing potassium intake; moderation of alcohol intake; and increased physical activity.
- Pharmacological therapy for patients with diabetes and hypertension should comprise a regimen that includes either an ACE inhibitor or an angiotensin receptor blocker (ARB) but not both. If one class is not tolerated, the other should be substituted.
- Multiple-drug therapy (including a thiazide diuretic and ACE inhibitor or angiotensin receptor blocker, at maximal doses) is generally required to achieve blood pressure targets.
- If ACE inhibitors, angiotensin receptor blockers, or diuretics are used, serum creatinine/eGFR and serum potassium levels should be monitored.
- In pregnant patients with diabetes and chronic hypertension, blood pressure targets of 110–129/65–79 mmHg are suggested in the interest of optimizing long-term maternal health and minimizing impaired fetal growth.

The new blood pressure goals related to diabetes according to the Joint National Committee (JNC 8) guidelines, published in the *Journal of the American Medical Association* (*JAMA*) in 2013, are:

- In adults sixty years or older without diabetes, the blood pressure goal is lower than 150/90 mmHg.
- In adults eighteen to fifty-nine years old and patients sixty years or older who have diabetes, chronic kidney disease, or both conditions, the blood pressure goal is lower than 140/90 mmHg.
- Medications to use for hypertension should be used in this order: thiazide-type diuretics, calcium channel blockers, ACE inhibitors,

and ARBs. Some other medications can also be added (beta-blockers, alpha-blockers, aldosterone antagonists, etc.).

Conventional Care for Hypertension: Medications

Antihypertensive drugs include ACE inhibitors (ACE-I), angiotension receptor blockers, diuretics, beta-blockers, and calcium channel blockers. I will discuss ACE-I and ARB in the section on kidneys, as they are used to help preserve kidney function in diabetic patients with or without hypertension.

DIURETICS

Diuretics help remove fluid from the body by stimulating glomerular filtration in the kidneys, which means more fluid passes through the kidney cells for excretion. Less fluid in the body is less of a strain on the heart and means the heart does not have to beat so hard. Thiazide diuretics, also known as "loop diuretics," are effective hypotension agents and are inexpensive. They have been around since the 1950s. They can also help reduce edema in limbs due to cardiac causes. They work on the distal convoluted tubules of the kidney tissue by stimulating diuresis, urination, which lowers the plasma volume and cardiac output. These diuretics can cause a loss of many vital minerals, such as potassium, magnesium, and zinc.

Although standard care physicians may place patients on potassium when they are on those types of diuretics, the fact is that diuretics that cause loss of potassium have been shown to raise glucose levels in patients. Moreover, it is rare for conventional medical practitioners to recommend magnesium or zinc replacement. Magnesium deficiency has devastating effects on muscles and is a mineral needed to absorb glucose into the cell membranes. Zinc is necessary to produce and secrete insulin from the pancreas and is required for cells to be sensitive to insulin, so it's not a good nutrient to urinate out every day! I have seen patients so depleted of magnesium due to their diuretic prescription that their muscles could not allow them to walk up a flight of stairs, turn over in bed, or get out of a car. Tell your alternative physician all the hypertensive agents you are on, so he or she can diagnose and correct nutritional deficiencies that may be occurring due to them. The thiazide diuretics may also increase triglycerides and uric acid (which causes gout).

COMMON DIURETICS

Thiazides. Microzide/hydrochlorothiazide: 12.5 mg tablets—1–4 tablets taken once per day

Common loop diuretic. Lasix/furosemide: 20, 40, 80 mg tablets—20–80 mg once per day

COMMON POTASSIUM-SPARING DIURETICS

These diuretics spare the kidneys from losing potassium.

Aldactone/spironolactone. 25, 50, 100 mg tablets: 50–100 mg once per day

Dyrenium/triamterene. 50, 100 mg tablets: 100 mg twice per day

COMMON POTASSIUM-SPARING DIURETIC/ CHLOROTHIAZIDE DIURETIC COMBINATIONS

These tend to have a neutral effect on elevating glucose levels, due to the potassium-sparing portion of the drug.

Dyazide (hydrochlorothiazide and triamterene). 25/37.5 mg—1 capsule once or twice per day

Maxzide-25 (triamterene and hydrochlorothiazide). 37.5/25 mg—1 tablet once or twice per day

Maxzide (triamterene and hydrochlorothiazide). 75/5 mg—1 tablet per day

Prinzide (lisinopril and hydrochlorothiazide). 10/12.5, 20/12.5 mg—1 tablet per day

Hyzaar (losartan potassium and hydrochloride). 50/12.5, 100/12.5, 100/25 mg—1 tablet once or twice per day

Lopressor HCT (metoprolol tartrate and hydrochlorothiazide). 50/25, 100/25, 100/50 mg—1 tablet once or twice per day (depending on the strength of tablet used)

BETA-BLOCKERS

These medications block beta receptors in the sympathetic nervous system, the part of our nervous system that is mainly designed for fight-or-flight reactions. In the cardiovascular system, beta receptors, when stimulated, increase the heart rate and the strength of the pumping action of the heart. Blocking those receptors slows down the heart rate and reduces the force of the heart's contractions, lowering the blood pressure. Beta-blockers can cause wheezing in asthmatic patients, and cold hands and feet by constricting the arteries in the limbs.

KEY TREATMENT NOTE

Insulin dependent patients with diabetes, both T1DM and T2DM, should ideally not use beta-blockers.

There are many different categories of beta-blocker medications, and they are usually prescribed to help control problematic cardiac arrhythmias and prevent the occurrence of a second heart attack. They are no longer recommended as a first choice medication for hypertension, and they do not protect the kidneys from diabetic damage.

The main concern with beta-blockers is that they block the action of epinephrine and norepinephrine on cell receptors that respond to those hormones. As a result, these drugs prolong, enhance, alter, and mask hypoglycemia reactions. These drugs can reduce the adrenal response symptoms of hypoglycemia, such as tremors and palpitations, so the hypoglycemic reaction can worsen until it causes a surprising and very dangerous unconsciousness. In fact, in twenty-six years of practice, only one T1DM patient of mine had a massive hypoglycemic reaction and needed a glucagon shot, and that was due to her mistakenly being diagnosed with hypertension and prescribed a beta-blocker by a cardiologist when she was in the hospital for a broken ankle. She had two significant hypoglycemic events while on the beta-blockers. I took her off the medication as soon as I saw her again, and she was fine without it, with normal blood pressure and no more hypoglycemic events. These are dangerous drugs for insulin dependent diabetic patients and should rarely be prescribed unless this class of drug is vital.

COMMON BETA-BLOCKER DRUG NAMES

Inderal/propranolol. 10, 20, 40, 60, 80 mg tablets—80–440 mg per day, usually divided into two doses per day

Lopressor/metoprolol. 50, 100 mg tablets—100–450 mg per day

Tenormin/atenolol. 25, 50, 100 mg tablets—50 or 100 mg once per day

COMMON DIURETIC COMBINATIONS WITH ACE-I OR ARB, OR BETA-BLOCKER

Benicar HCT (olmesartan nedocromil and hydrochlorothiazide). 20/12.5 mg; 40/12.5 mg; 40/25 mg—1 tablet once per day

Diovan HCT (valsartan and hydrochlorothiazide). 80/12.5 mg; 160/12.5 mg; 160/25 mg; 320/12.5 mg; 320/25 mg—1 tablet once per day

Hyzaar (losartan and hydrochlorothiazide). 50/12.5 mg; 100/12.5 mg; 100/25 mg—1 tablet usually once per day

Lopressor HCT (metoprolol and hydrochlorothiazide). 50/25 mg—2 tablets a day; 100/25 mg—1–2 tablets a day; 100/50 mg—1 tablet once per day

Lotensin HCT (benazepril and hydrochlorothiazide). 5/6.25mg; 10/12.5 mg; 20/12.5 mg; 20/25 mg—1 tablet once per day

Prinzide (lisinopril and hydrochlorothiazide). 10 or 20/12.5 mg—1 tablet once per day

CALCIUM CHANNEL BLOCKERS (CCBS)

These medications interfere with the movement of calcium through calcium channels in muscles. When calcium enters the heart muscles, it is responsible for contractions. CCBs reduce the contractions of the heart, and can slow down the heartbeat.

These medications are not used initially because they have many side effects affecting the heart, but also dizziness, headache, constipation, and edema.

COMMON CCBS

Dihydropyridine category.

Norvasc/amlodipine. 5–10 mg per day

Plendil/felodipine. 5–10 mg per day

Procardia/nifedipine. 30–60 mg per day

Phenylalkylamine category.

Calan/verapamil. 240–480 mg per day

Benzothiazepine category.

Cardizem/diltiazem. 120–360 mg per day

Medications are required for some patients at some times and integrative medical practitioners always have to ensure that the patient is being treated effectively and responsibly. Of course, patients interested in integrative care are often seeking alternatives to conventional medications or are trying to get off the ones they are on. This is a very valid desire and may be completely or partially achieved depending on the patient, their condition, their motivation, and their compliance with their diabetic regimen. I think a key point is to not demonize medications, but to use them judiciously, only when needed, when a medical condition is not being cleared expediently through only integrative care. We certainly will be talking about the entirety of a comprehensive protocol with alternatives to medications in following pages.

KEY TREATMENT NOTE

Most diabetic patients with hypertension are prescribed an ACE-I or ARB before a diuretic or calcium channel blocker.

Comprehensive Integrative Treatment of Hypertension

Of course, following all the diabetic basics, such as a low-carb diet, exercise, treating OSA if it exists, and stress management, is required to help reverse hypertension, especially if they successfully lead to weight loss and reduced glucose, A1C, and lipid panels. Some heavy metals are associated with causing hypertension, such as cadmium, and detoxification of those may indeed be helpful. And doing a vegetable juice fast has been successful for some of my patients in lowering their hypertension.

The seventh of The Eight Essentials is also important: supplementation. Botanicals such as rauwolfia, garlic, hawthorn berry, *Coleus forskhohili*, and *Gynostemma pentaphyllum* can often be found in hypertension specialty products or in an herbal liquid tincture. They may be used singly or mixed together.

Nutrients and nutraceuticals include magnesium and potassium; fish oils (at least 1,000 EPA/750 DHA per day); curcumin (200–3,000 mg per day); crystal-free CoQ10 (50–200 mg per day); L-arginine, an amino acid that can increase nitric oxide in the blood vessels, dilating them and lowering blood pressure (1,500 mg per day or more); and bonito peptides.

KEY TREATMENT NOTE

Integrative physicians have comprehensive protocols, lifestyle recommendations, and botanical and nutraceutical products that naturally can help lower blood pressure. I have also found that a vegetable juice fast for even ten days can significantly (and permanently) reduce blood pressure in many people.

Bonito peptides are fish peptides that have been shown to have effects similar to captopril, a blood pressure medication and ACE-I drug. They come in capsules and can also be eaten in dried fish if they are unsweetened. I ate bags of dried bonito fish during the year I spent living in Japan when I was in undergraduate school. In one study, bonito mixed with vinegar lowered blood pressure in those with mild to moderately high blood pressure but did not affect those with normal blood pressure. In another study, Japanese patients ingested dried bonito broth daily for one month. The patients had a significant lowering of their systolic blood pressure and reduced an oxidative stress marker, and it also helped their emotions. I have seen this product lower blood pressure up to 20 mmHg for both diastolic and systolic blood pressure. We know ACE-I are protective to the kidneys, so this product, which acts like an ACE-I, can be a simple way to lower blood pressure and protect the kidneys without using a prescription medication. It is available at Asian markets as a dried fish, but sweetened varieties should be avoided. It's best to treat it as a supplement, with a dosage of 1,500 mg per day.

Chronically elevated glucose levels in uncontrolled diabetes have been shown to increase the risk of fatal and nonfatal CVD, due to causing oxidative damage to the endothelial lining. Hyperglycemia can in and of itself damage the heart muscle. And, as confirmed by integrative cardiologist Dr. Stephen Sinatra, it is elevated glucose in the diet that causes cardiovascular disease, not fat or even cholesterol. A low-carb diet, which every person with diabetes should be on, is a great way to prevent and help reverse cardiovascular disease.

An integrative analysis of cardiovascular risk factors includes the following.

CLOTTING PROBLEMS

Elevated fibrinogen can increase the risk of developing a clot. Fibrinogen stimulates the creation of fibrin, which makes clots. T2DM patients have a high prevalence of high fibrinogen levels, and higher fibrinogen is associated with higher A1Cs, and higher BMI, total cholesterol, and LDL cholesterol. Fibrinogen is a marker for peripheral vascular disease in T1DM. Some nutrients that are helpful in reducing clotting risk and lowering fibrinogen and other indicators of increased clot risk include:

Fish oils. These can lower platelet activation, fibrinogen, and clotting factor V. Platelets are cells in our body that initiate a clotting sequence.

Nattokinase (and other enzymes, such as lumbrokinase and serraptadase). These have been shown to be very effective at lowering fibrinogen, and clotting factors VII and VIII. Nattokinase is a concentrated enzyme derived by fermenting soybeans (which should be from non-GMO soy). Blood clots account for 80 percent of strokes and can also cause deep vein thrombosis. Nattokinase has strong fibrinolytic activity; that means it breaks down and prevents clot formation. A good nattokinase product called Nattopine also contains 300 mg of pine bark extract, which has been shown to protect blood vessels from damaging free radicals. In one study, people taking Nattopine were shown to have 100 percent protection from developing deep vein thrombosis. Dosage is 3,650 FU (fibrinolytic units) per day.

Garlic. Garlic is a wonderful supplement as it can lower insulin resistance, lower hypertension, reduce lipid formation, reduce lipid oxidation, increase antioxidant status, and lower platelet aggregation and platelet thromboxane, which lowers the risk of clotting. Studies show eating more garlic reduces the risk of CVD. Eating garlic is the first place to start—it can be added to many meals, and it's also easy to simply eat cooked cloves. Peel cloves, wrap them in aluminum foil or put in a glass container and bake at 350° F for twenty minutes. The cloves become soft and sweet. Eat between one and six per day. There are also concentrated garlic capsules as supplements, too. The intensity of the allicin in the product, the most active component of garlic, will depend on the dosing.

Gingko biloba. This is a good antifibrinogen botanical.

APOE4 GENE

The APOE4 gene helps with the regulation of lipid metabolism. If there is a genetic mutation with this gene, it is an independent risk factor for a nearly sixfold increase in developing CVD in T2DM patients. APOE4 is also highly associated with Alzheimer's risk. Ideally, it seems that eating a lower fat diet and having an active lifestyle is most associated with preventing CVD in APOE4 patients. In fact, taking fish oils—generally considered protective for CVD and Alzheimer's—may work *against* these patients, since DHA is part of fish oils, and oxidized DHA is particularly harmful to APOE4 patients. If a person with the APOE4 gene eats a refined-sugar-free, lower fat diet that is drastically different from the standard American high-saturated-fat, pro-inflammatory diet, gets regular exercise, and takes a comprehensive supplementation protocol, including antioxidants such as curcumin, dosing some fish oils may be fine. I do suggest patients get tested to see if they have an APOE4 gene, and I work with a medical practitioner who is aware of working with that variant.

POOR DENTAL HYGIENE

Mild periodontal disease is common in the United States, affecting up to 75 percent of adults; 20–30 percent of those adults have moderate or severe periodontal disease. It is a chronic inflammatory condition and is the most common cause of tooth and bone loss. Diabetes is a risk factor for periodontal disease and periodontal disease is a risk factor for diabetes and increases the risk for diabetic complications to develop. Periodontal disease can lead to the formation of AGEs, causing damage to cells around the body, including the blood vessels. Bacteria in the mouth can translocate to the blood vessels, cause inflammation, and increase the risk of cardiovascular disease. The cleaner the mouth, the less the risk of bacteria getting to the blood vessels.

Brushing one's teeth twice a day with an electric toothbrush for two minutes, flossing or using a Waterpik once or twice a day, using mouthwash, and regular dental examinations are encouraged. Also, oil pulling is a good way to reduce bacteria in the mouth and prevent systemic inflammation. Oil pulling involves putting one to two tablespoons of an oil in your mouth and then swishing it around for twenty minutes, pushing it through the teeth and around the gums. The oil picks up bacteria in your oral cavity; you'll note that the oil becomes cloudy at the end of twenty minutes. Spit the oil out; do not swallow it.

Supplements for healthy gums include:

- 5-MTHF type folic acid.
- CoQ10. I recommend crystal-free CoQ10, which is much better absorbed than the crystalline form. 50–200 mg per day.
- Neem mouthwash.
- Probiotics. *Streptococcus salivarus* supports healthy oral microorganisms, reduces bad breath, and reduces the risk for ear infections, tonsillitis, and pharyngitis.
- Xylitol. One of the approved sweeteners for a patient with diabetes, xylitol also inhibits the growth of bacteria that release pro-inflammatory lipopolysaccharide toxin metabolites and thus reduces inflammatory markers.

POOR STRESS MANAGEMENT

When a person is feeing very stressed, cortisol levels increase, causing loss of potassium through the urine. Potassium is very useful for the cardiovascular system. Chronic stress may be an etiological factor for, and aggravate control of, diabetes, and it also predicts the occurrence of coronary heart disease.

SLEEP APNEA

As discussed in chapter 9, OSA is common in overweight and obese T2DM patients, found in nearly 40 percent of men with T2DM in one study. Untreated OSA can increase the risk for coronary artery disease, cardiac ischemia, cardiomyopathy, heartbeat irregularities (going too fast or too slow), and ventricular tachycardia. OSA treatment with a CPAP machine reduces systolic blood pressure, reduces the risk for clotting, and improves left ventricular systolic function.

INFLAMMATION

Diabetes is considered an inflammatory cardiovascular disease. Having an elevated A1C is associated with a higher HS-CRP inflammatory marker, and a higher risk of CVD. Another inflammatory marker, TNF-a, is associated both with the insulin resistance of T2DM and as a risk factor for CVD, as is IL-6 and other markers, elevated with high glucose in T2DM and a cause for atherosclerosis of blood vessels. Inflammation and the production of those markers can come from the oral cavity, belly fat, a poor diet, nutrient and antioxidant deficiencies, smoking, excessive drinking, damage to the gut, and environmental toxins.

The integrative protocol to reduce the risk of CVD or protect someone who has it includes investigating for and initiating treatment protocols for all of the above risk factors. If diabetes is excellently controlled, and there is no more metabolic syndrome or smoking, the risk for CVD is substantially lowered. Doing a specialty cardiovascular panel is helpful; your physician should do one through True Diagnostics, Cleveland Clinic, Boston Labs, Singulex, or another similar lab. At those labs, many of the most up to date and innovative tests can pinpoint risk for CVD and direct treatment. Also, both elevated random microalbuminuria and uric acid are associated with an increased risk for CVD.

Conventional treatment of CVD starts with statin drugs (please review my comments about them in chapter 5). The goals for integrative treatment are to reduce glucose levels, reduce inflammation, help heal from high blood pressure or at least excellently control it, increase cardiovascular fitness, remove unhealthy lifestyle habits, promote good sleep and stress management, and increase nutrition—all of these factors can help reduce CVD. Optimal treatment also addresses the second through sixth of The Eight Essentials. Recommendations include:

Stop smoking. This should be obvious!

Drink alcohol in moderation. For women, alcohol should be limited to seven or fewer drinks a week; for men, fewer than fourteen drinks a week. Anything above those limits should cause concern for alcoholism. Even still, alcohol contains calories that have to be burned off, and it is contraindicated in the case of fatty liver. For diabetic patients, it can lower glucose levels and that needs to be watched when on insulin to prevent a low. One alcoholic drink one to three times a week maximum seems best for diabetic patients and do not drink if you have fatty liver.

Eat a low-carb diet. Another obvious point! Other aspects to eating an anti-inflammatory diabetic diet include: avoid overeating; fast intermittently; watch animal protein intake and make sure all meat products are of the highest quality; increase fiber intake; eat lots of vegetables; use healthy and anti-inflammatory spices such as garlic, turmeric, thyme, oregano, ginger, and onions; drink green tea; and eat a lot of omega-3-rich foods: leafy greens, walnuts and walnut oil, healthy oily fish, omega-3 organic eggs, flax and chia seeds, grass-fed and grass-finished meat and organic poultry.

Exercise regularly. Even exercising for thirty minutes three times a week is better than nothing. The fitter one is, the less risk one has for cardiovascular disease, although overexercising can be a problem, too. Overexercising means doing an abundance of aerobic exercise in particular, such as running ten miles a day many days a week. Exercise as discussed in chapter 9.

Practice regular stress management and unplug. Spend less time on phones, computers, and tablets. Keep the adrenal hormones down, relax, chill out, be mellow. Whatever your generational term for keeping your stress level low, your cardiovascular system will reap huge benefits.

Encourage weight loss. Abdominal fat promotes increased glucose levels, lipid levels, insulin resistance, and inflammatory markers. All these are ripe to cause cardiovascular disease!

Do a detoxification protocol, both for hypertension and also for removing environmental chemicals released from fat cells during weight loss.

Practice excellent dental care.

Supplement to prevent or help reverse CVD:

- Multiple vitamin and mineral.
- Curcumin. Since inflammation drives the development of cardiovascular disease, dosing this safe and effective anti-inflammatory botanical is common. 200–3,000 mg per day.
- CoQ10. This supplement should be crystal-free; ensure your product is listed that way. Basic CoQ10 is a very large crystal molecule, and that significantly reduces its ability to be absorbed by the intestines. In a typical CoQ10 product, out of 100 mg, perhaps the gut can absorb 1–2 percent. When CoQ10 is crystal-free, absorption of the molecule can increase up to 8–15 percent. So, 50 mg of crystal-free CoQ10 may

have 4 mg absorption (8 percent absorption) equaling 200 mg of a crystalline CoQ10 (1 percent absorption). 50–200 mg per day.

- Taurine. Taurine is an inexpensive amino acid and the most plentiful amino acid in the heart muscle. Taurine is also helpful at reducing insulin resistance and lowering glucose levels in the body. Taurine is regularly prescribed by integrative physicians for patients who have heart ailments, particularly after heart attacks, with congestive heart failure or cardiomyopathy. 500–3,000 mg per day.
- Hawthorn. Hawthorn is a main botanical that is an all-around lovely toner for the heart. It is a gentle addition to any diabetic or CVD protocol. It comes in capsules, tinctures, or extracts. 200–600 mg per day.
- Ribose. This supplement is a sugar that specifically helps feed the heart muscle. It is indicated in patients who have had some heart damage, or even for athletes who wish to enhance heart functioning. It is safe and does not elevate glucose levels. 5 grams per day.
- Acetyl-l-carnitine. This nutrient is used for diabetic neuropathy, as a way to help prevent Alzheimer's disease, and to help the heart burn energy more easily. Acetyl-l-carnitine helps bring fats into cardiac cells for burning. It is dosed when the heart is not healthy, after a heart attack, or with congestive heart failure or cardiomyopathy. 1,500–3,000 mg per day.

What about using niacin to lower lipid levels? Niacin is vitamin B_3 and has been shown to lower total cholesterol and LDL cholesterol, raise HDL cholesterol, and lower lipids. That is more than a statin drug can do. Niacin is therefore often used by integrative medical practitioners with patients with elevated lipid panels, and low HDL cholesterol levels. The problem with niacin is that while it does affect lipids along those lines, niacin can also significantly increase glucose levels and promote the development of diabetes. In one study the use of niacin caused a 34 percent increased risk of developing diabetes versus the placebo. In patients who are already diabetic, one study showed that poorly controlled diabetic patients given immediate release niacin saw a 21 percent increase in their A1Cs and 16 percent increase in mean plasma glucose.

However, in a study called the Coronary Drug Project, 8,300 men who had previously had a heart attack were given either niacin or a placebo. In the niacin group, both fasting and one-hour plasma glucose levels increased, yet only niacin and not the placebo reduced the risk of CVD and mortality. So, each individual medical practitioner will have to analyze if niacin is or is not a supplement that is appropriate and safe enough to dose to patients for lowering lipids.

Cardiovascular disease is the typical reason uncontrolled diabetic patients die. Attaining excellent diabetic control, and following the lifestyle changes shown to significantly reduce the development of CVD means that a well-controlled diabetic patient can live a long, full life without ever having a blood clot, heart attack, or stroke.

Diabetic Eye Diseases

Diabetic eye diseases are unfortunately too common. Nearly 29 percent of diabetics over forty years old have diabetic retinopathy. Another 13 percent have diabetic macular edema, another type of serious eye damage. Someone who is diabetic for more than ten years has an elevenfold increased risk of developing macular edema, and every 1 percent increase in A1C corresponds with a 50 percent increased risk of diabetic macular edema.

Diabetic eye disease is higher in Mexican and African American populations, males in general, those who have had diabetes for longer, insulin dependent diabetics, patients with higher systolic blood pressure, and those with a higher A1C.

We will discuss the four main potential eye problems: diabetic retinopathy, diabetic macular edema, cataracts, and glaucoma.

Diabetic Retinopathy

Diabetic retinopathy occurs when the retina grows abnormal new blood vessels that are fragile, and they swell and leak. This is due to hyperglycemia, hypertension, and even hypercholesterolemia. There are several stages of diabetic retinopathy:

1. Mild nonproliferative retinopathy: This is the beginning of the pathological changes where microaneurysms, or out-pouchings of blood, occur in blood vessels.

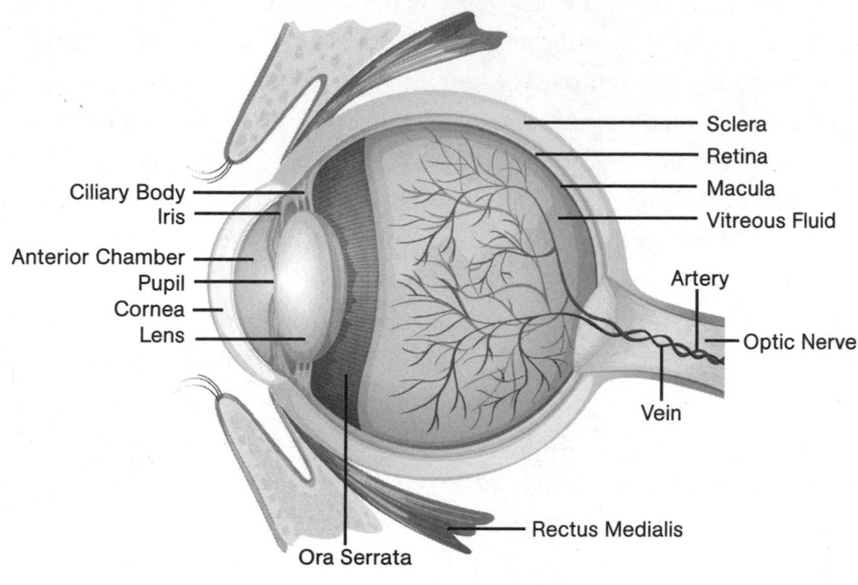

Figure 14.2. The anatomy of the eye. The parts affected by diabetes include the lens, the retina, the macula, the vitreous fluid, and all the blood vessels.

2. Moderate nonproliferative retinopathy: Retinal blood vessels are blocked from good blood flow.
3. Severe nonproliferative retinopathy: More areas of the retina start being deprived of blood, which signals new blood vessel growth as a result. This is promoted through a chemical called vascular endothelial growth factor (VEGF). VEGF is a natural protein that promotes angiogenesis in the body—new blood vessel formation. New blood vessel growth is vital when we need to heal a wound and require tissue repair. While VEGF is a normal protein, having it be used to make abnormal, unhealthy extra blood vessels in our eyes is a serious problem.
4. Proliferative retinopathy: This is the worst scenario. Many blood vessels are blocked, so larger areas of the retina are not getting oxygen. The new blood vessels growing are fragile and abnormal, since they should not be there to begin with. The vessels grow along the retina and into the surface of the vitreous fluid, which is the thick

> fluid in our eyes. The new vessels can leak, which causes vision loss, as light cannot pass through the bloodied vitreous gel and it cannot then strike our retinas. This can also lead to swelling of the macula, the place on the retina where our central vision is located. Blindness can occur, and the retina also has a higher risk of detachment. Lastly, proliferative retinopathy can lead to glaucoma, a higher pressure in the eye, which might damage the optic nerve.

A patient might not have any symptoms as diabetic retinopathy is occurring, because it is painless, but they might have floaters, blurred or lost vision, distortion of vision, or problems seeing at night. The eye is also at a higher risk for having a retinal detachment. This is why it is so important for a diabetic patient to have a yearly dilated eye exam, as there are many early signs of retinopathy that an ophthalmologist can detect, such as leaking blood vessels; retinal swelling; pale, fatty deposits on the retina; damaged nerve tissues; or other indications of abnormal blood vessel growth.

Aside from a dilated eye exam, an opthalmologist could also make use of the letter eye chart for analysis of vision acuity. It is typical for a yearly exam also to do tonometry, which measures the pressure in the eye, helping diagnose glaucoma. An ophthalmologist may take a picture of the retina, or even do a fluorescein angiogram, where dye is injected into the eye and pictures are taken as the dye passes through the retinal vessels.

DIABETIC RETINOPATHY TREATMENT

There is no conventional treatment for nonproliferative retinopathy, except trying to keep the glucose, cholesterol, and blood pressure under control.

Once proliferative retinopathy has developed, laser surgery is the main treatment. It is called pan retinal laser photocoagulation, also known as scattering laser treatment. The laser shrinks blood vessels, and usually two to three treatments are needed as the patient receives 1,000–2,000 laser burns in the retina. This works best before a bleed occurs. It carries with it some concerns: it can reduce peripheral vision, as well as color and night vision. Laser treatments are performed in the physician's office, with the eye being dilated and perhaps numbed; they do not hurt much but might cause a stinging sensation.

Another treatment is a vitrectomy, which is when the vitreous gel, full of blood from a serious blood vessel bleed, is removed from the center of the eye and is replaced with a salt solution under local or general anesthesia. While it sounds a bit creepy, this procedure can help return vision to an eye that was blinded by a significant bleed. Otherwise, it can take a long time for the blood to clear out and allow vision in that eye.

Macular Edema

Macular edema is when the macular part of the eye, our most valuable area for sight, swells due to leakage of the blood vessels. It is treated with focal laser treatment, where several hundred small laser burns are dosed around the retinal leakage, but not directly on the macula. This treatment is usually performed in one session.

There are also drugs that can be injected directly into the eye to help with diabetic macular damage (the same drugs are injected in nondiabetic macular eye disease), including Lucentis/ranibizumab, Avastin/bevacizumab, and Eylea/aflibercept, which are called VEGF inhibitors. They inhibit the VEGF protein that is signaling the overgrowth of blood vessels in the eye. The drugs are injected monthly or every two months (depending on the drug and how well the patient is doing). These drugs can be used with or without laser surgery. There are many possible side effects of these drugs, such as infection or retinal detachment, but overall, many patients handle them well.

Diabetic Cataracts

Diabetic cataracts occur due to lack of antioxidants protecting the lenses of the eyes. As discussed earlier, the sorbitol pathway, if overtaxed, causes the eye to become low in antioxidants and allows damage to occur in the eye, including in the lens.

Controlling glucose levels and adding antioxidants to the body can help prevent diabetic cataracts. I've never had a patient develop them. If a cataract does develop, and if it becomes severe, the patient can have surgery to remove the damaged lens and have a new lens inserted. This is a common surgery today in both diabetic and nondiabetic patients, and is usually, but not always, trouble-free.

Reentry Phenomenon

The eyes are very sensitive to changes in serum glucose. When glucose is high, vision can become blurry, as it also can when glucose levels decrease dramatically. It is good to know that beforehand, especially with lowering glucose, because comprehensive integrative care can cause rapid drops of glucose in the body, and the eyes can easily have problems as a result.

Especially in older patients, watch for vision changes when starting an integrative protocol, as vision changes can be so strong, reading may be difficult or impossible. This is not a positive experience, though it has only happened once to a senior patient of mine. But the rare risk of it occurring is something to note when setting up the treatment so a patient can be alerted to the possibility and call their physician if it starts happening. In that case, a gentler lowering of glucose is recommended by, for example, eliminating carbs from one's diet slowly, over several weeks, instead of all at once. If vision changes substantially and does not reverse with leveling of the glucose, the patient needs to visit their eye doctor. Sometimes eyeglass prescriptions have to be changed.

Another possible problem with the eyes is called reentry phenomenon. If a patient has proliferative diabetic retinopathy, and they embark upon an integrative protocol, glucose levels can decrease dramatically even in the first week. A patient might walk in with glucose levels in the 300s and within days have glucose levels in the low 100s. While that is an amazingly positive event, as a result, there may be something ominous working in their eyes.

When someone is insulin resistant, he tends to make more insulin and less insulin-like growth factor-1 (IGF-1). Insulin mainly has the body absorb glucose into fat and liver cells, where it is stored; IGF-1 is used to have glucose enter into muscle cells, where it is burned. However, a secondary action of IGF-1 is to promote angiogenesis, like the VEGF I've been discussing.

So, when a patient with retinopathy receives a comprehensive integrative protocol and lowers glucose levels and insulin resistance, their need for insulin significantly decreases. As insulin levels lower, the body naturally makes more IGF-1, to help glucose metabolize in muscle cells. If this happens and the patient's eyes are healthy, it does not cause any problems. If retinopathy exists, however, the increase in IGF-1 can stimulate increased fragile blood vessel growth in the eyes, significantly increasing the risk to have a bleed or worsening of the retinopathy. That is reentry phenomenon: eye bleeding as a result of sudden glucose lowering.

KEY TREATMENT NOTE

Each diabetic patient should have a dilated eye exam, or have had one at least within in the last year, before any integrative physician begins treating them, to uncover if they have any retinopathy. It is neither safe nor responsible to treat a new patient without that vital data.

I once saw a forty-eight-year-old man with high glucose levels. After only four years of being a T2DM patient he had diabetic retinopathy and had already suffered a heart attack. Some patients walk around with an A1C of 8.5 percent for thirty years and don't develop any complications; their bodies are resistant to damage from the high glucose numbers. Other patients, like this gentleman, have frail, weak bodies, and in a short amount of time, are suffering greatly from their hyperglycemia. This man followed my protocol, and his glucose came down as expected, but within a couple of weeks, he suffered a large bleed in one of his eyes, blinding him for six weeks until laser surgery and time cleared it up.

Naturally, I was devastated, and I turned to research, including reading Dr. Paul Chous's book *Diabetic Eye Disease*. Dr. Chous is an ophthalmologist who has T1DM. I highly recommend his book, which is where I learned about reentry phenomenon. I exchanged helpful emails with him on this condition.

I figured out that there are two main ways to initiate a comprehensive integrative regimen with patients who already have diabetic retinopathy. One is to reduce their glucose slowly, over a month or so, to prevent a sudden drop. The second is to dose them with supplements that will protect their eyes from the damage the temporary increase in IGF-1 can produce.

I have always chosen to do the latter, so I created a supplement regimen to use with patients with diabetic retinopathy, and it has allowed these patients to lower their glucose without suffering any bleeds. I also have patients do follow-up visits to their ophthalmologists two to three months after beginning the protocol to check in and ensure no damage is occurring from lowered glucose levels. I can proudly say no other patient has ever suffered this reentry phenomenon again under my care. I'll discuss the specific supplement regimen for patients with diabetic retinopathy below.

Comprehensive Integrative Treatments for Diabetic Eye Disease

First, of course, eat a low-carb diet, and allow your integrative physician to guide you through the second through eighth of The Eight Essentials.

To protect the eyes in general, but especially if diabetic retinopathy exists and the goal is to prevent reentry phenomenon, I have established a set of supplements that have worked for my patients. Most of these supplements have been proven in studies to prevent and treat diabetic retinopathy.

If there is no retinopathy, the entire protocol does not need to be taken, but if my patient has diabetic retinopathy, to prevent reentry phenomenon, this is the protocol I ensure they are on for two months. There is no guarantee this will prevent reentry phenomenon, so ensure you have the guidance and approval of your medical practitioner before using it:

Benfotiamine. Many studies support the benefit of using benfotiamine to protect the eyes. This is a key addition to any program to protect the eyes. 450 mg per day.

R-alpha-lipoic acid. 300–1,200 mg per day.

Alpha-lipoic acid plus genistein and vitamins. These supplements improved diabetic retinopathy after one month. 400 mg a day of alpha-lipoic acid.

Bilberry. There are some studies showing bilberry is protective to the eyes. 320–600 mg per day.

Taurine. Taurine is high in the retina, aids in retinal functioning, and has some antioxidative stress protection. 1,000–2,000 mg per day.

N-acetyl cysteine. This supplement may help to reduce VEGF, and reverses diabetic changes and decreases inflammatory markers and oxidative stress. 600–2,400 mg per day.

Selenium. This nutrient is key to forming glutathione, one of the best antioxidants made naturally in the human body. 200–600 mcg per day.

What about preventing the development of diabetic eye disease outside of reentry phenomenon? Integrative medicine may help. In one impressive animal study, diabetes was induced in rats. The researchers mixed many nutrients, and even in animals who had hyperglycemia occurring, retinopathy improved. They had decreased degenerative capillaries, significantly lowered reactive oxygen species, and increased antioxidant capacity. The protocol prevented DNA damage, mitochondrial damage, and retinal inflammatory cytokine development. Animal studies cannot always translate to similar human clinical results, but sometimes they can. Each kilogram of the nutrient product contained the below; the rats were given 50 grams a day:

Vitamin C: 300 mg
Vitamin E: 300 IU
Fish oils: 650 mg EPA/500 mg DHA
Vitamin D_3: 10,000 IU
Benfotiamine: 1 g (a very high dose!)
Alpha-lipoic acid: 750 mg
Tocomin: 200 mg
Zeaxanthin: 40 mg
Lutein: 20 mg
Mix of resveratrol, green tea, turmeric root, N-acetyl cysteine, pycnogenol, grapefruit extract, CoQ10, and zinc (2.65 mg): 300 mg

The study went for eleven months and at the end the rats on the nutrient mix had significantly less damage to the retinal vasculature and no retinopathy. They also had significantly less oxidative stress and mitochondrial damage in the retinas; the nutrient mix protected the eyes from inflammatory and DNA changes, and prevented an increase in VEGF, although it did not lower their levels of hyperglycemia.

Another nice mix of nutrients was found to be beneficial in another study, which examined the value of antioxidants in preventing oxidative damage in the diabetic retina: vitamin E, ascorbic acid, beta-carotene, zinc, copper, and lutein.

Using a comprehensive supplemental regimen, as well as a multiple vitamin/mineral, fish oils, and my Diamend product at full dose (seven capsules a day), my patients are well protected against reentry phenomenon, and also have a significantly lower risk of developing diabetic eye disease, if their glucose levels are well controlled. Putting patients on a comprehensive

KEY TREATMENT NOTE

Please do not self-treat yourself with these supplements on your own. Please always work with your physician and ophthalmologist.

supplemental regimen has assured I have not had any reentry phenomenon, or retinal bleeding, with any other patient with retinopathy who also experienced fairly rapid lowering of their glucose levels. I have also had patients report back to me, after a follow-up retinopathy analysis, that they were told their eyes looked healthier, stronger, and more stable.

In summary, diabetic eye disease can be prevented through excellent control of diabetes, and it can be treated if it does already exist. The Eight Essentials are key to follow to attain low A1Cs and superb glucose control. The seventh of The Eight Essentials, supplementation, is a key part of protecting the eyes from developing any diabetic damage, helping to reverse damage, and preventing reentry phenomenon.

Diabetic Nephropathy

Diabetic nephropathy is kidney disease due to elevated glucose over time causing oxidative damage to kidney cells. One's chance of death increases significantly the more kidney disease worsens.

About 20–30 percent of diabetic patients develop nephropathy, and 44 percent of patients in the United States with end-stage renal disease—the advanced disease, where patients have to be on dialysis—have diabetes. Diabetes is the number one reason people require dialysis. Hypertension is the second main cause and, of course, most T2DM patients have hypertension as well. T1DM progresses to end-stage renal disease more than T2DM, but because there are so many more T2DM patients, 50 percent of end-stage renal disease patients have T2DM. Unfortunately, as with most diabetic complications, Native Americans, Latinos, and African Americans have a higher risk of diabetic nephropathy.

The pathophysiology of diabetic kidney disease entails several processes: expansion of the mesangium, tissue in the kidneys with small blood vessels in it; thickening of the kidney cells' basement membrane; increased pressure in the kidney cells; scarring of the kidney cells; and hypertension and fluid retention.

The best, earliest test used to uncover kidney disease is called the random microalbuminuria test. This should be done at least once per year with diabetic patients, although newly diagnosed children with T1DM can wait five years before starting. An adult newly diagnosed with T1DM can wait five years too, but I like to do it yearly with them anyway. With T2DM patients, a physician should check for microalbuminuria right away upon diagnosis.

Albumin is a protein that is generally reabsorbed by the kidney cells and returned to our circulation. When we start seeing it in the urine, it indicates early kidney problems. This is a urine test, nonfasting, where you urinate in a cup either at your doctor's office or at the lab your physician uses. *Micro*albuminuria means that only a little bit of protein is found in the urine.

Microalbuminuria tests come with the albumin/creatinine ratio, where the albumin in the urine is compared to the concentration of creatinine (see chapter 4), and if that is within normal range, the test is more accurate. The test can be performed at any time of day, but it is commonly done in the morning when patients go to the lab fasting to have their blood work done.

If the microalbuminuria is elevated and continues to increase, it indicates the patient is likely developing nephropathy. What's also interesting is that a positive microalbuminuria test indicates the patient is at a higher risk for cardiovascular disease as well, because the hyperglycemia that is damaging the kidney cells is also likely damaging the endothelial lining of the blood vessels. Normal/negative test results show lower than 30 mg/g creatinine. Incipient nephropathy (early kidney disease) is diagnosed if the results show 30–300 mg/g creatinine. Lastly, overt nephropathy (worse kidney disease) is diagnosed with results showing higher than 300 mg/g creatinine.

A test can be repeated for verification two to three times within three to six months if it does not seem to be accurate given the patient's attention to their diabetic protocol, their general glucose levels, and their A1C. Elevated random microalbuminuria is associated with other causes of kidney disease, such as short-term hyperglycemia due to, for example, an acute illness or fever, exercise, urinary tract infection, significant hypertension, or congestive heart failure. So, for example, do not do a random microalbuminuria test the day after your diabetic patient runs a marathon! Smoking and environmental pollutants can also raise it.

It's not a very good scenario once a typical T1DM patient develops incipient nephropathy. Without care, 80 percent of T1DM patients can progress in ten to fifteen years to overt nephropathy; 50 percent of those people will develop end-stage renal disease within another ten years, and 75 percent within twenty-five years. Yes, we are talking decades—the kidneys are strong and hearty, but they can eventually fail.

In T2DM patients, microalbuminuria is found in a higher percentage upon diagnosis, mainly because these patients were prediabetic for up to ten to twelve years and damage was occurring to their kidneys during those prediabetic years. About 20–40 percent of T2DM patients will develop overt nephropathy and about 20 percent of those patients will wind up with end-stage renal disease. Around twenty million Americans have chronic kidney disease, and nearly half the cases are due to diabetes, so those are pretty big numbers we need to prevent.

I've had patients with test results all over the place, from normal to one patient who had a random microalbuminuria result of 3 million mg/g creatinine. What is good to know about this test is that it should never be used as a precursor to fear-based medicine, but it should be used to promote motivation and healing. Kidneys can and do heal, and learning early on that one's kidneys are starting to suffer damage can be a wonderful tool to help the patient embrace their comprehensive protocol, experience the vitality of their healing force, and witness their kidneys' return to health. Within three months, elevated microalbuminuria scores can oftentimes be greatly reduced or returned to normal.

Signs and Symptoms of Kidney Disease

There are usually no signs or symptoms accompanying a positive microalbuminuria test, but if the kidney disease continues to progress, a person might develop edema, leg cramps, frequent nighttime nausea or vomiting, paleness, anemia, itching, and reduced need for some oral hypoglycemic agents. For drugs that are excreted by the kidneys, if the kidneys are significantly damaged, they cannot excrete the drugs, so the drugs have a longer, stronger action in the body and their dosage would need to be reduced. Insulin is one of those drugs that might need to be reduced when a patient has significant kidney disease.

Chronic Kidney Disease

When kidney failure progresses, it is called chronic kidney disease (CKD). We base our stages of CKD on the estimated glomerular filtration rate (eGFR) of the kidneys. Glomeruli are tiny filters in the kidneys that filter waste from the blood. The eGFR measures how much blood passes through the kidneys each minute.

There is a natural decline in the eGFR reading in senior patients, and so it may not indicate any actual problematic kidney damage. Seniors can be misdiagnosed with CKD based on an eGFR lab result when they do not actually have that condition and the eGFR is low due to normal aging processes. In patients over sixty-five or seventy years old, eGFR rates lower than 60 mL/min/1.73 m^2 can be considered normal. This lab value should not be the entirety of analysis in diagnosing a diabetic senior with CKD.

Microalbuminuria can be an omen of kidney failure. Statin drugs that can raise glucose levels in diabetic patients have also been associated with raising microalbuminuria levels. In one analysis, patients not on statins had a microalbuminuria of 6.9, but for patients on statins, they had a microalbuminuria of 15, more than double the nonstatin group. Atorvastatin seemed to cause

Table 14.1. Stages of Chronic Kidney Disease

Stage	Description	Glomerular Filtration Rate (GFR) mL/min/1.73 m^2
1	Kidney damaged with normal GFR	> 90
2	Kidney damaged with slight decrease in GFR	60–89
3	Moderate decrease in GFR	30–59
4	Severe decrease in GFR	15–29
5	Kidney failure	< 15

Note: In stages 4 and 5, the patient requires kidney dialysis.
Source: http://www.kidney.org.

more microalbuminuria than simvastatin. What we do not know, however, is if this is a real problem for the kidneys, and studies so far have not wholly shown it is a concern in the long term. Still, it seems worrying and needs to be watched.

Some diabetic patients might have glomerular hyper filtration, which is also a very early sign of diabetic kidney disease. A 25 to 50 percent elevation in the eGFR is seen early in the course of up to 50 percent of patients with both T1DM and T2DM in comparison with the average of a control nondiabetic population. I mention this because you'll see that a simple diet change can correct problematic early elevated eGFR in T1DM (and, I also believe, T2DM) patients.

When should a primary care physician refer a patient to a nephrologist? A referral should occur if a patient's hypertension cannot be controlled, if there are high levels of serum potassium, or if their eGFR decreases to lower than 60 mL/min.

Conventional Treatment of Diabetic Kidney Disease—Diet

Historically, the conventional dietary approach for patients either developing kidney disease or with serious cases of kidney disease, has been to limit their protein intake. However, a Cochrane Database analysis of many studies done on diabetic patients with nephropathy did not show that protein restriction was beneficial in slowing the decline of kidney failure. In general, a dietary protein intake of 0.8 g/kg of body weight is an acceptable intake for a patient with any kidney disease. When patients require dialysis, it is potassium and phosphorous intake, rather, that *have* to be tightly monitored. However, if a patient with early kidney disease begins a comprehensive integrative protocol, there is a real chance to reverse the condition, preventing further kidney damage and the need for dialysis.

Conventional Treatment of Diabetic Kidney Disease—Medications

As noted, some of the medications given to diabetic patients need to be reduced as the eGFR decreases. I listed the medications that need to be stopped in chapter 5. A knowledgeable physician or nephrologist can guide patients through reducing or stopping them.

Protecting the Kidneys from Diabetic Kidney Disease (and Treating Hypertension)

The renin-angiotensin system (RAS), which is responsible for the secretion of aldosterone, is a key part of standard care to protect the kidneys from diabetic damage. Aldosterone is a hormone produced by the adrenals that prompts the body to save sodium and excrete potassium, the result being an increase in blood pressure. When the blood volume is low, the complicated RAS, with many components, kicks in. First, angiotensinogen is produced by the liver. Then, a chemical produced by the kidneys turns angiotensinogen into angiotensin 1. In turn, angiotensin 1 is turned into angiotensin 2 by an angiotensin-converting enzyme secreted by the lungs. Angiotensin 2 constricts blood vessels, increases blood pressure, and stimulates secretion of aldosterone from the adrenals.

In standard care, medications that interfere with this RAS, if it is abnormally active, can lower the blood pressure. Medical research has shown that interfering with the RAS can slow increases in creatinine, reduce microalbuminuria, and might also help slow the development of kidney failure. The two drugs used to affect the RAS consist of an angiotensin-converting enzyme inhibitor (ACE-I) or an angiotensin receptor blocker (ARB). If you are on one of those medications, it is not that concerning. I would rather remove a patient from a sulfonylurea or a TZD, or even a statin (if not indicated as discussed already), than be nervous or upset if they are on an ACE-I or an ARB.

ANGIOTENSIN-CONVERTING ENZYME INHIBITORS (ACE-IS)

These medicines work by interfering with the ACE enzyme so it cannot convert angiotensinogen to angiotensin 1. ACE-Is are valuable as antihypertensives and have been shown to decrease proteinuria, the spilling of protein into the urine. These are especially helpful in T1DM patients (ARBs are an alternative).

A big contraindication of ACE-I medications is not dangerous but is annoying; they can cause a dry, chronic cough. When someone develops that chronic ACE-I cough, switching to an ARB is helpful, as people usually do not cough as much with that type of medication.

ACE-Is should not be used during pregnancy. They can elevate potassium levels in patients with advanced renal failure, which is very dangerous, and they may worsen kidney function in advanced kidney disease.

An ACE-I is the hypertension medication to use first in a patient with congestive heart failure, followed by a beta-blocker. In patients with coronary artery disease, a beta-blocker is the first line and then an ACE-I.

COMMON ACE-1 MEDICATIONS AND DOSAGES FOR T1DM PATIENTS

Prinivil or Zestril/lisinopril. 2.5, 5, 10, 20, 40 mg (maximum 80 mg per day)
Lotensin/benazepril. 10–40 mg per day
Capoten/captropril. 12.5, 25, 50, 100 mg (maximum 450 mg per day)
Vasotec/enalapril. 2.5, 5, 10, 20 mg (maximum 40 mg per day)
Altace/ramipril. 1.25, 2.5, 5, 10 mg (maximum 20 mg per day)

ANGIOTENSIN RECEPTOR BLOCKERS (ARBS)

These medications work by blocking the receptors where angiotensin 2 adheres, so that angiotensin 2 cannot work and cannot lead to an elevation in blood pressure. These medicines have also been recognized as being helpful in decreasing the occurrence and progression of kidney disease. They are especially helpful in T2DM patients (an ACE-I would be an alternative).

COMMON ARBS AND DOSAGES FOR T2DM PATIENTS

Cozaar/losartan. 25, 50, 100 mg (maximum 100 mg per day)
Benicar/omesartan. 5, 20 40 mg (maximum 40 mg per day)
Diovan/valsartan. 40, 80, 160, 320 mg (maximum 320 mg per day)

A key, important note about these medications is that they should *never* be mixed together. Mixing them together can cause significant kidney damage.

The 2016 ADA medication guidelines for kidney disease treatment state that ACE-Is and ARBs are recommended for treating nonpregnant individuals with diabetes and modestly elevated microalbuminuria (30–299 mg/g) and are strongly recommended for patients with a microalbuminuria higher than 300 mg/g or who have an eGFR of lower than 60 mL/min/1.73m^2. ACE-I and ARB treatment is not recommended for primary prevention of diabetic kidney disease in individuals with diabetes who have normal blood pressure, microalbuminuria, and eGFR.

The National Kidney Foundation Kidney Disease Outcomes Quality Initiative guidelines include using these medications in patients with diabetes.

KEY TREATMENT NOTE

If you are on an ACE-1 inhibitor, don't worry; it is not a bad drug. If you have high blood pressure, you cannot stop the medication until your blood pressure is normalized and your physician agrees to its cessation. If you do not have hypertension, the drug was given to you no doubt at a low dose for kidney protection. It can be stopped if you are working with an integrative physician who has a valid protocol, including protective supplements, to recommend instead.

These guidelines are similar to the ADA's. They do not recommend using an ACE-I or ARB for the primary prevention of diabetic kidney disease in patients who have normal blood pressure and normal microalbuminuria with diabetes. They suggest an ACE-I or ARB in normotensive patients with diabetes and microalbuminuria levels equal to or higher than 30 mg/g who are at high risk of diabetic kidney disease or its progression. Hypertensive patients with diabetes and CKD (stages 1–4) should be treated with an ACE-I or ARB.

In African Americans, ACE-Is and ARBs are not as effective for lowering blood pressure. Thiazide diuretics and calcium channel blockers seem to work best. Unfortunately, those medications do not protect the kidneys from diabetic damage, except by lowering the blood pressure.

According to the *JAMA* 2014 evidence-based guidelines for the treatment of high blood pressure in adults, including those with diabetes, all adult patients with CKD should receive an ACE-I or ARB. However, African Americans should have their hypertension treated with CCBs or thiazide diuretics, unless they have chronic kidney disease with proteinuria, and then an ACE-I or ARB should be included. In patients over seventy-five years old with CKD, using CCBs, thiazides, ACE-Is, or ARBs is considered.

The ONTARGET study made clear that ACE-Is and ARBs should never be combined in patient use, as it seems to cause more renal problems.

Medications are required for some patients on occasion and integrative medical practitioners must always ensure that the patient is being treated effectively and responsibly. Of course, patients interested in integrative care are often

KEY TREATMENT NOTE

T1DM patients should be first dosed an ACE-I and T2DM patients should first be dosed an ARB. Never take these medications in combination. Patients on either medication should be regularly monitored for serum creatinine, eGFR, and potassium levels.

seeking alternatives to conventional medications or are trying to get off the ones they are on. This is a very valid desire and may be completely or partially achieved depending on the patient, their condition, their motivation and their compliance with their diabetic regimen. I think a key point is to not demonize medications, but to use them judiciously, only when needed, when a medical condition is not being cleared expediently solely through integrative care.

Conventional Treatment of Diabetic Kidney Disease—Lifestyle and Diet

A few key lifestyle and diet recommendations in conventional care are pragmatic and simply make good common sense. Any integrative physician should agree with these recommendations.

Lose weight. Any diet that promotes abdominal weight loss is helpful because central obesity promotes renal failure. Fat promotes renin and angiotensin secretion, raising the blood pressure. Fat also produces damaging inflammatory chemicals, and increases insulin resistance and glucose. Weight loss and reduction in insulin resistance can significantly help reduce or eradicate hypertension. Weight loss has also been shown in studies to reduce proteinuria significantly and to normalize creatinine.

Reduce alcohol intake. Alcohol can raise the blood pressure through several different physiological mechanisms.

Exercise. Obviously, a more healthy cardiovascular system has less hypertension.

Stop smoking. Toxins in cigarettes immediately raise blood pressure, and the chemicals can damage the endothelial lining, leading to chronic hypertension.

Lower salt intake. Reducing salt to around 2,000 mg per day can lower systolic blood pressure 4–8 mmHg. A high salt intake can increase the blood pressure, especially in seniors, African Americans, and the obese. High salt can also increase the risk of a stroke and kidney disease. Surprisingly, most of the salt ingested in America comes from bread. So, a low-carb diet is a win-win for reducing glucose-raising carbs and significantly lowering dietary salt intake.

Avoid radio-contrast materials. These are dyes sometimes injected into patients receiving certain imaging tests, such as MRIs or CT scans. If your kidneys are not wholly healthy, and you need that type of imaging, your physician should investigate whether the dye is safe for you.

Conventional Treatment of Diabetic Kidney Disease—Last Options

If chronic kidney disease has progressed to stage 4 or 5, the patient needs to begin kidney dialysis.

Comprehensive Integrative Prevention and Treatment of Diabetic Nephropathy—Removal of Kidney Irritants

Some things people ingest are irritating to the kidneys over time. These should be reduced or removed. Regarding fluid intake, do not under- or overhydrate the kidneys. In general, the basic rule for fluid intake is to drink half of one's body weight in ounces a day, of healthy beverages. So, if a patient weighs 150 pounds, that means 75 ounces of healthy fluids (particularly water!) each day. More fluid should be added if there is a lot of sweating or the patient is ill with vomiting or diarrhea.

Patients should also stop taking NSAIDs such as ibuprofen, naproxen, and aspirin, which can harm the kidneys over time, especially in higher doses. If you are in pain from some condition like arthritis or headaches, it is better to treat these naturally than to rely on kidney-irritating, temporary relief, and to remember that a healthy gut helps the systemic body be healthier, as well. Seek out an integrative physician who can treat any conditions requiring any regular NSAID intake, to get you off them as soon as possible.

Lastly, reduce caffeine intake. Although coffee is okay in general, as is green tea, I do not prefer patients to drink more than 12 ounces of coffee or 18 ounces of green tea a day.

Comprehensive Integrative Prevention and Treatment of Diabetic Nephropathy—Diet

As mentioned above, a diet of 0.8 g/kg of protein is safe for diabetic kidney patients. In fact, my patients who present with microalbuminuria eat up to 1 g/kg of their body weight because they are eating so little carbs, and they need to get some more calories in elsewhere. This works fine. Remember: Most Americans eat way too much protein. A man who is five feet ten inches tall and 170 pounds, for example, should eat around 12.8 ounces or 77 grams of protein a day. However, it is typical for the average man to eat three eggs and bacon for breakfast, a big 6 ounce chicken burger for lunch and an 8 ounce steak for supper, totaling 18 ounces / 108 grams of protein a day.

Low-carb ketogenic diets have been shown to help reverse impaired kidney function in both T1DM and T2DM patients. Moreover, another study showed that a low-carb diet reversed renal disease in T2DM patients.

Another type of diet, called the CR-LIPE or carbohydrate-restricted, low-iron, polyphenol-enriched diet, was shown in T2DM patients to reduce occurrence of death or renal transplant by nearly 50 percent, and reduced the doubling of serum creatinine by half. Iron is not a nutrient adults should ingest unless they are vegan or iron anemic. If a person has good stores of iron and is taking it in a supplement or is eating too much meat, this can increase iron levels in the body, and that can cause oxidative damage. And remember, the low-iron diet is beneficial for fatty livers, as well.

The CR-LIPE diet involves reducing one's carbohydrate intake by 50 percent; replacing iron-rich meats like pork and beef with white meats like fish and poultry; increasing fat intake; increasing iron-inhibitory proteins like eggs, soy, and dairy (a patient should also, of course, increase intake of vegetarian proteins such as nuts and seeds and protein powder); drinking only water, or iron inhibitors such as red wine (a maximum of 300 ml a day, if a patient does not have fatty liver), tea, and milk; and using good healthy oils (such as extra virgin olive oil) for dressings and cooking. The macronutrient breakdown of the diet is as follows: Carbs—35–65 percent less intake; protein—25–30 percent increased intake; fat—slightly increased intake.

This CR-LIPE is not too different from the other diets I've discussed earlier in this book—it seems to be very close to a modified vegan low-glycemic diet, or a modified omnivore low-carb diet. Although ketogenic advocates may disagree, in general it is a lot healthier to eat less red meat and pork. Regularly drinking a protein powder smoothie, and eating nuts, fish, soy, and dairy are all good choices for diabetic patients in general, as well as eating less meat overall.

OTHER DIETARY FACTORS

In one study on both T1DM and T2DM patients, eating more soy and less meat reduced urinary albumin excretion (in T2DM) and reduced eGFR in those with hyperfiltration eGFR rates. I imagine this relates to less iron in the diet, if nothing else.

Of course, all diabetic patients and the vast majority of everyone else need to avoid sugar. However, did you know that science proves that refined sugar, such as high fructose corn syrup, raises blood pressure? In one study, drinking 2.5 cans of regular soda pop a day increased hypertension by 30 percent (a key factor causing kidney damage). Avoiding sugar seems to be more important than avoiding salt, for hypertension control.

Diabetic patients should reduce their intake of advanced glycosylated end products (AGEs). You can eat AGEs, as well as make them by having too much glucose in your serum. When eating meat, if you fry, roast, or broil it, you increase serum AGEs by 24–29 percent. If you boil, poach, stew, or steam the meat, you can reduce serum AGEs by 34–35 percent. However, in real life, if we eat meat, we usually cook it in a way that elevates serum AGEs, so we should focus instead on regularly eating all the other dietary proteins, which do not create AGEs in their preparation.

In studies of IgA nephropathy, which is a condition whereby the kidney cells develop impaired filtration in a way similar to an uncontrolled diabetic patient, both low and high doses of omega-3 and omega-9 oils reduced the progression of these patients to end-stage renal failure. Foods that contain these healthy oils include oily fish (wild salmon, trout, sardines, herring), leafy greens, omega-3 eggs, grass-fed and grass-finished meat (although don't eat a lot of it!), organic soy, avocados and avocado oil, walnuts and walnut oil, organic unrefined flax seed oil, and organic unrefined extra virgin olive oil. Of course, omega-3 oils can also be supplemented, too.

Comprehensive Integrative Prevention and Treatment of Diabetic Nephropathy—Botanical Medicines

There are many botanical medicines that are protective to the kidneys and can help the kidneys heal. I do not tend to use these if the patient just has microalbuminuria, but if they come to me with more established kidney disease, then I always add in some mix of the following:

- *Rheum palmatum* / rhubarb root
- *Urtica* seed
- *Lespedeza capitata*
- *Parietaria*
- *Astragalus*
- *Codonopsis*
- *Gingko biloba*
- *Salvia miltorrhiza*
- *Cordyceps sinensis*
- *Tripterygium wilfordii*
- *Panax ginseng*

Many of these herbs have been shown in small animal and human studies to reduce nephropathy; reduce microalbuminuria; decrease AGEs in the serum and kidneys; decrease kidney tissue swelling; have antioxidant effects; decrease glucose; act as anti-inflammatories; and overall improve renal function.

A product called Two Treasures, from Heron Herbs, contains an excellent formula featuring several of these botanicals. Other botanical companies also have special kidney protective and healing formulas, including Saireito, a mix of twelve Asian herbs, with *Radix bupleuri* as the lead herb.

A simple combination of *Gingko biloba* and *Salvia miltorrhiza* can be valuable for kidney health. Gingko has been shown to help heal kidney capillaries and is considered a good protective herb for the kidneys. In a study on rats in which diabetes was induced, a gingko extract decreased creatinine, urine protein, fasting blood glucose, and AGE formation. *Salvia mitorrhiza* is considered a kidney protectant and an antioxidant. It decreases glucose, creatinine, and microalbuminuria, and improves kidney cell health.

Botanicals are wonderful at helping to heal the kidneys when combined with a comprehensive program to lower glucose. They will probably not be that effective if your glucose levels are regularly very high. These are also not common botanicals you can easily access at your local health food store, but an integrative physician should have these in their office if they treat diabetic or other kidney patients regularly.

Also, some botanicals can have some side effects or even be toxic. This is why all therapeutic botanicals should be prescribed and followed by a physician who practices integrative medicine and is well aware of the effects and possible dangers of long-term use of some of the aforementioned herbs. I often use them in a tincture, whereby herbs are macerated in alcohol for weeks, so all of their medicinal aspects enter into the alcohol. The herbs are then filtered out, and the tincture is dosed appropriately to the patient. I do not find a few droppers of alcohol tincture a day to be damaging to a fatty liver, unlike drinking entire glasses or shots of alcohol. I also use the botanicals in capsules, if the patient has severe fatty liver, is alcoholic, or really cannot stand the taste of the tincture. It is a general rule that sweet things make us sick, and bitter things make us well, and therapeutic herbal tinctures can be very bitter at times!

As described by Eric Yarnell, ND, a good method for mixing botanicals for the kidneys includes using herbs with different functions:

- Using adaptogens, including *Astragalus* or *Codonopsis* as a leading herb, can energize the body and stimulate healing.
- Synergizers like *Glycyrrhiza* are good herbs to help other herbs work better and also to reduce inflammation. Rarely, licorice can over time increase blood pressure, but this is not commonly seen. Nonetheless, any patient taking full licorice daily should be regularly monitoring his blood pressure for any increase.
- Lymphagogues are herbs that help stimulate blood and lymph flow through tissues to enable detoxification and support. *Ceanothus* and *Polymnia* are common herbs used in this manner.
- Nephroprotective herbs work specifically on enhancing kidney tissue health.

Please note that I did not list all the specific dosings of each botanical. Knowledgeable integrative physicians will often create tinctures in their offices that are specific to what each patient requires, or they will order established combinations from companies run by master herbalists. Seek appropriate dosing of all botanicals from your medical practitioner.

Comprehensive Integrative Prevention and Treatment of Diabetic Nephropathy—Supplements

There are many supplements that have solid scientific evidence showing they both protect and help heal damaged diabetic kidneys.

Benfotiamine. As we'll see with the preventive and therapeutic protocols for all diabetic complications, benfotiamine shows up as a key nutraceutical. We know it inhibits the formation of AGEs and reduces oxidative damage. In both animal and human studies, benfotiamine was shown to prevent diabetic nephropathy.

Benfotiamine + alpha-lipoic acid. This is a wonderful combination for all patients with diabetes. One study showed that these supplements together normalized pathways causing complications in T1DM patients.

Alpha-lipoic acid (by itself). In T1DM and T2DM patients at doses of 600 mg, ALA stopped the progression of urinary albumin concentration compared to a control group that did not take the supplements.

Antioxidants. ALA 600 mg *or* selenium 100 mcg *or* D-alpha tocopherol 1,200 IU per day. In each antioxidant group there was an improvement in diabetic kidney function.

Curcumin. This anti-inflammatory antioxidant had a very powerful effect in a study of rats with poorly functioning kidneys. Curcumin at 1,500–3,000 mg per day decreased microalbuminuria, and lowered creatinine levels, among many other benefits.

Quercitin. This strong bioflavonoid also decreased nephropathy in animal studies, at a dosage of 1,000–3,000 mg per day.

Omega-3 oils. There is solid evidence that omega-3 oils are a real boost to kidney health. O-3 oils have been shown to significantly lower macro and microalbuminuria.

Vitamin D_3. This simple vitamin has been shown to reduce proteinuria in diabetic nephropathy.

More antioxidants. Vitamin C 200 mg per day + vitamin E 100 IU per day *or* vitamin C 1,250 mg + vitamin E 680 IU *or* vitamin E 1,200 IU *or* vitamin C 500 mg twice per day: all were successful at reducing urinary microalbuminuria. Moreover, it was even better to add in some zinc and magnesium. These are simple, cheap antioxidants.

As you can see, it should not be very hard to prevent diabetic nephropathy in a compliant patient on a comprehensive integrative protocol. It is feasible to help reverse diabetic kidney damage using a low-carbohydrate diet, healthy lifestyle, and a properly prescribed mix of safe, responsible, pertinent, and effective supplements. You should allow your physician to choose the best mix for you, with your unique individual needs.

Diabetic Neuropathy

Diabetic neuropathy is defined as the progressive loss of nerve fiber function. It consists of symptoms and signs of nerve dysfunction in diabetic patients after other causes have been excluded. Diabetic neuropathy is the most common diabetic complication, with almost 50 percent of T1DM and T2DM patients developing it, and about 7.5 percent of patients having it upon diagnosis. It occurs after many years in T1DM patients and after just a few years in T2DM patients.

Diabetic neuropathy can easily lead to a greatly decreased quality of life due to constant and sometimes excruciating pain, numbness, and tingling in peripheral nerves, digestion or other body system damage, and the worst of the worst—patients developing foot ulcers that lead to amputations and then death. However, as with other complications, an expert in integrative diabetes management can be successful at preventing and reversing neuropathy. So, no need to give up hope!

There are three types of nerves that come out of our spinal cord or brain: motor nerves, which allow us to move our arms, hands, legs and feet; sensory nerves, which allow us to feel things through our skin; and autonomic nerves, which can be either sympathetic or parasympathetic. These control many of our organs and functions, such as our digestion, breathing, heartbeat, saliva production, and urination.

All of these nerves can be damaged by high glucose levels producing oxidative damage, as we've mentioned before. A nerve can also be damaged by nitric oxide, which can contribute to neuralgic pain and destroy vital parts of the nerve. Aside from high glucose levels, other risk factors for developing nerve damage include hypertension, the length of time one has had diabetes, being a senior, having high lipids/cholesterol, smoking, excessive alcohol intake, some genes, and being taller. Also, elevated arsenic levels found through integrative urinary testing can affect peripheral nerves.

Nerve symptoms of neuropathy include:

- Numbness or tingling in the feet or hands
- Pain in the feet or hands
- Muscle weakness
- Rapid or irregular heart rate
- Erectile dysfunction
- Nausea and vomiting
- Difficulty swallowing
- Constipation or diarrhea
- Orthostatic hypotension (that is, feeling dizzy and like you might black out when you stand up)
- Poor urinary stream, or feeling of incomplete voiding
- Heat intolerance, or heavy sweating

There are labs that should be run to ensure there is no other or additional reason for the above symptoms. Other conditions to investigate include pernicious anemia, an autoimmune condition that prevents vitamin B_{12} absorption from the gut. Alcoholism can cause neuropathy, as can vertebral disorders such as a herniated lumbar disk initiating sciatic pain, or carpal tunnel syndrome causing wrist and hand pain. Therefore a full lab workup should occur, to help uncover any possible other reasons aside from diabetes you may have neuropathy, including:

All the basic labs: CBC, CMP, fasting glucose, and A1C

Thyroid function tests: TSH, free T3, free T4

Inflammatory markers: erythrocyte sedimentation rate, high-sensitive c-reactive protein

Autoimmune panels: ANA, Anti-SSA/SSB, rheumatoid factor, cyclic citrullinated peptide

Functional vitamin B_{12} and folate: vitamin B_{12} and folic acid, but also methyl malonic acid and homocysteine. This is especially important for any patient on metformin, because 8–5 percent of patients on it develop vitamin B_{12} deficiency.

Serum B_1, which can be low in alcoholism and cause neuropathy; elevated GGT, a liver enzyme, can also point to alcoholism.

Serum B_6: elevation can cause neuropathy

Heavy metal toxicity (if the patient's past medical history indicates that they may be toxic in heavy metals, particularly arsenic)

HIV/AIDS testing, if pertinent

Spinal column vertebral or limb analysis through a naturopathic physician, osteopath, or chiropractor for nerve impingement. This is not a lab, but may be very helpful to check for, especially if the neuropathy is more one-sided.

In-Office Physical Exams

Any new patient to my office gets a thorough diabetic exam. I will check the patient's deep tendon reflexes, and I'll evaluate both their posterior tibialis and dorsal pedis arteries, which bring blood to the feet and toes. I'll do a skin check to ensure there are no wounds, ulcers, rashes, or toenail fungus, and to make sure there are no indents in their skin showing their shoes are not fitting right. I'll check for muscle atrophy and distortions to the foot like Charcot foot, which is a weakening of the bones of the foot that may cause fractures and resultant changes in its structure. Moreover, I'll do a vibratory and monofilament exam checking nerve function in the feet and toes.

The monofilament exam is a test whereby the physician very gently pokes your toes and the ball of your foot to see if you can feel those when your eyes are closed. The monofilament is a 5.07/10 gram standardized Semmes-Weinstein monofilament. I poke it until it bends in half—the standard poke pressure—against the patient's skin while their eyes are open. After they acknowledge they felt it, I then have them close their eyes, and test each foot separately. I poke the big toe and two other toes, two areas on the ball of their foot and the middle of their arch. On the second foot, I make the same points but in a different order. If a physician does not have a standard monofilament, they can use a very light touch of their fingers instead.

Unfortunately, many times the patient who reported no neuropathy during the intake cannot feel all the pokes, indicating they already have some neuropathy present and were unaware of it.

I do the vibratory test with a 128 Hz tuning fork, held against the bony prominence of the big toe, proximal to the nail bed. There are many variations on how to use the tuning fork test, but I like this simple one. I simply want to see if the patient can feel the vibration over a span of ten seconds. If not, that would show some large nerve damage.

More Involved Neuropathy Testing

Gastroparesis is an autonomic neuropathy that specifically affects the vagus nerve. This nerve is the key nerve that controls the functioning of the digestive organs. When it is damaged, people might start having problems digesting the food in their stomach and might experience a significant slowness of the food emptying into the small intestine. Gastroparesis can, as a result, cause nausea and vomiting, significant maldigestion, vomiting of undigested food, early feeling of fullness when eating, bloating, avoidance of food, weight loss, gastroesophageal reflux disease, spasms of the stomach wall, and small intestinal bacterial overgrowth. It can also, more dangerously, cause wildly fluctuating and erratic glucose numbers, particularly in patients on insulin. If you are on a rapid insulin injected fifteen minutes before your meal, and your food sits too long in your stomach, you might suffer a serious low. If the food is dumped into your intestine hours later after the insulin is no longer active, your glucose might rise precipitously. Wild fluctuations in glucose with digestive symptoms are excellent clues to investigate a diagnosis of gastroparesis.

There are two diagnostic tests for gastroparesis. The first is the barium swallow with video fluoroscopy. In this test, a patient eats a steak or scrambled egg meal that is coated with barium. It seems eating the eggs produces a more reliable test than the steak, so that is what I recommend a patient eats. Then, using an x-ray camera that measures the movement of the barium through the stomach and into the small intestine for up to four hours, we see how quickly food is digested in the stomach and moved into the small intestine. If this is done in proper time, the patient's vagus nerve is working fine. The average retention of a low-fat meal in a healthy person at one hour is 90 percent; at two hours is 60 percent; and at four hours is only 10 percent. Retention of greater than 10 percent of a meal after four hours is considered to be a diagnostic indication of gastroparesis.

However, the barium swallow can be inaccurate; it is typically only positive if the patient has already developed a rather severe case of delayed gastric emptying. If a patient only has mild or even moderate gastroparesis, which comes and goes and is not steady, then one meal might travel through the stomach fine, but other meals are problematic. If the test occurs when the food is well digested and efficiently secreted into the small intestine, the barium swallow might develop a "false negative," a mistaken analysis that the patient does not have this condition, when indeed there are times it does occur.

The heart rate variability test—also known as the R-R interval test—is the second designed to see if there is any damage to the vagus nerve, as the vagus nerve controls both the stomach and the heart. This is not done very often in clinical practice, as, in my experience, cardiologists are not well aware of the study. The R-R interval test is a simple and direct measurement of vagus nerve functioning. In this test, the heart rate is compared to the breathing rate of the patient. A normal heart varies with breathing; it goes faster with inhalation and quite slower with exhalation. If the vagus nerve is damaged, then the heart rate does not vary with breathing as it should, and there is not speeding up or slowing down with inhalations and exhalations.

In an R-R interval test, a patient lies down and EKG leads are attached to their body, so the patient is connected to a heart monitor. The patient is then led through a system of five-second inhalations and exhalations for a couple of minutes. Reading the EKG strip and analyzing the R-R interval of the heart rate can help make a diagnosis of vagus nerve dysfunction causing gastroparesis.

Aside from the barium swallow and R-R interval test there are even more complicated tests neurologists can perform, such as an MRI, electromyography, nerve conduction test, and so on.

Neuropathy Staging

Neuropathy is staged regarding its severity:

NO. No neuropathy.

N1a. Signs but no symptoms. This is what frequently happens in my office when the patient tells me they do not have any neuropathy sensations, but in my physical exam with the monofilament and tuning fork, I pick up nerve deficits.

N2a. The patient experiences symptoms of mild diabetic polyneuropathy in either sensory, motor, or autonomic nerves.

N2b. The patient experiences severe symptomatic diabetic polyneuropathy.

N3. The patient has disabling diabetic neuropathy.

Consequences of Diabetic Neuropathy

Consequences of progressive diabetic neuropathy are devastating, particularly as it is commonly associated with peripheral vascular disease. Peripheral vascular disease (PVD), also known as peripheral artery disease (PAD), is like atherosclerosis but in smaller blood vessels than those of the heart and brain. It produces blood vessel dysfunction, and causes inflammation and hypercoagulability (blood clot risk). PVD reflects a likely overall cardiovascular ischemic disease process in the body. With neuropathy, PVD decreases blood flow to body parts, like the feet, and so if they are injured, it is much harder for them to heal and instead they may worsen. In patients with neuropathy and PVD, skin lesions can ulcerate and get infected. If the infection develops into cellulitis (infection of fat tissue under the skin), and spreads into deep skin and soft tissue, and into the bones, then the part will likely need to be amputated. If a person has one amputation, then within a year, according to statistics, they will have another. As I noted previously, diabetes is the number one reason for amputations of limbs outside of trauma care. Patients having cardiovascular autonomic neuropathy (heart rate irregularities, postural hypotension, exercise intolerance, and heart attacks) and lower extremity amputation are the two most common reasons people with diabetes are hospitalized in Western countries.

Once a body part is amputated, the risk of dying over the next five years significantly increases; there is a 30–80 percent increased risk of death after one's first amputation. So, this complication is chilling in the reality of its effect on patients.

CHARCOT FOOT

Charcot foot is an uncommon but devastating side effect of poorly controlled diabetes. In general, it only occurs in 0.1 percent of the general diabetic population, but that can increase to 13 percent in the high-risk diabetic population. It tends to occur eight to twelve years after diabetes is diagnosed in a person, and it occurs more in men than in women. It is usually seen in the fifth and sixth decades of life. Moreover, 30 percent of the time it occurs in both feet at the same time.

Charcot foot was first described in 1883. Its formal name is Charcot neuropathic osteoarthropathy, and it affects the bones, joints, and soft tissues of the foot and ankle. Charcot foot mostly develops in diabetic patients and only in those with neuropathy. It also occurs more often in patients with metabolic abnormalities of the bones, especially low bone mass density, that is, osteopenia or osteoporosis.

When a bone fractures in people with normal nerves, inflammatory cytokines are released. This produces pain, alerting the person an injury has occurred, and thus, treatment is sought, and the bone is immobilized, reducing the inflammatory reaction. In a person with diabetes who suffers from sensory-motor and autonomic neuropathy, if trauma occurs and especially if the bone has less bone mass, the inflammation that develops continues, because the patient cannot feel the pain and thus does not immobilize the foot or ankle. This can lead to repetitive trauma, bone destruction, joint subluxation and dislocation, and deformity. That is medicine's best understanding of the etiology, but Charcot foot is not wholly understood.

The classic deformity is called "rocker bottom," where the sole is rounded like the curved leg on which a rocking chair moves forward and back. Charcot foot can be diagnosed with a foot x-ray, and if that is not definitive, an MRI or nuclear imaging can be performed. Conventional treatment consists of "offloading," which is immobilization of the foot and ankle in an irremovable total contact cast. Antiresorptive therapy drugs given to build up low bone mass and prevent further degeneration of the bone may be prescribed. The only other treatment is surgery.

I do not know natural methods for treating established Charcot foot. Often, diabetic patients are tested for vitamin D_3 levels. But, if a patient also has osteopenia or osteoporosis, found through a DEXA scan, it is very important to check their vitamin K levels. Vitamin D_3, among other things, helps absorb calcium from the gut. Vitamin K activates osteocalcin in the bone by carboxylating it. Then, the bone is "sticky" and will absorb the calcium. If a patient is deficient in vitamin K, calcium won't be able to enter the bone, and even with wonderful levels of serum vitamin D, fractures can still easily occur. There is, as far as I know, only one lab in the country that does functional vitamin K testing, as well as testing for undercarboxylated osteocalcin—Genova Labs—and that is the lab I use. There are many ways to strengthen bones, even in patients with osteopenia and osteoporosis, and in all diabetic patients with one of those conditions, ensuring bone strengthening protocols are added into diabetic control protocols makes excellent sense.

Otherwise, I am not aware of natural treatments to help reverse the extensive damage of Charcot foot deformities; luckily, it is rare. However, I do feel that following the comprehensive integrative protocol in this book gives a diabetic patient the best chance of never developing this condition in the first place.

Conventional Treatment of Neuropathy: Foot Care

Prevention of neuropathy relies on managing glucose and taking good care of your feet. Do not go into hot baths if you have any serious neuropathy, and, as I constantly tell diabetic patients here in the Valley of the Sun, do not wear thong sandals but wear supportive sandals and shoes instead. Do not walk barefoot outside. Try to keep your feet from having any injury at all.

Engaging in physical or occupational therapy might be helpful for some patients at times. Considering foot orthotics is a good idea if feet are flat. In my opinion, the best orthotic is made when the person is seated, not standing, and the orthotic specialist conforms the foot in the kit.

One good way to help reduce neuropathy damage is to check your feet every day for any wound. If you notice one, notify your physician immediately. Going to a podiatrist regularly to have nails cut (especially in elderly patients) and to deal with ingrown nails is also helpful. Refer to chapter 3 for more information on foot care.

Conventional Care of Neuropathy: Medications

Reversing neuropathy can be achieved through excellent glucose control and integrative treatments, but if glucose control is not attained, neuropathy will continue and likely will progress. In conventional care, treatment of neuropathy attempts to reduce symptoms, but if a patient cannot tightly control their glucose levels and reduce systemic inflammation, neuropathy tends to continue to progress. The most commonly known medications to deal with the symptoms are anticonvulsants, which may help reduce the agonizing pain some people develop with their diabetic neuropathy. These include:

Lyrica/pregabalin. 50 to 200 mg three times per day (every eight hours)
Neurontin/gabapentin. 300 mg at bedtime or 300–1,200 mg three times per day
Depakote/sodium valproate. 500 mg per day
Tegretol/carbamazepine. 200–600 mg per day

Tricyclic antidepressants, older antidepressants not used for depression anymore, are also sometimes tried, such as:

Elavil/amitriptyline. 25–150 mg at bedtime
Tofranil/imipramine. 25–200 mg per day
Pamelor/nortriptyline HCL, aventyl HCL. 25–50 mg at bedtime

Physicians might also prescribe a selective serotonin/norepinephrine reuptake inhibitor. There are two of these used for neuropathic pain:

Cymbalta/duloxetine. 60 or 120 mg per day or 30 mg twice per day
Effexor XR/venlafaxine. 150–225 mg per day. We've all seen TV commercials for this medication for nerve pain, as we have for Lyrica.

There are topical creams used as well:

Lidoderm/lidocaine gel 5 percent. Apply 1–3 ml for fifteen to twenty minutes or a patch for up to twelve hours per day

Capsaicin/cayenne pepper cream (Zostrix/Capsin/Dolorac). Can be bought over the counter. Follow the directions exactly for applying the capsaicin cream, and after you apply it to your skin, do not touch your eyes or your genitals!

Lastly, opioids might be used, if necessary, but this is a very problematic choice and should always be avoided if possible. These are terribly addictive and are causing numerous problems in patients in the United States.

The American Association of Family Practitioners guidelines state that in the treatment of diabetic peripheral neuropathic pain first try tricyclic antidepressants, then anticonvulsants and SSRIs, and then opiates. Topical antipain meds can be used at any time, with any medicine.

As you might expect, there are numerous other medicines prescribed for various other, much rarer manifestations of diabetic neuropathy—there are drugs for orthostatic hypotension, bladder stimulation, erectile dysfunction, slowing diarrhea, aiding defecation, and so forth. There are drugs that promote stomach stimulation like the antibiotic erythromycin, Miralax/polyethylene glycol, domperidone, nitric oxide agonists, and Reglan/metoclopramide. Metoclopramide and domperidone can have extremely serious hormonal, intestinal, and central nervous system side effects, and I do not use them. Antiemetics are also used at times if nausea and vomiting are serious symptoms the patient has regularly. Medications may help, but they can also stop working over time, too.

If things continue to worsen, inserting a gastric neurotransmitter, similar to a heart pacemaker, might be suggested, and in the worst case scenarios, a patient might need to use a feeding tube that bypasses the stomach. A newer treatment of injecting botulinum toxin into the pyloric sphincter, the sphincter between the bottom of the stomach and the entrance into the duodenum, may be attempted.

Many patients use medications such as Lyrica or Cymbalta and do have some palliation of their neuropathic pain. However, let's discuss the other ways to consider addressing neuropathy.

Comprehensive Integrative Treatment of Neuropathy—ReBuilder Medical Machine

I have no financial association with this company, but I have used their machine with patients with success. The ReBuilder Medical machine is a highly rated machine used in diabetic clinics all around the country. It is a NeuroElectric Therapy device that is not a TENS unit, but instead actually seems to help calm down painful and overactive nerves, increase blood flow to the area, and stimulate nerves to heal.

The machine is expensive, currently around $535, though some insurances may help cover it. You can talk to the company representatives about that. If you suffer from bad neuropathy, this is an investment to seriously consider making. Patients do a treatment with the machine one to two times a day, and when I have patients add this machine into their comprehensive protocol, it has often added a noticeable synergy of healing. I've used this with patients with neuropathy in a comprehensive protocol and have had patients regain full sensitivity, who could not feel their lower limbs previously. You can check it out at www.rebuildermedical.com.

Comprehensive Integrative Prevention and Treatment of Neuropathy—Supplements

Treating a patient to help heal painful diabetic neuropathy requires a comprehensive focus on all of the pertinent comprehensive integrative treatment modalities. There are numerous supplements that are backed by good scientific evidence of being of key value in patients with diabetic neuropathy.

Acetyl-l-carnitine. I will always add this supplement into my patient's protocol if they have any signs or symptoms of neuropathy. This supplement has been shown to lessen pain, increase nerve regeneration (in many aspects of nerve anatomy rebuilding), and increase vibratory perception. ALC can be deficient in diabetic patients, too. 1,500–3,000 mg per day.

Benfotiamine. Well, there is our old friend again! At higher doses it can reduce the pain of diabetic neuropathy. 450 mg per day.

R-alpha-lipoic acid. Another old friend! R-ALA can also reduce pain, odd sensations, and numbness. It can improve blood circulation to nerves. It can delay and reverse diabetic peripheral neuropathy. 300–1,200 mg per day.

Lion's mane. This water-extracted botanical is called "nature's nutrient for the neurons." It stimulates the production of nerve growth factor and has been shown to help with nerve repair and regeneration. 250 mg once or twice a day.

Vitamin B_{12} alone *or* B complex *or* vitamin B_{12} + benfotiamine. There are medical studies showing the neurological benefit of these supplements to diabetic patients.

Fish oils. It seems that patients low in omega-3 oils lose nerve function quicker than those with higher omega-3 status in their bodies. Omega-3 oils can prevent neuropathy by maintaining nerve conduction velocity.

Curcumin. In an animal study, curcumin was shown to be helpful at 1,500–3,000 mg per day.

Comprehensive Integrative Treatment of Diabetic Gastroparesis

The goal of treating gastroparesis is to eliminate physical complaints of the condition, try to help heal the vagus nerve, and smooth out the erratic high and low glucose levels. Aside from an aggressive combination of the first through sixth of The Eight Essentials, there are a few other ideas to consider if you have gastroparesis.

Chewing gum may help to promote digestive juices, and I recommend using a gum called PUR. It has very clean ingredients, and although the flavor does not last a long time, it does not contain any nasty sweeteners or GMO soy. I like the mint pomegranate flavor.

Patients should eat slowly, chewing very well, making sure food is totally broken down well in the mouth before swallowing. Some foods, such as meats, should be ground up rather than eaten as steaks or chops, which are harder to break down. It may be good to eat more protein during the morning and lunch and a little less at night, when stomach activity is less. Avoiding heavy fats and high fiber foods is helpful because those foods slow stomach emptying.

For patients with more severe gastroparesis, eating soups, protein powders, cooked vegetables, and other easier-to-digest foods is a good idea. In patients with mild gastroparesis, a low-carb diet, as well as following the rest of The Eight Essentials, including the supplements listed below, may work. I've had patients do just fine that way. But what do we do about insulin in moderate to severe gastroparesis patients, when the stomach is not emptying with any regularity, and glucose numbers are consistently high and low? Figuring out how to dose insulin at meals is a step-by-step process.

In general, rapid insulins should not be used for patients with established gastroparesis, though they can be used to correct highs before meals. The best insulin for gastroparesis is regular insulin. Options include doing regular before meals, which is less strong than rapid but lasts significantly longer, so if the meal is delayed, the low might not be so severe and the insulin might last long enough to cover it. Other strategies include dosing regular after the meal, if stomach emptying is significantly and regularly delayed. Or, of course, there is always the middle area—dose half the regular before and half after the meal. Since, however, many patients do not want to dose regular, experimenting with rapid dosing can be tried. Perhaps dose half before and half after the meal and see if that works.

There are some natural products, medications, and other therapies we can use to help the stomach empty on time:

Nervinum vagum. Homeopathic vagus nerve may help strengthen the nerve that directs the stomach to digest and excretes the food into the small intestine.

Iberogast. This nine-herb combination is backed by positive studies specifically for helping patients with gastroparesis. It contains *Iberis amara*, *Matricaria*, *Angelica*, caraway, lemon balm, celandine, licorice, and peppermint.

Other promising herbal combinations. The following do not seem to have the studies behind them that Iberogast does: Astratin, Gastrotab, Pranofax, Trenical, and Perteton.

Low-dose naltrexone (LDN). Another focus of my medical practice is gastrointestinal disorders, and I appreciate using LDN as a prokinetic for patients who have small intestine bacterial overgrowth (SIBO). There are studies showing that LDN helps empty the stomach and move food through the small intestine. LDN is a compounded prescription medication. It may cause grogginess, vivid dreams, or hallucinations in some patients. 1–5 mg per day at bedtime (typically), away from food.

6-gentleman herbal formula. This Chinese formula has been shown in studies to be a good prokinetic. However, traditional Chinese medicine works best when the patient is analyzed by a practitioner and the specific herbs they need are discerned. This product can irritate patients who do not match the herbal prescription.

Ginger. 1,000 mg per day can help with stomach emptying although it may upset some stomachs.

Tryptophan or 5-HTTP. This amino acid can help with stomach emptying, as it makes serotonin; 95 percent of serotonin is made in the intestines to push food forward. Both should be taken away from food or only with carbohydrates, and vitamin B_6 helps them work.

- Tryptophan: 500–3,000 mg per day
- 5-HTTP: 50–600 mg per day (may cause agitation in patients, but that is rare)

Digestive enzymes. Low stomach acid can slow stomach digestion. I would suggest HCL/pepsin and pancreatic enzymes, but dose the HCL/pepsin carefully. There is an old myth that says you should take HCL capsules one by one until the stomach burns, and then decrease to the highest nonburn dose. This is not in any way scientifically accurate. Nigel Plummer, PhD, a British researcher, has figured out how much HCL needs to be given in patients with low or no hydrochloric acid production. Patients need to take 600–2,400 mg HCL per meal maximum.

Aloe vera juice. Up to 4–8 ounces before eating.

Apple cider vinegar. Apple cider vinegar has also been shown to lower carbohydrate excursions after meals, so it's a win-win for patients with diabetes. 1 tablespoon before meals.

Gentian and scutellaria capsules. This formula is a very old naturopathic formula designed to help stimulate stomach digestion, and also reduce inflammation. Gentian is one of the best stomachics—an herb that specifically promotes the production of stomach acid and digestion. This form of scutellaria is used to decrease intestinal inflammation.

Acupuncture may be helpful.

Constitutional hydrotherapy may be helpful. This is an old and highly respected modality in naturopathic medicine that is designed solely to increase the functioning of the gastrointestinal tract.

Yoga positions. For both stress relaxation and to enhance the functioning of nerves and organ health, yoga classes might be helpful.

Magnetty magnets. These are 1,000 gauss therapeutic magnets you can order from Austin Medical Supply, which can be placed over the stomach to help it energetically work more efficiently. They should be taken off for an MRI and going through security at the airport.

Vertebral manipulations and deep massage of muscles. The nerves from the thoracic area of the spine energize the stomach, so it is good to ensure that there are no ergonomic or vertebral blocks to proper nerve function in the end organ. Seeing a naturopathic physician, chiropractor, or osteopathic doctor for analysis is recommended, and seeing a good massage therapist may be helpful.

Finding a knowledgeable integrative physician can help guide you through the supplements and tools to use that seem best for you and your situation.

Comprehensive Integrative Treatment of Diabetic Ulcers

In twenty plus years of treating diabetic patients, I've only had one patient develop an ulcer. My patient got a new job, and they required him to wear specific shoes. The shoes did not fit well, and he developed an ulcer on his foot.

I used Amerigel on my patient, as per their ulcer healing directions on their website. I also wrote the patient's company a letter stating that he had to be allowed to wear shoes that would protect his feet from further damage, and the company agreed. Amerigel is used at diabetic clinics all over the country. I can highly recommend their product. It is made with natural tannins from oak trees and worked fantastically with my patient. His ulcer was healed up entirely in eight days. I did hear from another practitioner that one patient had an allergic reaction to Amerigel. It seems best to use a little on the skin and test for allergy before using it on an ulcer.

Other topical treatments useful in healing ulcers include botanical salves with calendula, comfrey, hypericum, chickweed, mullein, and plantain leaf.

Neuropathy Patient Case

I once saw an eighty-year-old African American woman with diabetes. She came in heavily dependent on a walker. Due to twelve years of poorly controlled diabetes, and also a stroke, she could not feel her feet or legs up to her knees, and she also had poor circulation. I could not palpate the two main pulses checked in the feet. Her skin was darker, as if the blood was not circulating well. As a result, walking was a very shaky procedure, as it is when one cannot feel the ground upon which one walks. She also had a speech impediment from the stroke.

She was very receptive to making any changes I thought might help her. I set her up on a low-carb diet, good multiple vitamin/mineral, fish oils, R-alpha-lipoic acid, benfotiamine, and a diabetes specialty product. She bought a ReBuilder Medical machine and used it daily as I prescribed.

Two weeks after her first treatment visit the patient returned. Her neuropathy was already 50 percent better. She could feel her lower legs and felt steadier when walking. Those two pulses in her feet were now both palpable and strong. She also had an improvement in her speech. I continued the entire protocol without any changes.

Two weeks later she returned again. Her neuropathy was 80 percent better, and she walked very well with the walker; she felt she had significantly improved balance. She could feel her feet and legs and had good results on monofilament and vibratory tests. Her skin color was looking more normal.

Two months after her first treatment visit, she was able to walk down the hall with just a cane. She had good energy, was happy with the diet, and felt the best she had for years.

Getting onto a comprehensive integrative protocol kicked in a healing capacity that had been stagnant due to a high-carb diet and poor diabetes control. Thus, she was able, even at her age, to experience a truly healing regimen. We are never too old to heal!

If not in the salve, it's helpful to also open up and add in vitamin E and vitamin A capsules.

Gentle hydrotherapy may be helpful to increase blood flow to the feet. Hydrotherapy is done by putting the foot into a container of warm water for three minutes, *not above 95° F*, followed by immediately placing the foot in a container of cool water, *not below 50° F*. Repeat that two more times for a total of three times. Always end with the cooler water. This hydrotherapy is excellent for moving the circulation in the body part treated. If insertion into water is not possible, using warm and cool towel applications can suffice.

Summary

Diabetic complications are the bane of uncontrolled diabetic patients. They are common and too frequently devastating. Isn't it great to learn that diabetic control can be attained, and that diabetic complications can be fully avoided, and even, if not too far advanced, reversed and healed?

This isn't magic; this is scientifically based medicine combined with decades of clinical experience. Controlling diabetes and preventing and reversing complications is the goal of this book. It is time to end this tragic epidemic. It is time for integrative medicine to get the respect it deserves and to be used by all diabetic patients to get their lives and their health back into their own hands. It is time for patients to go from being victims of diabetes to being victors over it.

— CHAPTER FIFTEEN —

Diabetic Case Studies and Concluding Summary

Here are six case studies to show that what I've been talking about really works. I have changed the names of patients and abbreviated the visits and the labs for easy reading.

Case Study #1

Tom was a thirty-three-year-old, high-functioning adult male patient with Down syndrome. He was brought to me by his parents because he had recently been diagnosed with T2DM. He was pleasant and easy to talk to. His mother was an advocate of integrative care, and she wished to avoid having her son take prescription medications.

I took his blood sugar in my office, as he had eaten two hours prior; it was 368, a very seriously high blood sugar level. His parents had put him on alpha-lipoic acid, vitamin B_{12} drops, chromium, and a One-A-Day vitamin. It's obvious that only taking supplements is not enough for patients with diabetes. He was totally out of control. This patient craved carbohydrates and ate a lot of them, both grains and sweets. He also had no exercise regimen.

His weight was 160 pounds at five feet six inches, with a BMI of 26, showing he was overweight. I did a physical exam on him and everything was normal.

Here were his initial pertinent blood work results:

- A1C: 10.9 (which means his glucose was about 330 mg/dL on average for the last three months)
- Fasting insulin: 15 mg/dL (high)
- Fasting blood sugar: 325 (very high)
- Total cholesterol: 288 (high)
- Triglycerides: 688 (very high)
- HDL (good cholesterol): 26 (low)
- LDL (bad cholesterol): could not determine due to high triglycerides

Any conventional practitioner would understandably have immediately placed Tom on one, if not two, oral hypoglycemic agents. I was willing to educate Tom on a comprehensive integrative diabetic protocol and wait two to three weeks, and if his glucose levels were decreasing, I would not prescribe medications. I put him on the omnivore low-carb diet. I gave him an excellent multiple vitamin/mineral, fish oils, flax seed oil, and a diabetic supplement including *Gymnema sylvestre*, vanadium, alanine, glutamine, chromium, and vitamin C. I kept him on the alpha-lipoic acid. I told him how to exercise five days a week, getting him out walking, which he stated he liked to do. He was willing to be compliant.

He came back two months later. He had followed everything well: the diet, exercising, and taking his supplements. He had more energy and was sleeping better. He was eager to follow the protocol. He had lost twenty pounds.

These were his pertinent blood results:

- A1C: 6.0 (average blood sugar levels of around 126)
- Fasting glucose: 98 mg/dL
- His cholesterol and triglycerides had all reduced to normal levels

I followed Tom for a year. I saw him every two to three months and he continued to do amazingly well. With his parents' support and because he was happy weighing less and not having to take medications, Tom was committed to following the protocol. His weight dropped to 135 pounds and then stabilized. At his height and new weight, Tom's new BMI was 21.78, which is absolutely perfect.

A year after my first visit with Tom, his A1C was 4.8 percent, and his cholesterol and lipid levels were all within normal ranges. If Tom had gone to a physician at that point, he would not have even been diagnosed with diabetes. When a patient is committed and has family support, diabetes can be totally controlled. Instead of going on oral medicines, and maybe even insulin, Tom used diet, exercise, and supplementation to enable weight loss and glucose control and successfully reversed his diabetes. Tom was a victor over diabetes!

Case Study #2

Ed, a forty-six-year-old already diagnosed T2DM patient, came to my clinic. This patient had suffered a hypoglycemic diabetic coma due to overmedication of oral hypoglycemic agents: Amaryl, metformin, and Actos. He was only on Actos when I first saw him. Ed weighed 310 pounds at five feet nine inches, so he had a BMI of 46, a score indicating morbid obesity. He was also on two medications for hypertension. Coming in he had his most recent lab work with him and his A1C was 8.2 percent.

This patient welcomed a new treatment paradigm, and I put him on the comprehensive integrative protocol I've talked about in this book: omnivore low-carb diet, multiple vitamin/mineral, fish oils, diabetes specialty supplement, and vitamin E. I recommended he begin aerobic and resistance exercise. Soon after our first visit he got a new security job that entailed him walking around a mall numerous times a night, so that helped.

Things improved rapidly with Ed.

- Two weeks after his first visit his glucose was so low he had to be taken off Actos.
- One month after his first visit his blood pressure was coming down, and I had to remove one hypertensive medication.
- Two months after his first visit I was able to safely and responsibly remove his second hypertensive medication, as his blood pressure was now normal.
- Three months after his first visit his A1C had reduced to 5.0 percent.

- Four months after his first visit he had lost 57 pounds, and his A1C was 5.0 percent. His new BMI was 36 percent, still obese, but better nonetheless.

I worked with Ed for five years. In our time together his A1C was always at 5.0 percent, his blood pressure was normal, he did not gain back any of the weight he had lost, and he also had normal lipid panels. He did not need any diabetic or blood pressure medications. Ed was a victor over diabetes!

Case Study #3

Sam was a sixty-two-year-old man with T2DM. His A1C was 8.4 percent, and his fasting glucose was usually around 159 mg/dL. He was fifty pounds overweight and was frustrated that he could not lose any weight, even doing some moderate exercise.

Sam injected 44 units of Lantus a night into one area of his abdomen. He was also on a statin drug for elevated cholesterol, as well as a blood pressure medicine. He had all the metabolic syndrome factors.

Measuring his c-peptide, I found it was completely normal, so Sam had the ability to make all the insulin his body needed. He did not need injectable insulin due to uncontrolled T2DM pancreatic damage causing insulin deficiency. His pancreas was still strong.

I put Sam on an omnivore low-carb diet, multiple vitamin/mineral, fish oils, a diabetes specialty supplement, and R-alpha-lipoic acid. I added in CoQ10 because he was on statin medication; whenever someone is on a statin medication, they need to be supported with CoQ10. Sam began an exercise routine with his active son: a little aerobics and a lot of weightlifting.

Right away I decreased Sam's Lantus to 22 units a night, as a practitioner needs to do when a patient on insulin starts a low-carb diet, and asked him to inject his insulin into three separate areas—7 units, 7 units, and 8 units—to maximize the effectiveness of insulin. Remember that injecting more than 7–10 units in one area can significantly reduce the effectiveness of the insulin's action.

Three weeks after his first treatment visit, Sam was able to stop all his Lantus insulin: His glucose levels had come down dramatically, and his basal insulin was no longer needed. Three months after Sam's treatment visit he had lost 25 pounds. He could lose weight now, due to less insulin in his system. Insulin prevents fat metabolism so injecting 44 units had interfered with his ability to lose weight even with exercise. He was on the diet and supplements, and working out regularly.

Sam's lab work showed his A1C had reduced to 6.3 percent, and his fasting glucose was 93 mg/dL. His A1C was not ideal, but it was 2.2 percent better than when he had been on 44 units of Lantus!

Eight months after his first treatment visit, Sam was still losing weight, was still off insulin, and had been able to stop his blood pressure medicine, as well. He was still fully compliant with the protocol. His A1C was now down to 5.8 percent. He had continued his statin medication by choice.

Not every T2DM patient can get off basal insulin, but some can when following a comprehensive integrative protocol. Sam was a victor over diabetes!

Case Study #4

Edith was a fifty-year-old female. I first saw her for hypertension and gastroesophageal reflux disease, and treated her for a year for those conditions. Her blood pressure normalized without medications and her GERD was eradicated.

Three years later, in early April, Edith called my office and explained that each March she developed bronchitis and typically called her primary care physician and got antibiotics ordered without an office visit, and those antibiotics would cure it. With her bout of bronchitis this year, her first antibiotic had not worked, so her PCP had called in a second antibiotic, and it had not worked, either. Edith was calling to see if I treated bronchitis. When I said yes, she asked if she could just pick something up, and I told her she had to come in for an office visit.

I wondered, before I saw her, what was the "obstacle to cure" with this patient? After all, I was not happy about her taking two antibiotics for her upper respiratory infection, as integrative protocols and supplements usually cure those without the need for drugs. But, the main question was: If each year an antibiotic easily cured her March bronchitis, why did it not work this year? Why did her body still have the infection after two doses of antibiotics? What was keeping her body from healing this infection?

When Edith came in, I realized right off the bat what the obstacle was. In the three years since I had seen her, she had become morbidly obese, gaining 60 pounds all around her abdomen. I intuitively grabbed my in-office glucose meter and asked for a finger to poke—her glucose was 308 mg/dL. She had T2DM and had had no idea. That was why her immune system was so faulty and she could not overcome her yearly bronchitis; high glucose numbers severely decrease the immune system function.

Edith was on Toprol, a beta-blocker, for hypertension. She had put herself on the following supplements: multiple vitamin/mineral, fish oil, shark liver oil, CoQ10, and garlic pills.

Edith's blood pressure was 200/100 mmHg (very high blood pressure). She was 240 pounds at five feet four inches, with a BMI of 41. She had some sounds in her lungs indicating bronchitis. Otherwise, her physical exam was normal. I treated her aggressively for the bronchitis with natural medicines, sent her home with a diet diary and glucose graph, and did lab work.

Here are some pertinent results of her blood tests:

- Fasting plasma glucose: 126 mg/dL (high)
- A1C: 8.3 percent
- Fasting insulin: 23 uIU/mL (high)
- Cholesterol: 332 mg/dL (high)
- Triglycerides: 340 mg/dL (high)
- HDL (good cholesterol): 34 mg/dL (low)
- LDL (bad cholesterol): 241 mg/dL (high)

On the treatment visit, I discussed the omnivore low-carb diet and suggested Edith drink three cups a day of green tea. I updated her regimen to a multiple vitamin/mineral, fish oils, diabetes specialty supplement, lecithin (to lower lipids), N-acetyl cysteine, and R-alpha-lipoic acid. I also suggested she begin an exercise regimen with aerobic and resistance exercise. Edith was 100 percent committed to reversing her diabetes.

Three months after the treatment visit Edith came back in. She had followed the plan. Her blood pressure had lowered and she had been able to stop the Toprol. She had lost 40 pounds and now weighed 200 pounds.

Her labs had markedly improved:

- BMI: 29 (lowered to overweight status from morbidly obese)
- Fasting plasma glucose: 75 mg/dL (reduced)
- A1C: 4.8 percent (reduced)
- Fasting insulin: 8 uIU/mL (reduced)
- Cholesterol: 226 mg/dL (reduced)
- Triglycerides: 158 mg/dL (reduced)
- LDL cholesterol: 166 mg/dL (reduced)

So, without any diabetic medications, this patient lowered her A1C from 8.3 to 4.8 percent in three months! There is no limit to how far an A1C can drop in three months. Edith had gone from totally out of control diabetes to totally in control diabetes.

Seven months after Edith's first treatment visit, her weight was down to 149 pounds, a BMI of 26, only slightly overweight. In seven months, Edith had lost nearly 100 pounds. Her blood pressure was well controlled without any medications.

Here were a few of her labs (her lipids were a little higher since she had been sneaking sugary candies):

- A1C: 4.8 percent
- Cholesterol: 251 mg/dL
- HDL cholesterol: 45 mg/dL
- LDL cholesterol: 185 mg/dL

Patients fall off the diet now and then, and blood work and a diet diary will usually uncover that right away.

I changed Edith's supplement regimen somewhat: multiple vitamin/mineral, R-alpha-lipoic acid, a green powder (chlorella, spirulina, etc.), lecithin granules, natural cholesterol product, diabetes specialty supplement, folic acid, vitamin E, garlic, and fish oils. This sounds like a lot, but we had a good goal. Edith was adamant about not going on a statin drug, which I didn't want to prescribe anyway, and she had an extensive family history of cardiovascular disease.

Ten months after Edith's first treatment visit, and with no more sugary candies, her labs were perfect:

- A1C: 4.7 percent
- Fasting plasma glucose: 95 mg/dL

- Cholesterol: 211 mg/dL
- Triglycerides: 86 mg/dL
- HDL cholesterol: 56 mg/dL
- LDL cholesterol: 141 mg/dL

Edith's improvement was stable and steady; she had reversed her diabetes, her obesity, and her hypertension. Nearly two years into treating Edith, she was down to 140 pounds, with a BMI of 24, a completely normal weight for her height. Her blood pressure without any medications was 138/78 mmHg.

Her labs were still excellent:

- A1C: 4.6 percent
- Fasting plasma glucose: 76 mg/dL
- Cholesterol: 221 mg/dL
- Triglycerides: 74 mg/dL
- HDL cholesterol: 60 mg/dL
- LDL cholesterol: 142 mg/dL

Three years after first visit, Edith's weight was down to 132 pounds, her BMI was at 23, and her blood pressure was 138/74 mmHg. Her labs were *still* perfect:

- A1C: 4.8 percent
- Cholesterol: 196 mg/dL
- LDL cholesterol: 129 mg/dL
- HDL cholesterol: 51 mg/dL

This patient continued to do well. It is lovely to see that an integrative protocol truly does work in motivated patients. Edith is another who if she went to a new physician today, would never be diagnosed with diabetes. Edith was a victor over diabetes!

Case Study #5

Joseph was a teen who came to see me in July of 2013; he had been diagnosed with T1DM in February of that year. A school exam had uncovered glucose in his urine in June of 2012, but that unusual finding, a warning sign, had been ignored. Things had slowly progressed so that symptoms began developing in December of 2012, and he was diagnosed in the emergency room in February.

Joseph was told to eat whatever he wanted and cover it with insulin, as the vast majority of children are told to do. He began Lantus and Humalog insulins. He went into a honeymoon period within weeks, and when he saw me he was only taking one unit of Lantus in the morning. His A1C was 6.2 percent, fasting glucose was 112 mg/dL, and his c-peptide was 2.2 ng/mL, still showing a functional pancreas. Although his A1C was not ideal, the majority of teens with T1DM have A1Cs averaging 9.0 percent, so he was certainly in much better control overall.

Joseph was only checking his glucose levels before meals, not after, so he did not know how his food was affecting his glucose levels. He had never had a serious low, and he had a T1DM bracelet ID. His celiac and thyroid panels were negative. He was already five feet ten inches and weighed 131 pounds. Joseph exercised weekly in school swim club, skateboarding, and by being a golf caddy. His mother was very supportive of him and involved in his diabetes care.

A diet diary showed that Joseph was eating bread, ketchup, applesauce, honey, burritos, and bean soups, foods that are in general going to raise glucose levels significantly in diabetic patients.

My comprehensive protocol with Joseph began with a grain-free, low-carb diet, with adequate protein and fat, and I switched his Lantus to evening. I added in a multiple vitamin/mineral, fish oils, R-alpha-lipoic acid, a diabetes specialty supplement, niacinamide, and vitamin D_3.

Three months later his A1C was 5.7 percent, his fasting glucose was 99 mg/dL, his c-peptide was down to 1.35, and he was still only on 1 unit of Lantus at bedtime. His diet diary showed that he was following the diet very well, drinking healthy smoothies, eating salads, and enjoying nut flour based "grain" products. He knew how to manage his diet so that when out with his friends, he could modify menu items and still feel full, so he didn't miss out on having an active social life.

Nearly a year later, in 2014, Joseph was losing his honeymoon period. His c-peptide was down to 0.6 ng/mL, and he had to increase his Lantus dosing at night. By the end of 2014, Joseph required 16 units of Lantus at night, and

2 units in the morning, and finally needed to start adding in mealtime bolus insulin. So, Joseph had gone almost two years only needing basal insulin, which is a good, long honeymoon period. Once he was on full basal and bolus dosing, Joseph got a CGMS to monitor his glucose better.

Since growth hormone and sexual hormones, both of which are plentiful during adolescence and puberty, cause insulin resistance, even in teens with T1DM, Joseph's A1C snuck up to 6.5 percent, which we discovered when we were together figuring out how much insulin he needed to keep injecting. He also had stopped exercising for many months, and Joseph realized that exercising really helped lower his glucose numbers. However, he had no serious lows.

Joseph embraced his diabetes with a supportive mom and a good comprehensive protocol that made sense to him. He had good energy, the ability to be active, and could handle eating out with nondiabetic friends. By returning to an exercise regimen, he got his A1C down, and he is now at college. Joseph is happy to share his story and to help other teens feel inspired and motivated to live life well with diabetes.

Case History #6

I had been treating Lisa for T1DM for twelve years when she married and became pregnant with her first child in May of 2014. She was thirty-four years old. Lisa was on a pump, and I had her basals under good control; her A1Cs for the vast majority of our time together were nearly always lower than 5.5 percent. Lisa also had a CGMS, and that was helpful for me to reset a basal dose here and there.

It's best for a woman with T1DM to be in excellent control before she becomes pregnant, and be committed to having excellent glucose monitoring during the pregnancy. During pregnancy, due to elevated estrogen levels, insulin resistance develops and the mother with T1DM will require a lot more insulin dosing. I explained all this to Lisa, who was fully prepared and excited.

Lisa had some nausea until week fifteen, which is common in pregnancy. Of course, in general we tell pregnant women who are nauseous to eat crackers and, frequently, to eat inbetween meals, but this is problematic for a T1DM patient, who has to work hard to control glucose numbers. Ginger capsules helped for a while, but the nausea eventually turned very serious, so Lisa was put on antinausea medications for a time. But by week fifteen she was off them and feeling much better.

Lisa followed her typical low-carb diet, "cheating" now and then on higher carb foods. I had prescribed a prenatal vitamin/mineral, fish oils, and vitamin D_3 (with vitamins A and K). I had her stop her diabetes specialty supplement because it contained berberine, and that is not considered a safe drug for pregnancy.

Lisa was considered a high-risk pregnancy due to her T1DM, so her gynecologist had her A1C drawn each month. They started at 5.6 percent, and then were 5.1–5.3 percent for the rest of her pregnancy. As the pregnancy progressed, Lisa started seeing insulin resistance appear, and she realized how much more insulin she needed to inject, even eating her low-carb diet. When she was not pregnant, she injected a total of 24–30 units of insulin a day. Meals could be covered with 2–4 units. When she was thirty weeks pregnant, however, her total daily insulin dosing was 60 units, and she needed to inject 8–10 units with the same meal.

Lisa and I worked to create her birth plan, so she could instruct the delivery staff on her labor and childbirth guidelines. She wanted to keep using her insulin pump as long as possible through labor, delivery, and birth, even though hospitals prefer to put diabetic patients on IVs to monitor glucose levels and dose insulin. Lisa was adamant that she did not want to be on an IV glucose drip combined with a sliding scale of insulin. She also wrote in her plan she would wear her CGMS, and she did allow the hospital staff to check her glucose via her glucose monitor kit.

Lisa explained how she would manage hypoglycemic events, including what she would do at different levels of low and high glucose. She and I created specific instructions so the hospital staff would know exactly what treatment would occur if hypoglycemia or hyperglycemia occurred. Lisa also explained other details of the birth, in relation to her newborn.

Lisa delivered a healthy baby boy in January of 2015. Immediately after the delivery, Lisa had significantly reduced insulin needs.

Having T1DM means one can marry, have children, and be a wonderful mother. Well controlled T1DM allows for life to be lived to its fullest, and for all the joys and wonders to be equally experienced.

Summary

Instead of treating diabetes as a progressive condition where a person needs more and more medicines and insulin, and then develops complications, we can instead control it amazingly well. Weight can be lost. Lipids and blood pressure can return to normal. Medicines at times can be avoided, or removed.

There should be nothing scary about diabetes. When diabetes is well controlled a person can anticipate living a long, healthy life doing everything they wish with joy—having children, being physically active, having the energy to do what they wish when they want.

Diabetes is a potentially dangerous condition *only* when it is poorly controlled. It does not have to ever be poorly controlled if the physician is knowledgeable about comprehensive integrative care and takes the time to educate and support every single patient. Yes, T1DM and T2DM patients need to make necessary changes to their diet and lifestyle and take well-prescribed supplements. Bread is exchanged for healthy eyes, kidneys, and nerves and the avoidance of cardiovascular disease, fatty liver, and Alzheimer's. Who wouldn't agree to that exchange?

This protocol *works*. I have been using it for nearly thirty years in my practice with consistent and remarkable success. I formed the nonprofit Low Carb Diabetes Association to be able to spread the word to more patients, caregivers, and medical practitioners. Please join at lowcarbdiabetes.org to further your learning and join with others to give and get support, motivation, and inspiration.

This protocol is the truth about diabetes and the way for all diabetic patients to become empowered. There *is* hope. There *are* answers. You are not helpless against this disease. It is yours to control. It is yours to gain victory over.

— APPENDIX A —

Resources

Diabetes Organizations, Associations, and Groups

American Diabetes Association: This is a conventional diabetes organization designed to prevent and cure diabetes and to improve the lives of all people affected by diabetes. (www.diabetes.org)

International Diabetes Federation: The IDF is an umbrella organization of over 230 national diabetes associations in 170 countries and territories. (www.idf.org)

Juvenile Diabetes Research Foundation: The JDRF is the leading global organization funding T1DM research. (www.jdrf.org)

Low Carb Diabetes Association: The author's nonprofit organization. (www.lowcarb diabetes.org)

Diabetes Information and Support Websites

In addition to the following websites, there are also several groups on Facebook where a diabetic person interested in integrative care and in eating low carb can find camaraderie, support, recipes, and advice, including the *Low Carb Diabetes Association, The Vegetarian Low Carb Diabetic Healthy Diet Society,* and *Dr. Richard K. Bernstein's Diabetes Solution Advocates.*

Children with Diabetes: An online community for kids, families, and adults with diabetes. It is conventionally based but has a wide variety of diabetes information and resources. (www.childrenwithdiabetes.org)

Diabetes and the Environment: A website by Sarah Howard that is a leading source of information regarding studies and information on environmental toxins as potential etiological factors in T1DM and T2DM. (www.diabetesandenvironment.org)

Diabetes.co.uk: A global community of people with diabetes, family members, friends, supporters, and caregivers, offering support and firsthand knowledge. (www.diabetes .co.uk)

Diabetes in Control: A conventionally based website designed to give news and information to medical professionals. (www.diabetesincontrol.com)

diaTribe: An organization designed to "make sense of diabetes," discussing a wide variety of topics regarding diabetes. (www.diatribe.org)

Diet Doctor: A very popular and highly respected ketogenic based website run by Dr. Andreas Eenfeldt, rich with information on low-carb, ketogenic diets and intermittent fasting. (www.dietdoctor.com)

Health-e-Solutions: This website contains very helpful training courses on eating low carb, and I also recommend their ebooks, which cover vegan low-glycemic diets, low-carb diets with animal products, and smoothie recipes. (www.healthesolutions.com)

Books

300 15-Minute Low-Carb Meals by Dana Carpender (Beverly, MA: Fair Winds Press, 2003).

The 30-Day Ketogenic Cleanse by Maria Emmerich (Las Vegas, NV: Victory Belt Publishing, 2016).

The Art and Science of Low Carbohydrate Living by Jeff S. Volek, PhD, RD, and Stephen D. Phinney, MD, PhD (Miami, FL: Beyond Obesity, 2011).

The Art and Science of Low Carbohydrate Performance Living by Jeff S. Volek, PhD, RD, and Stephen D. Phinney, MD, PhD (Miami, FL: Beyond Obesity, 2012).

The Case against Sugar by Gary Taubes (New York, NY: Alfred A. Knopf, 2016).

The Complete Guide to Fasting by Jimmy Moore and Dr. Jason Fung (Las Vegas, NV: Victory Belt Publishing, 2016).

The Complete Low-Carb Cookbook by George Stella (Brandon, MS: Quail Ridge Press, 2014).

Diabetes Burnout by William H. Polonsky, PhD (Alexandria, VA: American Diabetes Association, 1999). A classic book, designed to help people with diabetes better handle the stresses of having diabetes.

Dr. Bernstein's Diabetes Solution by Richard K. Bernstein, MD (Boston, MA: Little Brown and Company, 1997). The original bible of low-carb diets and correct insulin dosing. It remains a classic book.

The Ketogenic Diet for Type 1 Diabetes by Ellen Davis, MS, and Keith Runyan, MD (www.ketogenic-diet-resource.com, 2015). A self-published ebook full of recipes for diabetic patients eating a low-carb ketogenic diet.

The Obesity Code by Dr. Jason Fung (Vancouver, BC: Greystone Books, 2016).

The World Turned Upside Down by Richard David Feinman, PhD (Brooklyn, NY: NMS Press-Duck-in-a-Boat, 2014).

Alternative Food Purchasing

Nota Bene: I am not a fan of using sucralose, except now and then in products such as fruit jam or barbecue sauce, when the typical sugary product should not be used.

DaVinci Gourmet: Sugar-free syrups and flavorings (www.davincigourmet.com).

Frontier Co-op: Organic spices, herbs, and flavorings (www.frontiercoop.com).

Gerbs Allergen Friendly Foods: Raw pumpkin, sunflower, chia, flax, and hemp seed meal (www.mygerbs.com).

Nature's Hollow: Products made with xylitol (www.natureshollow.com).

Nuts.com: A wide variety of nuts and seeds for making flours (www.nuts.com).
Walden Farms: Products made with sucralose (www.waldenfarms.com).

Recipes

There are many recipes online—any quick search for a low-carb recipe will bring up thousands of choices. Skinny on Low Carb (margeburkell.com), for example, contains lots of recipes, including twenty-one ways to make oopsie rolls. In addition, there are many groups on social media where people share recipes. Pinterest (www.pinterest.com), for example, lets users post pictures and recipes, and features many groups, including Low Carb, and Low Carb High Fat, where you can find innovative low-carb recipes and helpful hints for maintaining a low-carb diet.

Nutrition and Diet Trackers and Apps

Carb Manager: An internet and smartphone app for recording one's daily diet, and for analyzing macronutrients (www.carbmanager.com).

CarbProtein Insulin Calculator: It is the only calculator that includes protein at meals for insulin dosing, since proteins also raise glucose levels. It will accurately report mealtime and correction insulin dosage either in rapid or regular insulin. It is very simple to use.

Doc's Diabetes Diary: This free phone app, available in Apple's iTunes store, is designed to be both a diet diary and a glucose graph. It can be emailed to your physician before your office visit (www.itunes.apple.com).

MyFitnessPal: An internet and smartphone app for recording one's daily diet, and for analyzing macronutrients (www.myfitnesspal.com).

SELF Nutrition Data: Analyzes carb and protein content in food per serving (www.nutritiondata.self.com).

SuperTracker: Provides diet information for adults and pediatrics, including micronutrients such as omega-3 oils, zinc, and chromium (supertracker.usda.gov).

— APPENDIX B —

Diet Diary

DIET DIARY GUIDELINES: The purpose of this diary is not to judge your eating habits, but to learn more about your nutritional, biochemical, and hormonal needs and strengths. Write down **EVERYTHING** you eat and drink for meals and snacks and **AMOUNTS**. List **BRAND NAMES** of foods you bought in a supermarket. List **EXACT INGREDIENTS** of homemade foods. Under the SYMPTOM column please record any problematic symptoms you experienced and the time of day any occurred. Under BM, please list the time you had a bowel movement and if it was D (diarrhea) or C (constipation). **Record type and amount of insulin injected (if pertinent).**

Patient Name: ______________________________

Date to Begin: ______________________________

	BREAKFAST Times	LUNCH Times
Day One		
Day Two		
Day Three		
Day Four		
Day Five		
Day Six		
Day Seven		

SUPPER Times	SYMPTOMS Times	BM Times

— APPENDIX C —

Glucose Graph

Record Time and Glucose	Fasting	After Breakfast	Before Lunch	After Lunch	Before Supper
Day One					
Day Two					
Day Three					
Day Four					
Day Five					
Day Six					
Day Seven					

FULL RECORD FOR PATIENTS

Patient Name: ______________________________ Dates of Graph: ____________

Dr.'s Phone #: __________________________ / _____________________________

GUIDELINES: Record blood sugars at listed times. **After a meal means 1.5 hours after eating**. Record times, too. Also record time of exercise, length of exercise, and type of exercise.

After Supper	Bedtime	Middle of the Night	Before Exercise	During Exercise	After Exercise

Bibliography

ACR Committee on Drugs and Contrast Media. *ACR Manual on Contrast Media, Version 10.2*. American College of Radiology;2016. http://www.acr.org/~/media/37D84428BF1D4E1B9A3A2918DA9E27A3.pdf. Accessed June 7, 2017.

Action to Control Cardiovascular Risk in Diabetes Study Group. Effects of intensive glucose lowering in Type 2 diabetes. *N Engl J Med*. 2008;358:2545–2559. doi:10.1056/NEJMoa0802743.

ADA: Teenagers with Type 1 diabetes not even close to meeting goals. Diabetes in Control. http://www.diabetesincontrol.com/articles/53-/16557-ada-teenagers-with-type-1-diabetes-not-even-close-to-meeting-goals. Published July 4, 2014. Accessed November 28, 2016.

Afkhami-Ardekani M, Shojaoddiny-Ardekani A. Effect of vitamin C on blood glucose, serum lipids and serum insulin in Type 2 diabetes patients. *Indian J Med Res*. 2007;126(5):471–474. http://www.ncbi.nlm.nih.gov/pubmed/18160753.

Ahn S, Song R. Effects of Tai Chi exercise on glucose control, neuropathy scores, balance, and quality of life in patients with Type 2 diabetes and neuropathy. *J Altern Complement Med*. 2012;18(12):1172–1178. doi:10.1089/acm.2011.0690.

Aigner E, Weiss G, Datz C. Dysregulation of iron and copper homeostasis in nonalcoholic fatty liver. *World J Hepatol*. 2015;7(2):177–188. doi:10.4254/wjh.v7.i2.177.

Alisi A, Ceccarelli S, Panera N, Nobili V. Causative role of gut microbiota in non-alcoholic fatty liver disease pathogenesis. *Front Cell Infect Microbiol*. 2012;2:132. doi:10.3389/fcimb.2012.00132.

Aljabri KS, Bokhari SA, Kahn MJ. Glycemic changes after vitamin D supplementation in patients with Type 1 diabetes mellitus and vitamin D deficiency. *Ann Saudi Med*. 2010;30(6):454–458. doi:10.4103/0256-4947.72265.

Allen RW, Schwartzman E, Baker WL, Coleman CI, Phung OJ. Cinnamon use in Type 2 diabetes: An updated systematic review and meta-analysis. *Ann Fam Med*. 2013;11(5):452–459. doi:10.1370/afm.1517.

American Diabetes Association. Classification and diagnosis of diabetes. *Diabetes Care*. 2015;38(suppl 1):S8–S16. doi:10.2337/dc15-S005.

———. Diabetes care at diabetes camps. *Diabetes Care*. 2006;29(suppl 1):s56–s58. https://www.ncbi.nlm.nih.gov/pubmed/16373934.

———. Implications of the United Kingdom Prospective Diabetes Study. *Diabetes Care*. 2002;25(suppl 1):s28–s32. doi:10.2337/diacare.25.2007.S28.

———. Introduction. *Diabetes Care*. 2015;38 (suppl 1). doi:10.2337/dc15-S001.

———. Standards of medical care in diabetes—2016. *Diabetes Care*. 2016;39(suppl 1). http://care.diabetesjournals.org/content/suppl/2015/12/21/39.Supplement_1.DC2/2016-Standards-of-Care.pdf.

American Diabetes Association releases new nutritional guidelines. American Diabetes Association. http://www.diabetes.org/newsroom/press-releases/2013/american-diabetes-association-releases-nutritional-guidelines.html. Published October 9, 2013. Accessed June 9, 2017.

Arab JP, Candia R, Zapata R, et al. Management of nonalcoholic fatty liver disease: An evidence-based clinical practice review. *World J Gastroenterol*. 2014;20(34):12182–12201. doi:10.3748/wjg.v20.i34.12182.

Babaei-Jadidi R, Karachalias N, Ahmed N, Battah S, Thornalley PJ. Prevention of incipient diabetic nephropathy by high-dose thiamine and benfotiamine. *Diabetes*. 2003;52(8):2110–2120. doi:10.2337/diabetes.52.8.2110.

Bakris GL, Glassock RJ. Microalbuminuria: Is it even a word anymore? Medscape. http://www.medscape.com/viewarticle/804835. Published June 3, 2013.

Balsells M, García-Patterson A, Solà I, Roqué M, Gich I, Corcoy R. Glibenclamide, metformin, and insulin for the treatment of gestational diabetes: A systematic review and meta-analysis. *BMJ*. 2015;350:h102. doi:10.1136/bmj.h102.

Baltatzi M, Cavopoulos C, Hatzitolios A. Role of angiotensin converting enzyme inhibitors and angiotensin receptor blockers in hypertension of chronic kidney disease and renoprotection. *Hippokratia*. 2011;15(suppl 1):27–32. https://www.ncbi.nlm.nih.gov/pmc/articles/PMC3139675.

Barbagallo M, Dominguez LJ. Magnesium and Type 2 diabetes. *World J Diabetes*. 2015;6(10):1152–1157. doi:10.4239/wjd.v6.i10.1152.

———. Type 2 diabetes mellitus and Alzheimer's disease. *World J Diabetes*. 2014;5(6):889–893. doi:10.4239/wjd.v5.i6.889.

Barbour L, McCurdy CE, Hernandez TL, Kirwan JP, Catalano PM, Friedman JE. Cellular mechanisms for insulin resistance in normal pregnancy and gestational diabetes. *Diabetes Care*. 2007;30(suppl 2):S112–S119. doi:10.2337/dc07-s202.

Bash LD, Selvin E, Steffes M, Coresh J, Astor BC. Poor glycemic control in diabetes and the risk of incident chronic kidney disease even in the absence of albuminuria and retinopathy: Atherosclerosis Risk in Communities (ARIC) Study. *Arch Intern Med*. 2008;168(22):2240–2247. http://www.natap.org/2008/HIV/120908_05.htm. Accessed November 28, 2016.

Bauman WA, Shaw S, Jayatilleke E, Spungen AM, Herbert V. Increased intake of calcium reverses vitamin B12 malabsorption induced by metformin. *Diabetes Care*. 2000;23(9):1227–1231. doi:10.2337/diacare.23.9.1227.

Bell DS. Metformin-induced vitamin B12 deficiency presenting as a peripheral neuropathy. *South Med J*. 2010;103(3):265–267. doi:10.1097/SMJ.0b013e3181ce0e4d.

Benbrook C, Zhao X, Yáñez J, Davies N, Andrews P. New evidence confirms the nutritional superiority of plant-based organic foods. The Organic Center. https://www.organic-center.org/reportfiles/5367_Nutrient_Content_SSR_FINAL_V2.pdf. Published March 2008. Accessed June 9, 2017.

Bender M, Rader JI. Guidance for industry: Nutrition labeling manual—a guide for developing and using data bases. FDA. https://www.fda.gov/Food/GuidanceRegulation/GuidanceDocumentsRegulatoryInformation/LabelingNutrition/ucm063113.htm. Published March 17, 1998. Updated July 5, 2016.

Bener A, Alsaied A, Al-Ali M, et al. High prevalence of vitamin D deficiency in Type 1 diabetes mellitus and healthy children. *Act Diabetol*. 2009;46(3):183–189. doi:10.1007/s00592-008-0071-6.

Bhattacharyya A, Brown S, Hughes S, Vice PA. Insulin lispro and regular insulin in pregnancy. *QJM*. 2001;94(5):255–260. http://www.ncbi.nlm.nih.gov/pubmed/11353099.

Blair SN, Kohl HW, Paffenbarger RS, Clark DG, Cooper KH, Gibbons LW. Physical fitness and all-cause mortality: A prospective study of healthy men and women. *JAMA*. 1989;262(17):2395–2401. https://www.ncbi.nlm.nih.gov/pubmed/2795824.

Borcea V, Nourooz-Zadeh J, Wolff SP, et al. Alpha-lipoic acid decreases oxidative stress even in diabetic patients with poor glycemic control and albuminuria. *Free Radic Biol Med*. 1999;26(11–12):1495–1500. doi:10.1016/S0891-5849(99)00011-8.

Bordia A, Verma SK, Srivastava KC. Effect of garlic (*Allium sativum*) on blood lipids, blood sugar, fibrinogen and fibrinolytic activity in patients with coronary artery disease. *Prostaglandins Leukot Essent Fatty Acids*. 1998;58(4):257–263. http://www.ncbi.nlm.nih.gov/pubmed/9654398.

Bosi E, Molteni L, Radaelli MG, et al. Increased intestinal permeability precedes clinical onset of Type 1 diabetes. *Diabetologia*. 2006;49(12):2824–2827. doi:10.1007/s00125-006-0465-3.

Bredesen DE. Reversal of cognitive decline: A novel therapeutic program. *Aging (Albany NY)*. 2014;6(9):707–717. https://www.ncbi.nlm.nih.gov/pubmed/25324467.

Brooks M. SGLT2 inhibitor diabetes drugs may cause ketoacidosis: FDA. Medscape. http://www.medscape.com/viewarticle/844754. Published May 15, 2015. Accessed November 29, 2016.

Brown M, Ferruzzi MG, Nguyen Minhthy, et al. Carotenoid bioavailability is higher from salads ingested with full-fat than with fat-reduced salad dressings as measured with electrochemical detection. *Am J Clin Nutr*. 2004;80(2):396–403. http://www.ajcn.org/cgi/content/abstract/80/2/396.

Bryden KS, Dunger DB, Mayou RA, Peveler RC, Neil AW. Poor prognosis of young adults with Type 1 diabetes. *Diabetes Care*. 2003;26(4):1052–1057. doi:10.2337/diacare.26.4.1052.

Busko M. High-fat diet best for diabetes prevention in obesity prone. Medscape. http://www.medscape.com/viewarticle/865525. Published June 29, 2016.

———. Safety of incretin-based therapies hotly debated. Medscape. http://www.medscape.com/viewarticle/803794. Published May 8, 2013. Accessed November 29, 2016.

Busse N, Paroni F, Richardson SJ, et al. Detection and localization of viral infection in the pancreas of patients with Type 1 using short fluorescently-labelled oligonucleotide probes. *Oncotarget*. 2017;8:12620–12636. doi:10.18632/oncotarget.14896.

Canner PL, Furberg CD, Terrin ML, McGovern ME. Benefits of niacin by glycemic status in patients with healed myocardial infarction. *Am J Cardiol*. 2005;95(2):254–257. doi:10.1016/j.amjcard.2004.09.013.

Cardwell CR, Stene LC, Ludvigsson J, et al. Breast-feeding and childhood-onset Type 1 diabetes. *Diabetes Care*. 2012;35(11):2215–2225. doi:10.2337/dc12-0438.

Caricilli AM, Saad MJ. The role of gut microbiota on insulin resistance. *Nutrients*. 2013;5(3):829–851. doi:10.3390/nu5030829.

Castenada C, Layne JE, Munoz-Orians L, et al. A randomized controlled trial of resistance exercise training to improve glycemic control in older adults with Type 2 diabetes. *Diabetes Care*. 2002;25(12):2335–2341. http://faculty.ksu.edu.sa/hazzaa/Resources/Resistance Exercise Training and diabetes - Diab Care 2002.pdf.

Celmer L. CPAP improves glycemic control in Type 2 diabetics with sleep apnea. American Academy of Sleep Medicine. http://www.aasmnet.org/articles.aspx?id=3932. Published June 3, 2013.

Centers for Disease Control and Prevention (CDC). A1c distribution among adults with diagnosed diabetes, United States, 1988–1994 to 1999–2006. *Diabetes Public Health Resource*. http://www.cdc.gov/diabetes/statistics/a1c/a1c_dist.htm. Updated October 2, 2014. Accessed November 28, 2016.

———. *CDC's Second Nutrition Report: A Comprehensive Biochemical Assessment of the Nutrition Status of the U.S. Population*. National Center for Environmental Health: Division of Laboratory Sciences; 2012. https://www.cdc.gov/nutritionreport.

———. *Fourth National Report on Human Exposure to Environmental Chemicals*. National Center for Environmental Health, Division of Laboratory Sciences. 2015. http://www.cdc.gov/biomonitoring/pdf/FourthReport_UpdatedTables_Feb2015.pdf.

Chalasani N, Younossi Z, Lavine JE, et al. The diagnosis and management of non-alcoholic fatty liver disease. *Hepatology*, 2012;55(6):2005–2023. https://www.aasld.org/sites/default/files/guideline_documents/NonalcoholicFattyLiverDisease2012.pdf.

Chausmer AB. Zinc, insulin and diabetes. *J Am Coll Nutr*. 1998;17(2):109–115. https://www.ncbi.nlm.nih.gov/pubmed/9550453.

Cheng YJ, Gregg EW, Geiss LS, et al. Association of A1C and fasting plasma glucose levels with diabetic retinopathy prevalence in the U.S. population: Implications for diabetes diagnostic thresholds. *Diabetes Care*. 2009;32(11):2027–2032. doi:10.2337/dc09-0440.

Chevrier J, Dewailly É, Ayotte P, Mauriege P, Despres J-P, Tremblay A. Body weight loss increases plasma and adipose tissue concentrations of potentially toxic pollutants in obese individuals. *Int J Obes*. 2000;24(10):1272–1278. http://www.nature.com/ijo/journal/v24/n10/full/0801380a.html.

Chuengsamarn S, Rattanamongkolgul S, Luechapudiporn R, Phisalaphong C, Jirawatnotai S. Curcumin extract for prevention of Type 2 diabetes. *Diabetes Care*. 2012;35(11):2121–2127. doi:10.2337/dc12-0116.

Classen B. Vaccines and T1DM. *N Z Med J*. 1996.

Colberg SR, Grieco CR, Somma CT. Exercise effects on postprandial glycemia, mood, and sympathovagal balance in Type 2 diabetes. *J Am Med Dir Assoc*. 2014;15(4):261–266. doi:10.1016/j.jamda.2013.11.026.

Copeland KC, Silverstein J, Moore KR, et al. Management of newly diagnosed Type 2 diabetes mellitus (T2DM) in children and adolescents. *Am Acad Ped*. 2013;131(2):364–382. http://pediatrics.aappublications.org/content/131/2/364.full.pdf.

Cordain L, Watkins BA, Florant GL, Kelher M, Rogers L, Li Y. Fatty acid analysis of wild ruminant tissues: Evolutionary implications for reducing diet-related chronic disease. *Eur J Clin Nutr*. 2002;56(3):181–191. http://www.nature.com/ejcn/journal/v56/n3/full/1601307a.html.

Crinò A, Schiaffini R, Manfrini S, et al. A randomized trial of nicotinamide and vitamin E in children with recent onset Type 1 diabetes. *Eur J Endocrinol*. 2004;150(5):719–724. http://www.ncbi.nlm.nih.gov/pubmed/15132730.

Cuellar NG. A comparison of glycemic control, sleep, fatigue, and depression in Type 2 diabetes with and without restless legs syndrome. *JCSM*. 2008;4(1):50–56. http://www.aasmnet.org/JCSM/Articles/040109.pdf.

Cusi K, Cukier S, DeFronzo RA, Torres M, Puchulu FM, Pereira Redondo. Vanadyl sulfate improves hepatic and muscle insulin sensitivity in Type 2 diabetes. *J Clin Endocrinol Metab*. 2001;86(3):1410–1417. doi:10.1210/jcem.86.3.7337.

Czupryniak L, Wolffenbuttel BHR. Patient ethnicity alters A1c goals. Medscape. http://www.medscape.com/viewarticle/773265. Published October 25, 2012.

D'Alessandro ME, Lombardo YB, Chicco A. Effect of dietary fish oil on insulin sensitivity and metabolic fate of glucose in the skeletal muscle of normal rats. *Ann Nutr Metab*. 2002;46(3–4):114–120. https://www.ncbi.nlm.nih.gov/pubmed/12169854.

Dalgård C, Petersen MS, Weihe P, Grandjean P. Vitamin D status in relation to glucose metabolism and Type 2 diabetes in septuagenarians. *Diabetes Care*. 2011;34(6):1284–1288. http://care.diabetesjournals.org/content/34/6/1284.full.

Dashti HM, Methew TC, Hussein T, et al. Long-term effects of a ketogenic diet in obese patients. *Exp Clin Cardiol*. 2004;9(3):200–205. https://www.ncbi.nlm.nih.gov/pmc/articles/PMC2716748.

Davidson J. Should postprandial glucose be measured and treated to a particular target? Yes. *Diabetes Care*. 2003;26(6):1919–1921. doi:10.2337/diacare.26.6.1919.

DCCT and EDIC: The Diabetes Control and Complications Trial and Follow-Up Study. U.S. Department of Health and Human Services; 2008. https://www.niddk.nih.gov/about-niddk/research-areas/diabetes/dcct-edic-diabetes-control-complications-trial-follow-up-study/Documents/DCCT-EDIC_508.pdf.

de Goffau MC, Luopajarvi K, et al. Fecal microbiota composition differs between children with B-cell autoimmunity and those without. *Diabetes*. 2013;62(4):1238–1244. doi: 10.2337/db12-0526.

De Jager J, et al. Long term treatment with metformin in patients with Type 2 diabetes and risk of vitamin B-12 deficiency: Randomised placebo controlled trial. *BMJ*. 2010;340:c2181. doi:10.1136/bmj.c2181.

Dean L, McEntyre J. *The Genetic Landscape of Diabetes*. Bethesda, MD: National Center for Biotechnology Information (US); 2004.

DeFeyter HM, Praet SF, van den Broek NM, et al. Exercise training improves glycemic control in long-standing insulin-treated Type 2 diabetic patients. *Diabetes Care*. 2007; 30(10):2511–2513. doi:10.2337/dc07-0183.

Delanaye P, Schaeffner E, Ebert N, et al. Normal reference values for glomerular filtration rate: What do we really know? *Nephrol Dial Transplant*. 2012;27(7):2664–2672. doi:10.1093/ndt/gfs265.

Demmer RT, Jacobs DR, Desvarieux M. Periodontal disease and incident of Type 2 diabetes. *Diabetes Care*. 2008;31(7):1373–1379. doi:10.2337/dc08-0026.

Devaraj S, Hemarajata P, Versalovic J. The human gut microbiome and body metabolism: Implications for obesity and diabetes. *Clin Chem*. 2013;59(4):617–628. doi:10.1373/clinchem.2012.187617.

Diabetes Control and Complications Trial Research Group. The effect of intensive treatment of diabetes on the development and progression of long-term complications in insulin dependent diabetes mellitus. *N Engl J Med*. 1993;329:977–986. doi:10.1056/NEJM199309303291401.

Diabetes and prediabetes tests. National Institute of Diabetes and Digestive and Kidney Diseases. https://www.niddk.nih.gov/health-information/health-topics/diagnostic-tests/comparing-tests-diabetes-prediabetes/Pages/index.aspx. Published April 2014. Accessed November 28, 2016.

Diabetes Prevention Program Research Group. Intensive lifestyle intervention or metformin on inflammation and coagulation in participants with impaired glucose tolerance. *Diabetes*. 2005;54(5):1566–1572 https://www.ncbi.nlm.nih.gov/pmc/articles/PMC1314967.

———. The 10-year cost-effectiveness of lifestyle intervention or metformin for diabetes prevention. *Diabetes Care*. 2012;35(4):723–730. doi: 10.2337/dc11-1468.

Donadio JV, Larson TS, Bergstralh EJ, Grande JP. A randomized trial of high-dose compared with low-dose omega-3 fatty acids in severe IgA nephropathy. *J Am Soc Nephrol*. 2001; 12(4):791–799. https://www.ncbi.nlm.nih.gov/pubmed/11274240.

DuBroff RJ. The statin diabetes conundrum: Short-term gain, long-term risk or inconvenient truth? *Evid Based Med*. 2015;20(4):121–123. doi:10.1136/ebmed-2015-110236.

Einhorn D. American Association of Clinical Endocrinologists. American College of Endocrinology statement on the use of hemoglobin A1c for the diagnosis of diabetes. *Endocr Pract*. 2010;16(2):155–156. https://www.aace.com/files/position-statements/a1c positionstatement.pdf. Accessed November 28, 2016.

Ersoz G, Günsar F, Karasu Z, Akay S, Batur Y, Akarca US. Management of fatty liver disease with vitamin E and C compared to ursodeoxycholic acid treatment. *Turk J Gastroenterol*. 2005;16(3):124–128. https://www.ncbi.nlm.nih.gov/pubmed/16245220.

Faccini FS, Saylor KL. A low-iron-available, polyphenol-enriched, carbohydrate-restricted diet to slow progression of diabetic nephropathy. *Diabetes*. 2003;52(5):1204–1209. doi:10.2337/diabetes.52.5.1204.

Fang F, Kang Z, Wong C. Vitamin E tocotrienols improve insulin sensivity through activating peroxisome proliferator-activated receptors. *Mol Nutr Food Res*. 2010;54(3):345–352. http://www.ncbi.nlm.nih.gov/pubmed/19866471.

Feinman R, Pogozelski WK, Astrup A, et al. Dietary carbohydrate restriction as the first approach in diabetes management: Critical review and evidence base. *Nutrition*. 2015;31(1):1–13. doi: 10.1016/j.nut.2014.06.011.

Filippi CM, von Herrath MG. Viral triggers for Type 1 diabetes: Pros and cons. *Diabetes*. 2008;57(11):2863–2871. doi:10.2337/db07-1023.

Flack JM, Nasser SA, Levy PD. Therapy of hypertension in African Americans. *Am J Cardiovasc Drugs*. 2011;11(2):83–92. doi:10.2165/11586930-000000000-00000.

Foster GD. Obstructive sleep apnea and diabetes: What we know and what can be done? Diabetes Care.net. http://www.diabetescare.net/flash_article.asp?id=444835. Published June 21, 2010. Accessed June 7, 2017.

Fraser DA, Diep LM, Hovden IA, et al. The effects of long-term oral benfotiamine supplementation on peripheral nerve function and inflammatory markers in patients with Type 1 diabetes. *Diabetes Care*. 2012;35(5):1095–1097. doi:10.2337/dc11-1895.

Fujita N, Takei Y. Iron overload in nonalcoholic steatohepatitis. *Adv Clin Chem*. 2011;55: 105–132. https://www.ncbi.nlm.nih.gov/pubmed/22126026.

Gangswisch JE, Malaspina D, Boden-Albala B, Heymsfield SB. Inadequate sleep as a risk factor for obesity: Analyses of the NHANES I. *Sleep*. 2005;28(10)1289–1296. http://www.journalsleep.org/Articles/281017.pdf.

Gao Z, Yin J, Zhang J, et al. Butyrate improves insulin sensitivity and increases energy expenditure in mice. *Diabetes*. 2009;58(7):1509–1517. doi:10.2337/db08-1637.

Gill HK, Wu GY. Non-alcoholic fatty liver disease and the metabolic syndrome: Effects of weight loss and a review of popular diets. Are low carbohydrate diets the answer? *World J Gastroenterol*. 2006;12(3):345–353. doi:10.3748/wjg.v12.i3.345.

Glassock RJ, Winearls C. Ageing and the glomerula filtration rate: Truths and consequences. *Trans Am Clin Climatol Assoc*. 2009;120:419–428. https://www.ncbi.nlm.nih.gov/pmc/articles/PMC2744545.

Goldfine AB, Patti ME, Zuberi L, et al. Metabolic effects of vanadyl sulfate in humans with non-insulin-dependent diabetes mellitus: In vivo and in vitro studies. *Metabolism*. 2000;49(3):400–410. https://www.ncbi.nlm.nih.gov/pubmed/10726921.

Goldie C, Taylor AJ, Nguyen P, McCoy C, Zhao X-Q, Preiss D. Niacin therapy and the risk of new-onset diabetes: A meta-analysis of randomised controlled trials. *Heart*. 2016;102(3):198–203. http://heart.bmj.com/content/102/3/198.

Goldman E. When questioning clinical dogma is a doctor's duty. Holistic Primary Care. http://www.holisticprimarycare.net/topics/topics-a-g/cardiovascular-health/1494-when-questioning-clinical-dogma-is-a-doctors-duty. 2013;15(2). Published June 5, 2013. Accessed November 29, 2016.

Gomes MB, Negrato CA. Alpha-lipoic acid as a pleiotropic compound with potential therapeutic use in diabetes and other chronic diseases. *Diabetol Metab Syndr*. 2014;6:80. doi:10.1186/1758-5996-6-80.

Gonzales AM, Orlando RA. Curcumin and resveratrol inhibit nuclear factor-kappaB-mediated cytokine expression in adipocytes. *Nutr Metab*. 2008;5:17. doi:10.1186/1743-7075-5-17.

Goran MI, Gower BA. Longitudinal study on pubertal insulin resistance. *Diabetes*. 2001;50(11):2444–2450. doi:10.2337/diabetes.50.11.2444.

Graves DE, White JC, Kirk JK. The use of insulin glargine with gestational diabetes mellitus. *Diabetes Care*. 2006;29(2):471–472. doi:10.2337/diacare.29.02.06.dc05-2042.

Gross LS, Li L, Ford ES, Liu S. Increased consumption of refined carbohydrates and the epidemic of Type 2 diabetes in the ecologic assessment. *Am J Clin Nutr*. 2004;79(5):774–779. http://ajcn.nutrition.org/content/79/5/774.full.

Gu Y, Scarmeas N, Cosentino S, et al. Change in body mass index before and after Alzheimer's disease onset. *Curr Alzheimer Res*. 2014;11(4):349–356. https://www.ncbi.nlm.nih.gov/pmc/articles/PMC4026350.

Hajiana E, Hashemi SJ. Comparison of therapeutic effects of silymarin and vitamin E in nonalcoholic fatty liver disease: Results of an open-labeled, prospective, randomized study. *Jundishapur J Nat Pharm Prod*. 2007;4(1):8–14. http://jjnpp.com/?page=article&article_id=3213.

Hammes HP, Du X, Edelstein D, et al. Benfotiamine blocks three major pathways of hyperglycemic damage and prevents experimental diabetic retinopathy. *Nat Med*. 2003;9(3):294–299. http://www.ncbi.nlm.nih.gov/pubmed/12592403.

Hand L. Diabetes linked to phthalates. *Diabetes Care*. http://www.medscape.com/viewarticle/761957. Published April 12, 2012.

Handelsman Y. Potential place of SGLT2 inhibitors in treatment paradigms for Type 2 diabetes mellitus. *Endocr Pract*. 2015;21(9):1054–1065. doi:10.4158/EP15703.RA.

Handelsman Y, Bloomgarden ZT, Grunberger G, et al. American Association of Clinical Endocrinologists and American College of Endocrinology—Clinical practice guidelines for developing a diabetes mellitus comprehensive care plan. *Endocr Pract*. 2015;21(suppl 1). https://www.aace.com/files/dm-guidelines-ccp.pdf.

Harman J, Walker ER, Charbonneau V, Akylbekova EL, Nelson C, Wyatt SB. Treatment of hypertension among African Americans: The Jackson Heart Study. *J Clin Hypertens (Greenwich)*. 2013;15(6):367–374. doi:10.1111/jch.12088.

Harris SS. Vitamin D in Type 1 diabetes prevention. *J Nutr*. 2005;135(2):323–325. https://www.ncbi.nlm.nih.gov/pubmed/15671235.

Harrison L. High-intensity training no better than conventional training. Medscape. http://www.medscape.com/viewarticle/845794. Published June 2, 2015.

Haupt E, Ledermann H, Köpcke W. Benfotiamine in the treatment of diabetic polyneuropathy—a three-week randomized, controlled pilot study (BEDIP study). *Int J Clin Pharmacol Ther*. 2005;43(2):71–77. https://www.ncbi.nlm.nih.gov/pubmed/15726875.

Health benefits of grass-fed products. Eat Wild. http://www.eatwild.com/healthbenefits.htm. Accessed June 7, 2017.

Hegde S, Adhikari P, Kotian S, Pinto VJ, D'Souza S, D'Souza V. Effect of 3-month yoga on oxidative stress in Type 2 diabetes with or without complications: A controlled clinical trial. *Diabetes Care*. 2011;34(10):2208–2210. doi:10.2337/dc10-2430.

Heiman ML. OR40-5 improved oral glucose tolerance in prediabetics and Type 2 diabetics (T2D) in a pilot clinical trial testing a novel gastrointestinal (GI) microbiome modulator. Talk presented at: ICE/ENDO 2014. https://endo.confex.com/endo/2014endo/webprogram/Paper14546.html.

Hijikata Y, Yamada S. Walking just after a meal seems to be more effective for weight loss than waiting for one hour to walk after a meal. *Int J Gen Med*. 2011;4:447–450. doi:10.2147/IJGM.S18837.

How much sugar do you eat? You may be surprised! NH DHHS-DPHS-Health Promotion in Motion. http://www.dhhs.nh.gov/dphs/nhp/documents/sugar.pdf. Published August 2014. Accessed June 9, 2017.

Howard SG, Lee DH. What is the role of human contamination by environmental chemicals in the development of Type 1 diabetes? *J Epidemiol Community Health*. 2012;66(6):479–481. doi:10.1136/jech.2011.133694.

Hsia CH, Shen MC, Lin JS, et al. Nattokinase decreases plasma levels of fibrinogen, factor VII, and factor VIII in human subjects. *Nutr Res*. 2009;29(3):190–196. doi:10.1016/j.nutres.2009.01.009.

Hsieh F-C, Lee C-L, Chai C-Y, Chen W-T, Lu Y-C, Wu C-S. Oral administration of *Lactobacillus reuteri* GMNL-263 improves insulin resistance and ameliorates hepatic steatosis in high fructose-fed rats. *Nutr Metab (Lond)*. 2013;10(1):35. doi:10.1186/1743-7075-10-35.

Huebschmann AG, Regensteiner JG, Vlassara H, Reusch JEB. Diabetes and advanced glycoxidation end products. *Diabetes Care*. 2006;29(6):1420–1432. doi:10.2337/dc05-2096.

Hughes S. ONTARGET: Clear messages from well-conducted study. Medscape. http://www.medscape.com/viewarticle/572393. Published April 1, 2008.

Hviid A, Stellfeld M, Wohlfahrt J, Melbye M. Childhood vaccination and Type 1 diabetes. *NEJM*. 2004;350:1398–1404. doi:10.1056/NEJMoa032665.

Hyman MA. Environmental toxins, obesity, and diabetes: An emerging risk factor. *Altern Ther Health Med*. 2010;16(2):56–58. https://www.ncbi.nlm.nih.gov/pubmed/20232619.

———. Systems biology, toxins, obesity, and functional medicine. 13th International Symposium of the Institute for Functional Medicine. S134–S139. http://drhyman.com/downloads/Toxins-and-Obesity.pdf.

Ito T, Schaffer SW, Azuma J. The potential usefulness of taurine on diabetes mellitus and its complications. *Amino Acids*. 2012;42(5):1529–1539. doi:10.1007/s00726-011-0883-5.

Jacob S, Henriksen EJ, Schiemann AL, et al. Enhancement of glucose disposal in patients with Type 2 diabetes by alpha-lipoic acid. *Arzneimittelforschung*. 1995;45(8):872–874. http://www.ncbi.nlm.nih.gov/pubmed/7575750.

Jacob S, Ruus PR, Hermann R, et al. Oral administration of RAC-alpha-lipoic acid modulates insulin sensitivity in patients with Type-2 diabetes mellitus: A placebo-controlled pilot trial. *Free Radic Biol Med*. 1999;27(3–4):309–314. doi:10.1016/S0891-5849(99)00089-1.

James PA, Oparil S, Carter BL, et al. 2014 evidence-based guideline for the management of high blood pressure in adults. *JAMA*. 2014;311(5):507–520. doi:10.1001/jama.2013.284427.

Jayawardena R, Ranasinghe P, Galappatthy P, Malkanthi RLDK, Constantine GR, Katulanda P. Effects of zinc supplementation on diabetes mellitus: A systematic review and meta-analysis. *Diabetol Metab Syndr*. 2012;4:13. doi: 10.1186/1758-5996-4-13.

Ji S. Research confirms sweating dangerous metals, petrochemicals. GreenMedInfo. http://www.greenmedinfo.com/blog/research-confirms-sweating-detoxifies-dangerous-metals-petrochemicals. Published July 23, 2013. Accessed June 9, 2017.

Joergensen C, Hovind P, Schmedes A, Parving HH, Rossing P. Vitamin D levels, microvascular complications, and mortality in Type 1 diabetes. *Diabetes Care*. 2011;34(5):1081–1085. doi:10.2337/dc10-2459.

Joffe DL. Effect of extended release *Gymnema sylvestre* leaf extract (Beta Fast GXR). Diabetes in Control. http://www.diabetesincontrol.com/articles/uncategorized/10355-effect-of-extended-release-gymnema-sylvestre-leaf-extract-beta-fast-gxr. Published January 6, 2011. Accessed June 9, 2017.

Johnson JF. Drug interactions with diabetes. *Endocrine Today*. http://www.healio.com/endocrinology/diabetes/news/print/endocrine-today/%7B5b64b6a4-1cfa-4fc5-b916-e8284a7945aa%7D/drug-interactions-with-diabetes. Published March 2009. Accessed June 9, 2017.

Jung S-P, Lee KM, Kang JH, et al. Effect of *Lactobacillus gasseri* BNR17 on overweight and obese adults: A randomized, double-blind clinical trial. *Korean J Fam Med*. 2013;34(2):80–89. doi:10.4082/kjfm.2013.34.2.80.

Kähler W, Kuklinski B, Rühlmann C, Plötz C. Diabetes mellitus—a free radical-associated disease. Results of adjuvant antioxidant supplementation. *Z Gesamte Inn Med*. 1993;48(5):223–232. https://www.ncbi.nlm.nih.gov/pubmed/8390768.

Kasznicki J, Sliwinska A, Drzewoski J. Metformin in cancer prevention and therapy. *Ann Transl Med*. 2014;2(6):57. doi:10.3978/j.issn.2305-5839.2014.06.01.

Kayaniyil S, Vieth R, Retnakaran R, et al. Association of vitamin D with insulin resistance and beta-cell dysfunction in subjects at risk for Type 2 diabetes. *Diabetes Care*. 2010;33(6):1379–1381. doi:10.2337/dc09-2321.

Kidney Disease Outcomes Quality Initiative (NKF KDOQI). The National Kidney Foundation. http://www.kidney.org/professionals/kdoqi/guidelines.cfm. Accessed June 7, 2017.

Kim HM, Kim J. The effects of green tea on obesity and Type 2 diabetes. *Diabetes Metab J*. 2013;37(3):173–175. doi:10.4093/dmj.2013.37.3.173.

Kim KS, Oh DH, Kim JY, et al. Taurine ameliorates hyperglycemia and dyslipidemia by reducing insulin resistance and leptin level in Otsuka Long-Evans Tokushima fatty (OLETF) rats with long-term diabetes. *Exp Mol Med*. 2012;44:665–673. doi:10.3858/emm.2012.44.11.075.

King P, Peacock I, Donnelly R. The UK Prospective Diabetes Study (UKPDS): Clinical and therapeutic implications for Type 2 diabetes. *Br J Clin Pharmacol*. 1999;48(5):643–648. doi:10.1046/j.1365-2125.1999.00092.x.

Knowler WC, Barrett-Connor E, Fowler SE, et al. Reduction in the incidence of Type 2 diabetes with lifestyle intervention or metformin. *N Engl J Med*. 2002;346(6):393–403. https://www.ncbi.nlm.nih.gov/pubmed/11832527.

Kouno K, Hirano S, Kuboki H, Kasai M, Hatae K. Effects of dried bonito (katsuobushi) and captopril, an angiotensin l-converting enzyme inhibitor, on rat isolated aorta: A possible mechanism of antihypertensive action. *Biosci Biotechnol Biochem*. 2005;69(5):911–915. https://www.ncbi.nlm.nih.gov/pubmed/15914909.

Kowluru RA, Odenbach S. Effect of long-term administration of alpha-lipoic acid on retinal capillary cell death and the development of retinopathy in diabetic rats. *Diabetes*. 2004;53(12):3233–3238. http://www.ncbi.nlm.nih.gov/pubmed/15561955.

Kowluru RA, Zhong Q, Santos JM, Thandampallayam M, Putt D, Gierhart DL. Beneficial effects of the nutritional supplements on the development of diabetic retinopathy. *Nutr Metab*. 2014;11:8. http://www.nutritionandmetabolism.com/content/11/1/8.

Lain K. First-trimester levels of sex hormone binding globulin predict gestational diabetes. *OBG Manag*. 2004;16(10):16–23. http://www.mdedge.com/obgmanagement/article/61670/first-trimester-levels-sex-hormone-binding-globulin-predict-gestational.

Lalau JD. Lactic acidosis induced by metformin: Incidence, management and prevention. *Drug Saf*. 2010;33(9):727–740. doi:10.2165/11536790-000000000-00000.

Langer O, Yogev Y, Xenakis EM, Rosenn B. Insulin and glyburide therapy: Dosage, severity level of gestational diabetes, and pregnancy outcome. *Am J Obstet Gynecol*. 2005;192(1):134–139. http://www.ncbi.nlm.nih.gov/pubmed/15672015?dopt=Abstract.

Lautatzis ME, Goulis DG, Vrontakis M. Efficacy and safety of metformin during pregnancy in women with gestational diabetes mellitus or polycystic ovary syndrome: A systematic review. *Metabolism*. 2013;62(11):1522–1534. doi:10.1016/j.metabol.2013.06.006.

Lee D-H. Persistent organic pollutants and obesity-related metabolic dysfunction: Focusing on Type 2 diabetes. *Epidemiol Health*. 2012;34:e2012002. doi:10.4178/epih/e2012002.

Lee SW, Ng KY, Chin WK. The impact of sleep amount and sleep quality on glycemic control in Type 2 diabetes: A systematic review and meta-analysis. *Sleep Med Rev*. 2017;31:91–101. doi:10.1016/j.smrv.2016.02.001.

Li S-Y, Fu ZJ, Lo ACY. Hypoxia-induced oxidative stress in ischemic retinopathy. *Oxid Med Cell Longev*. 2012;10. doi:10.1155/2012/426769.

Light DW. New prescription drugs: A major health risk with few offsetting advantages. Edmond J. Safra Center for Ethics. http://ethics.harvard.edu/blog/new-prescription-drugs-major-health-risk-few-offsetting-advantages. Published June 27, 2014. Accessed June 9, 2017.

Lim SS, Jung SH, Ji J, Shin KH, Keum SR. Synthesis of flavonoids and their effects on aldose reductase and sorbitol accumulation in streptozotocin-induced diabetic rat tissues. *J Pharm Pharmacol*. 2001;53(5):653–668. http://www.ncbi.nlm.nih.gov/pubmed/11370705.

Lindsay T, Rodgers BC, Savath V, Hettinger K. Treating diabetic peripheral neuropathic pain. *Am Fam Physician*. 2010;82(2):151–158. http://www.aafp.org/afp/2010/0715/p151.html.

Lloyd C, Smith J, Weinger K. Stress and diabetes: A review of the links. *Diabetes Spectrum*. 2005;18(2):121–127. doi:10.2337/diaspect.18.2.121.

Low vitamin D levels may raise death risk in Type 1 diabetes. American Diabetes Association. http://www.diabetes.org/research-and-practice/patient-access-to-research/low-vitamin-d-levels-may.html. Updated October 7, 2013. Accessed June 9, 2017.

Luchsinger JA, Tang M-X, Shea S, Mayeux R. Caloric intake and the risk of Alzheimer disease. *Arch Neurol*. 2002;59(8):1258–1263. doi:10.1001/archneur.59.8.1258.

Ludvigsson JF, Ludvigsson J, Ekbom A, Montgomery SM. Celiac disease and risk of subsequent Type 1 diabetes. *Diabetes Care*. 2006;29(11):2483–2488. doi:10.2337/dc06-0794.

Maiorana A, O'Driscoll G, Goodman C, Taylor R, Green D. Combined aerobic and resistance exercise improves glycemic control and fitness in Type 2 diabetes. *Diabetes Res Clin Pract*. 2002;56(2):115–123. https://www.ncbi.nlm.nih.gov/pubmed/11891019.

Mäkinen M, Simell V, Mykkänen J, et al. An increase in serum 25-hydroxyvitamin D concentrations preceded a plateau in Type 1 diabetes incidence in Finnish children. *J Clin Endocrionol Metab*. 2014;99(11):E2353–E2356. doi:10.1210/jc.2014-1455.

Malik VS, Popkin BM, Bray GA, Després J-P, Hu FB. Sugar sweetened beverages, obesity, Type 2 diabetes and cardiovascular disease risk. *Circulation*. 2010;121(11):1356–1364. doi:10.1161/CIRCULATIONAHA.109.876185.

Mamtani R, Haynes K, Bilker WB, et al. Association between longer therapy with thiazolidinediones and risk of bladder cancer: A cohort study. *J Natl Cancer Inst*. 2012;104(18):1411–1421. http://www.ncbi.nlm.nih.gov/pubmed/22878886.

Mann D. Diabetes drug Actos again linked to bladder cancer. WebMD. http://www.webmd.com/cancer/news/20120531/diabetes-drug-actos-again-linked-to-bladder-cancer. Published May 31, 2012. Accessed November 29, 2016.

Mann J. Sugar revisited—again. *Bulletin of the World Health Organization*. 2003;81(8):552. http://www.who.int/bulletin/volumes/81/8/editorial2.pdf.

Manning PJ, Sutherland WH, Walker RJ, et al. Effect of high-dose vitamin E on insulin resistance and associated parameters in overweight subjects. *Diabetes Care*. 2004;27(9):2166–2171. http://www.ncbi.nlm.nih.gov/pubmed/15333479.

Markell MS. Herbal therapies and the patient with kidney disease. EnCognitive.com http://www.encognitive.com/node/4622. Accessed July 20, 2015.

Martins AR, Nachbar RT, Gorjao R, et al. Mechanisms underlying skeletal muscle insulin resistance induced by fatty acids: Importance of the mitochondrial function. *Lipids Health Dis*. 2012;11:30. doi:10.1186/1476-511X-11-30.

Mathieu C, Gysemans C, Giuletti A, Bouillon R. Vitamin D and diabetes. *Diabetologia*. 2005;48(7):1247–1257. https://www.ncbi.nlm.nih.gov/pubmed/15971062.

Mathurin P, Hollebecque A, Amalsteen L, et al. Prospective study of the long-term effects of bariatric surgery on liver injury in patients without advanced disease. *Gastroenterology*. 2009;137(2):532–540. doi:10.1053/j.gastro.2009.04.052.

Meneghini L. Using target glucose goals and self-titration for improved glycemic control. Medscape. http://www.medscape.org/viewarticle/726962. Published August 20, 2010.

Miller KM, Foster NC, Beck RW, et al. Current state of Type 1 diabetes treatment in the US: Updated data from the T1D Exchange Clinic Registry. *Diabetes Care*. 2015;38(6):971–978. doi:10.2337/dc15-0078.

Mishra S, Palanivelu K. The effect of curcumin (turmeric) on Alzheimer's disease: An overview. *Ann Indian Acad Neurol*. 2008;11(1):13–19. doi:10.4103/0972-2327.40220. Accessed November 30, 2016.

Moore TR, et al. Diabetes mellitus and pregnancy. Medscape. http://emedicine.medscape.com/article/127547-overview-a17. Updated February 14, 2017.

Moretti ME, Rezvani M, Koren G. Safety of glyburide for gestational diabetes: A meta-analysis of pregnancy outcomes. *Ann Pharmacother*. 2008;42(4):483–490. doi:10.1345/aph.1K577.

Morgan E, Halliday SR, Campbell GR, Cardwell CR, Patterson CC. Vaccinations and childhood Type 1 diabetes mellitus: A meta-analysis of observational studies. *Diabetologia*. 2016;59(2):237–243. doi:10.1007/s00125-015-3800-8.

Morris MC, Tangney CC, Wang Y, Sacks FM, Bennett DA, Aggarwal NT. MIND diet associated with reduced incidence of Alzheimer's disease. *Alzheimer's Dement*. 2015;11(9):1007–1014. doi:10.1016/j.jalz.2014.11.009.

Muldoon MF, Erickson KI, Goodpaster BH, et al. Concurrent physical activity modifies the association between n3 long-chain fatty acids and cardiometabolic risk in midlife adults. *J Nutr*. 2013;143(9):1414–1420. doi:10.3945/jn.113.174078.

Muntoni S, Cocco P, Aru G, Cucca F. Nutritional factors and worldwide incidence of childhood Type 1 diabetes. *Am J Clin Nutr*. 2000;71(6):1525–1529. https://www.ncbi.nlm.nih.gov/pubmed/10837294.

Naderi GA, Asgary S, Jafarian A, Askari N, Behagh A, Aghdam RH. Fibrinolytic effects of *Gingko biloba* extract. *Exp Clin Cardiol*. 2005;10(2):85–87. http://www.ncbi.nlm.nih.gov/pmc/articles/PMC2716226.

Nainggolan L. BMJ digs deep into incretins and pancreatic cancer debate. Medscape. http://www.medscape.com/viewarticle/805541. Published June 10, 2013.

Nelson JE, Klintworth H, Kowdley KV. Iron metabolism in nonalcoholic fatty liver disease. *Curr Gastroenterol Rep*. 2012;14(1):8–16. doi:10.1007/s11894-011-0234-4.

Nelson RG, Tuttle KR. KDOQI clinical practice guideline for diabetes and CKD: 2012 update. *Am J Kidney Dis*. 2012;60(5):850–886. https://www.kidney.org/sites/default/files/docs/diabetes-ckd-update-2012.pdf.

Ngwa EN, Kengne A-P, Tiedei-Atogho B, Mofo-Mato E-P, Sobngwi E. Persistent organic pollutants as risk factors for Type 2 diabetes. *Diabetol Metab Syndr*. 2015;7:41. doi:10.1186/s13098-015-0031-6.

Nichols GA. Are statins worth the diabetes risk? Medscape. http://www.medscape.com/viewarticle/781684. Published April 8, 2013.

Nielsen JV, Westerlund P, Bygren P. A low-carbohydrate diet may prevent end-stage renal failure in Type 2 diabetes. A case report. *Nutr Metab*. 2006;3:23. doi:10.1186/1743-7075-3-23.

Nielsen SF, Nordestgaard BG. Statin use before diabetes diagnosis and risk of microvascular disease: A nationwide nested matched study. *Lancet*. 2014;2(11):894–900. doi:10.1016/S2213-8587(14)70173-1.

Norouzy A, Salehi M, Philoppou E, et al. Effect of fasting in Ramadan on body composition and nutritional intake: A prospective study. *J Hum Nutr Diet*. 2013;26(suppl 1):97–104. doi:10.1111/jhn.12042.

Norris JM, Yin X, Lamb MM, et al. Omega-3 polyunsaturated fatty acid intake and islet autoimmunity in children at increased risk for Type 1 diabetes. *JAMA*. 2007;298(12):1420–1428. doi:10.1001/jama.298.12.1420.

Ntuk UE, Celis-Morales CA, Mackay DF, Sattar N, Pell JP, Gill JMR. Association between grip strength and diabetes prevalence in black, South-Asian, and white European ethnic groups: A cross-sectional analysis of 418,656 participants in the UK Biobank study. *Diabet Med*. 2017. doi:10.1111/dme.13323.

O'Connell BS. Select vitamins and minerals in the management of diabetes. *Diabetes Spectrum*. 2001;14(3):133–148. http://spectrum.diabetesjournals.org/content/diaspect/14/3/133.full.pdf.

O'Riordan M. Niacin reduces cardiovascular events and total mortality in MI patients, regardless of glycemic status. Medscape. http://www.medscape.com/viewarticle/787240. Published January 12, 2005.

———. JUPITER analysis helps assuage fears about diabetes risk with statins. Medscape. http://www.medscape.com/viewarticle/769024. Published August 13, 2012.

Odetti P, Pesce C, Traverso N, et al. Comparative trial of N-acetyl-cysteine, taurine, and oxerutin on skin and kidney damage in long-term experimental diabetes. *Diabetes*. 2003;52(2):499–505. doi:10.2337/diabetes.52.2.499.

Ogbera A, Ezeobi E, Unachukwu C, Oshinaike O. Treatment of diabetes mellitus-associated neuropathy with vitamin E and Eve primrose. *Indian J Endocrinol Metab*. 2014;18(6):846–849. doi:10.4103/2230-8210.140270.

Ohara T, Doi Y, Ninomiya T, et al. Glucose tolerance status and risk of dementia in the community: The Hisayama study. *Neurology*. 2011;77(12):1126–1134. doi:10.1212/WNL.0b013e31822f0435.

Ozkilic AC, Cengix M, Ozaydin A, Cobanoglu A, Kanigur G. The role of N-acetylcysteine treatment on anti-oxidative status in patients with Type II diabetes mellitus. *J Basic Clin Physiol Pharmacol*. 2006;17(4):245–254. https://www.ncbi.nlm.nih.gov/pubmed/17338280.

Palomer X, González-Celemente JM, Bianco-Vaca F, Mauricio D. Role of vitamin D in the pathogenesis of Type 2 diabetes mellitus. *Diabetes Obes Metab*. 2008;10(3):185–197. doi:10.1111/j.1463-1326.2007.00710.x.

Pani L, Korenda L, Meigs JB, et al. Effect of aging on A1C levels in individuals without diabetes. *Diabetes Care*. 2008;31(10):1991–1996. doi:10.2337/dc08-0577.

Papanikolaou Y, Brooks J, Reider C, Fulgoni VL. US adults are not meeting recommended levels of fish and omega-3 fatty acid intake: Results of an analysis using observational data from NHANES 2003–2008. *Nutr J*. 2014;13:31. doi:10.1186/1475-2891-13-31.

Parker VG, Mayo RM, Logan BN, Holder BJ, Smart PT. Toxins and diabetes mellitus: An environmental connection? *Diabetes Spectrum*. 2002;15(2):109–112. doi:10.2337/diaspect.15.2.109.

Peters KG, Davis MG, Howard BW, et al. Mechanism of insulin sensitization by BMOV (bis maltolato oxo vanadium); unliganded vanadium (VO4) as the active component. *J Inorg Biochem*. 2003;96(2–3):321–330. https://www.ncbi.nlm.nih.gov/pubmed/12888267.

Pilichiewicz AN, Horowitz M, Russo A, et al. Effects of Iberogast on proximal gastric volume, antropyloroduodenal motility and gastric emptying in healthy men. *Am J Gastroenterol*. 2007;102(6):1276–1283. https://www.ncbi.nlm.nih.gov/pubmed/17378904.

Pizzorno L. Omega-3s, ApoE genotype and cognitive decline. Longevity Medicine Review. http://www.lmreview.com/articles/view/omega-3s-apoe-genotype-and-cognitive-decline. Accessed May 12, 2016.

Popov VB, Lim JK. Treatment of nonalcoholic fatty liver disease: The role of medical, surgical, and endoscopic weight loss. *J Clin Transl Hepatol*. 2015;3(3):230–238. doi:10.14218/JCTH.2015.00019.

Porrata C, Sánchez J, Correa V, et al. Ma-Pi 2 macrobiotic diet intervention in adults with Type 2 diabetes mellitus. *MEDICC Rev*. 2009;11(4):29–35. http://www.medicc.org/mediccreview/articles/mr_119.pdf.

Porrata-Maury C, Hernández-Triana M, Ruiz-Álvarez V, et al. Ma-Pi 2 macrobiotic diet and Type 2 diabetes mellitus: Pooled analysis of short-term intervention studies. *Diabetes Metab Res Rev*. 2014;30 (suppl 1):55–66. doi:10.1002/dmrr.2519.

Pullen LC. Environmental toxins associated with diabetes, obesity. Medscape. http://www.medscape.com/viewarticle/827282. Published June 24, 2014.

Putnam W, Buhariwalla F, Lacey K, et al. Drug management for hypertension in Type 2 diabetes in family practice. *Can Fam Physician*. 2009;55(7):728–734. http://www.ncbi.nlm.nih.gov/pmc/articles/PMC2718608.

Rahman K, Lowe GM. Garlic and cardiovascular disease: A critical review. *J Nutr*. 2006;136(3):736S–740S. http://jn.nutrition.org/content/136/3/736S.full.

Rasmussen OW, Lauszus FF, Hermansen K. Effects of postprandial exercise response in IDDM subjects: Studies at constant insulinemia. *Diabetes Care*. 1994;17(10):1203–1205. doi:10.2337/diacare.17.10.1203.

Reis de Azevedo F, et al. Effects of intermittent fasting on metabolism in men. *Rev Assoc Med Bras*. 2013;59(2):167–173. http://www.sciencedirect.com/science/article/pii/S0104423013000213.

Rewers M, Gottlieb P. Immunotherapy for the prevention and treatment of Type 1 diabetes: Human trials and a look into the future. *Diabetes Care*. 2009;32(10):1769–1782. doi:10.2337/dc09-0374.

Riddle M, Umpierrez G, DiGenio A, Zhou R, Rosenstock J. Contributions of basal and postprandial hyperglycemia over a wide range of A1C levels before and after treatment intensification in Type 2 diabetes. *Diabetes Care* 2011;34(12):2508–2514. doi:10.2337/dc11-0632.

Robertson L, Waugh N, Robertson A. Protein restriction for diabetic renal disease. *Cochrane Database Syst Rev*. 2007;(4): CD002181. doi:10.1002/14651858.CD002181.pub2.

Robles NR, Velasco J, Mena C, Polo J, Angulo E, Espinosa J; for MICREX Group Investigators. Increased frequency of microalbuminuria in patients receiving statins. *Clin Lipidol*. 2013;8(2):257–262. doi:10.2217/clp.13.5.

Rodríguez-Morán M, Guerrero-Romero F. Oral magnesium supplementation improves insulin sensitivity and metabolic control in Type 2 diabetic subjects. *Diabetes Care*. 2003;26(4):1147–1152. doi:10.2337/diacare.26.4.1147.

Rosenstock J, Ferrannini E. Euglycemic diabetic ketoacidosis: A predictable, detectable, and preventable safety concern with SGLT2 inhibitors. *Diabetes Care*. 2015;38(9):1638–1642. doi:10.2337/dc15-1380.

Rowan JA, Hague WH, Gao W, Battin MR, Moore P; for MiG Trial Investigators. Metformin versus insulin for the treatment of gestational diabetes. *N Engl J Med*. 2008;358:2003–2015. doi:10.1056/NEJMoa0707193.

Ruan Y, Sun J, He J, Chen F, Chen R, Chen H. Effect of probiotics on glycemic control: A systematic review and meta-analysis of randomized, controlled trials. *PLOS ONE*. 2015;10(7):e0132121. doi:10.1371/journal.pone.0132121.

Rubino F, Nathan DM, Eckel RH, et al; for Delegates of the 2nd Diabetes Surgery Summit. Metabolic surgery in the treatment algorithm for Type 2 diabetes: A joint statement by international diabetes organizations. *Diabetes Care*. 2016;39(6):861–877. doi:10.2337/dc16-0236.

Russell WR, Gratz SW, Duncan SH, et al. High-protein, reduced-carbohydrate weight-loss diets promote metabolite profiles likely to be detrimental to colonic health. *Am J Clin Nutr*. 2011;93(5):1062–1072. doi:10.3945/ajcn.110.002188.

Sacks DB. A1C versus glucose testing: A comparison. *Diabetes Care*. 2011;34(2):518–523. doi:10.2337/dc10-1546.

Salas-Salvadó J, Bulló M, Babio N, et al. Reduction in the incidence of Type 2 diabetes with the Mediterranean diet. *Diabetes Care*. 2011;34(1):14–19. doi:10.2337/dc10-1288.

Samuelson U, Oikarinen S, Hyöty H, Lidvigsson J. Low zinc in drinking water is associated with the risk of Type 1 diabetes in children. *Pediatr Diabetes*. 2011;12(3, pt 1):156–164. doi:10.1111/j.1399-5448.2010.00678.x.

Sanyal AJ, Chalasani N, Kowdley KV, et al. Pioglitazone, vitamin E, or placebo for nonalcoholic steatohepatitis. *N Engl J Med*. 2010;362(18):1675–1685. doi:10.1056/NEJMoa0907929.

Sapone A, de Magistris L, Pietzak M, et al. Zonulin upregulation is associated with increased gut permeability in subjects with Type 1 diabetes and their relatives. *Diabetes*. 2006;55(5);1443–1449. https://www.ncbi.nlm.nih.gov/pubmed/16644703.

Schmid S, Buuck D, Knopff A, Bonifacio E, Ziegler AG. BABYDIET, a feasibility study to prevent the appearance of islet autoantibodies in relatives of patients with Type 1 diabetes by delaying exposure to gluten. *Diabetologia*. 2004;47(6):1130–1131. doi:10.1007/s00125-004-1420-9.

Selvin E, Zhu H, Brancati FL. Elevated A1C in adults without a history of diabetes in the U.S. *Diabetes Care*. 2009;32(5):828–833. doi:10.2337/dc08-1699.

Shanmugasundaram ER, Rajeswari G, Rajesh Kumar BR, Radha Shanmugasundaram K, Kizar Ahmath B. Use of *Gymnema sylvestre* leaf extract in the control of blood glucose in insulin-dependent diabetes mellitus. *J Ethnopharmacol*. 1990;30(3):281–294. https://www.ncbi.nlm.nih.gov/pubmed/2259216.

Sherifali D, Nerenbreg K, Pullenayegum E, Cheng JE, Gerstain HC. The effect of oral antidiabetic agents on A1C levels: A systematic review and meta-analysis. *Diabetes Care*. 2010;33(8):1859–1864. doi:10.2337/dc09-1727.

Short, KR. Regulation of glycemic control by physical activity: A role for mitochondria? *Diabetes*. 2013;62(1):34–35. doi:10.2337/db12-1209.

Sima AAF, Calvani M, Mehra M, Amato A. Acetyl-l-carnitine improves pain, nerve regeneration, and vibratory perception in patients with chronic diabetic neuropathy: An analysis of two randomized placebo-controlled trials. *Diabetes Care*. 2005;28(1):89–94. doi:10.2337/diacare.28.1.89.

Sleep apnoea and Type 2 diabetes. International Diabetes Federation. http://www.idf.org/sleep-apnoea-and-type-2-diabetes.

Smith JM. *State-of-the-Science on the Health Risks of GM Foods*. Institute for Responsible Technology. http://responsibletechnology.org/irtnew/docs/state_science_gmo.pdf. Accessed June 9, 2017.

Snyder MJ, Gibbs LM. Treating painful diabetic peripheral neuropathy: An update. *Am Fam Physician*. 2016;94(3):227–234. http://www.aafp.org/afp/2016/0801/p227.html.

Song Y, Xu Q, Park Y, Hollenbeck A, Schatzkin A, Chen H. Multivitamins, individual vitamin and mineral supplements, and risk of diabetes among older U.S. adults. *Diabetes Care*. 2011;34(1):108–114. doi:10.2337/dc10-1260.

Sørensen IM, Joner G, Jenum PA, Eskild A, Torjesen PA, Stene LC. Maternal serum levels of 25-hydroxy-vitamin D during pregnancy and risk of Type 1 diabetes in the offspring. *Diabetes*. 2012;61(1):175–178. doi:10.2337/db11-0875.

Sprague JE, Arbeláez AM. Glucose counterregulatory responses to hypoglycemia. *Pediatr Endocrinol Rev*. 2011; 9(1): 463–475. http://www.ncbi.nlm.nih.gov/pmc/articles/PMC3755377.

St Peter WL, Odum LE, Whaley-Connell AT. To RAS or not to RAS? The evidence for and cautions with renin-angiotensin system inhibition in patients with diabetic kidney disease. *Pharmacotherapy*. 2013;33(5):496–514. doi:10.1002/phar.1232.

Statistics about diabetes. American Diabetes Association. http://www.diabetes.org/diabetes-basics/statistics. Updated December 12, 2016. Accessed November 28, 2016.

Stene LC, Hongve D, Magnus P, Rønningen KS, Joner G. Acidic drinking water and risk of childhood-onset Type 1 diabetes. *Diabetes Care*. 2002;25(9):1534–1538. doi:10.2337/diacare.25.9.1534.

Stene LC, Ulriksen J, Magnus P, Joner G. Use of cod liver oil during pregnancy associated with lower risk of Type 1 diabetes in the offspring. *Diabetologia*. 2000;43(9):1093–1098. doi:10.1007/s001250051499.

Stiles S. Cutting intake of sugar-sweetened drinks lowers BP in observational study. MedScape. http://www.medscape.com/viewarticle/722534. Published May 26, 2010.

Stirban A, Negrean M, Stratmann B, et al. Benfotiamine prevents macro- and microvascular endothelial dysfunction and oxidative stress following a meal rich in advanced glycation end products in individuals with Type 2 diabetes. *Diabetes Care*. 2006;29(9):2064–2071. doi:10.2337/dc06-0531.

Sugars Intake for Adults and Children. World Health Organization; 2015. http://www.who.int/nutrition/publications/guidelines/sugars_intake/en.

Sukhija R, Prayaga S, Marashedeh M, et al. Effect of statins on fasting plasma glucose in diabetic and nondiabetic patients. *J Investig Med*. 2009;57(3):495–499. doi:10.2310/JIM.0b013e318197ec8b.

Sun Q, van Dam RM, Willett WC, Hu FB. Prospective study of zinc intake and risk of Type 2 diabetes in women. *Diabetes Care*. 2009;32(4):629–634. doi:10.2337/dc08-1913.

Sundram K, Karupaiah T, Hayes KC. Stearic acid-rich interestified fat and trans-rich fat raise the LDL/HDL ratio and plasma glucose relative to palm olein in humans. *Nutr Metab (Lond)*. 2007;4:3. doi:10.1186/1743-7075-4-3.

Surwit RS, van Tilburg M, Zucker N, et al. Stress management improves long-term glycemic control in Type 2 diabetes. *Diabetes Care*. 2002; 25(1):30–34. https://www.ncbi.nlm.nih.gov/pubmed/11772897.

Svitil K. Diet and exercise can reduce protein build-ups linked to Alzheimer's, UCLA study shows. UCLA Newsroom. http://newsroom.ucla.edu/releases/diet-and-exercise-can-reduce-protein-build-ups-linked-to-alzheimers-ucla-study-shows. Published August 16, 2016. Accessed February 6, 2017.

Swanson N, Leu A, Abrahamson J, Wallet B. Genetically engineered crops, glyphosate and the deterioration of health in the United States of America. *Journal of Organic Systems*. 2014;9(2). http://www.organic-systems.org/journal/92/abstracts/Swanson-et-al.html.

Tanaka H, Watanabe K, Ma M, et al. The effects of gamma-aminobutyric acid, vinegar, and dried bonito on blood pressure in normotensive and mildly or moderately hypertensive volunteers. *J Clin Biochem Nutr*. 2009;45(1):93–100. doi:10.3164/jcbn.09-04.

Taylor JR. Use of niacin in patients with diabetes. *Endocrine Today*. http://www.healio.com/endocrinology/diabetes/news/print/endocrine-today/%7Bfd45c706-7eda-433a-9e6f-529e229af4fd%7D/use-of-niacin-in-patients-with-diabetes. Published June 2010. Accessed June 9, 2017.

Taylor SI, Blau JE, Rother KI. Possible adverse effects of SGLT2 inhibitors on bone. *The Lancet: Diabetes & Endocrinology*. 2015;3(1):8–10. doi:10.1016/S2213-8587(14)70227-X.

TEDDY: The environmental determinants of diabetes in the young. http://teddy.epi.usf.edu. Accessed June 9, 2017.

Thorsdottir I, Brigisdottir BE, Johannsdottir IM, et al. Different β-casein fractions in Icelandic versus Scandinavian cow's milk may influence diabetogenicity of cow's milk in infancy and explain low incidence of insulin-dependent diabetes mellitus in Iceland. *Pediatrics*. 2000;106(4):719–724. http://pediatrics.aappublications.org/content/106/4/719.full.

Tilgner S. The contented kidney. HerbalTransitions.com. http://www.herbaltransitions.com/Newsletters%20and%20other%20goodies/Kidney%20Health.pdf. Published 2005. Accessed November 30, 2016.

Toiba R. Gestational diabetes. *Today's Dietician*. 2013;15(8):48. http://www.todaysdietitian.com/newarchives/080113p48.shtml.

Tolhurst G, Heffron H, Lam YS, et al. Short-chain fatty acids stimulate glucagon-like peptide-1 secretion via the g-protein–coupled receptor FFAR2. *Diabetes*. 2012;61(2):364–371. doi:10.2337/db11-1019.

Trafton A. Nutrient mixture improves memory in patients with early Alzheimer's. *MIT News*. http://news.mit.edu/2012/alzheimers-nutrient-mixture-0709. Published July 9, 2012. Accessed June 7, 2017.

Tsai YW, Kann NH, Tung TH, et al. Impact of subjective sleep quality on glycemic control in Type 2 diabetes mellitus. *Fam Pract*. 2012;29(1):30–35. doi:10.1093/fampra/cmr041.

Tucker ME. Pioglitazone use not linked to bladder cancer at 10 years. Medscape. http://www.medscape.com/viewarticle/848390. Published July 21, 2015.

Turnbaugh PJ, Ley RE, Mahowald MA, Margrini V, Mardis ER, Gordon JI. An obesity-associated gut microbiome with increased capacity for energy harvest. *Nature*. 2006;444:1027–1031. doi:10.1038/nature05414.

Tuvemo T, Gebre-Medhin M. The role of trace elements in juvenile diabetes mellitus. *Pediatrician*. 1983–1985;12(4):213–219. http://www.ncbi.nlm.nih.gov/pubmed/6400452.

Umeki Y, et al. The effect of the dried-bonito broth on blood pressure, 8-hydroxydeoxyguanosine (8-OHdG), an oxidative stress marker, and emotional states in elderly subjects. *J Clin Biochem Nutr*. 2008;43(3):175–184. doi:10.3164/jcbn.2008061.

University of Exeter Medical School. Genetic types of diabetes including maturity-onset diabetes of the young (MODY). Diabetes Genes. http://www.projects.ex.ac.uk/diabetesgenes. Accessed November 28, 2016.

Unlu NZ, Bohn T, Clinton SK, Schwartz SJ. Carotenoid absorption from salad and salsa by humans is enhanced by the addition of avocado or avocado oil. *J Nutr*. 2005;135(3):431–436. http://jn.nutrition.org/cgi/content/abstract/135/3/431.

Use of metformin in gestational diabetes. Diabetes in Control. http://www.diabetesincontrol.com/articles/diabetes-news/15367-use-of-metformin-in-gestational-diabetes. Published October 25, 2013. Accessed November 29, 2016.

Vaarala O. The gut as a regulator of early inflammation in Type 1 diabetes. *Curr Opin Endocrinol Diabetes Obes*. 2011;18(4):241–247. doi:10.1097/MED.0b013e3283488218.

Vaarala O, Atkinson MA, Neu J. The "perfect storm" for Type 1 diabetes: The complex interplay between intestinal microbiota, gut permeability, and mucosal immunity. *Diabetes*. 2008;57(10):2555–2562. doi:10.2337/db08-0331.

Vajro P, Mandato C, Licenziati MR, et al. Effects of *Lactobacillus rhamnosus* strain GG in pediatric obesity-related liver disease. *J Pediatr Gastroenterol Nutr*. 2011;52(6):740–743. doi:10.1097/MPG.0b013e31821f9b85.

Vallianou N, Evangelopoulos A, Koutalas P. Alpha-lipoic acid and diabetic neuropathy. *Rev Diabet Stud*. 2009;6(4):230–236. doi:10.1900/RDS.2009.6.230.

Van Buren PN, Toto R. Hypertension in diabetic nephropathy: Epidemiology, mechanisms, and management. *Ady Chronic Kidney Dis*. 2011;18(1):28–41. doi:10.1053/j.ackd.2010.10.003.

van de Ven KCC, van der Graaf M, Tack CJ, Heerschap A, de Galan BE. Steady-state brain glucose concentrations during hypoglycemia in healthy humans and patients with Type 1 diabetes. *Diabetes*. 2012;61(8):1974–1977. doi:10.2337/db11-1778.

Van Proeyen K, Szlufcik K, Nielens H, et al. Training in the fasted state improves glucose tolerance during fat-rich diet. *J Physiol*. 2010;588(pt 21):4289–4302. doi:10.1113/jphysiol.2010.196493.

Vanschoonbeek K, et al. Variable hypocoagulant effect of fish oil intake in humans: Modulation of fibrinogen level and thrombin generation. *Arterioscler Thromb Vasc Biol*. 2004;24(9):1734–1740. doi:10.1161/01.ATV.0000137119.28893.0b.

Varma SD, Mikuni I, Kinoshita JH. Flavonoids as inhibitors of lens aldose reductase. *Science*. 1975;188(4194):1215–1216. http://www.ncbi.nlm.nih.gov/pubmed/1145193.

Varshney R, Budoff MJ. Garlic and heart disease. *J Nutr*. 2016. doi:10.3945/jn.114.202333.

Vasquez A. Diabetes: Are toxins to blame? *Naturopathy Digest*. http://www.naturopathydigest.com/archives/2007/apr/diabetes.php. Published 2007. Accessed June 9, 2017.

Vessby B, Uusitupa M, Mermansen K, et al. Substituting dietary saturated for monounsaturated fat impairs insulin sensitivity in healthy men and women: The KANWU Study. *Diabetologia*. 2001;44(3):312–319. https://www.ncbi.nlm.nih.gov/pubmed/11317662.

Vincent JB. The biochemistry of chromium. *J Nutr*. 2000;130(4):715–718. http://jn.nutrition.org/cgi/content/full/130/4/715.

Virtanen SM, Knip M. Nutritional risk predictors of ß cell auto-immunity and Type 1 diabetes at a young age. *Amer J Clin Nutr*. 2003;78(6):1053–1067. http://ajcn.nutrition.org/content/78/6/1053.full.

Vitamin E and fatty liver. Lancaster General Health. http://www.lancastergeneralhealth.org/LGH/ECommerceSite/media/LGH-Media-Library/Healthcare%20Professionals/Nurses/Events/7-Nutriceuticals-Handout.pdf. Accessed June 7, 2017.

Volta U, Tovoli F, Caio G. Clinical and immunological features of celiac disease in patients with Type 1 diabetes mellitus. *Expert Rev Gastroenterol Hepatol*. 2011;5(4):479–487. doi:10.1586/egh.11.38.

von Arnim U, Peitz U, Vinson B, Gundermann KJ, Malfeertheiner P. STW 5, a phytopharmacon for patients with functional dyspepsia: Results of a multicenter, placebo-controlled double-blind study. *Am J Gastroenterol*. 2007;102(6):1268–1075. doi:10.1111/j.1572-0241.2006.01183.x.

von Frankenberg AD, Marina A, Song X, Callahan HS, Kratz M, Utzschneider KM. A high-fat, high-saturated fat diet decreases insulin sensitivity without changing intra-abdominal fat in weight-stable overweight and obese adults. *Eur J Nutr*. 2015:1–13. doi:10.1007/s00394-015-1108-6.

Wang J, Persuitte G, Olendzki BC, et al. Dietary magnesium intake improves insulin resistance among non-diabetic individuals with metabolic syndrome participating in a dietary trial. *Nutrients*. 2013;5(10):3910–3919. doi:10.3390/nu5103910.

Weng J, Li Y, Xu W, et al. Effect of intensive insulin therapy on β-cell function and glycaemic control in patients with newly diagnosed Type 2 diabetes: A multicentre randomised parallel-group trial. *Lancet*. 2008;371(9626):1753–1760. doi:10.1016/S0140-6736(08)60762-X.

Whyte J, Mohr C. Exercise can improve glycemic control: How to get patients started. Consultant 360. http://www.consultant360.com/Exercise-Improve-Glycemic-Control-diabetes-Get-Patients-Started. Published January 16, 2013. Accessed June 9, 2017.

Winkler G, Pál B, Nagybéganyi E, Ory I, Porochnavec M, Kempler P. Effectiveness of different benfotiamine dosage regimens in the treatment of painful diabetic neuropathy. *Arzneimittelforschung*. 1999;49(3):220–224. doi:10.1055/s-0031-1300405.

Woodford KB. *Devil in the Milk: Illness, Health and Politics of A1 and A2 Milk*. White River Junction, VT: Chelsea Green Publishing; 2009.

World Gastroenterology Organisation. Nonalcoholic fatty liver disease and nonalcoholic steatohepatitis. World Gastroenterology Organisation Global Guidelines. http://www.worldgastroenterology.org/assets/export/userfiles/2012_NASH%20and%20NAFLD_Final_long.pdf. Published June 2012. Accessed June 9, 2017.

Yancy WS, Foy M, Chalecki AM, Vernon MC, Westman EC. A low-carbohydrate, ketogenic diet to treat Type 2 diabetes. *Nutr Metab (Lond)*. 2005;2:34. doi:10.1186/1743-7075-2-34.

Yeung WC, Rawlinson WD, Craig ME. Enterovirus infection and Type 1 diabetes mellitus: Systemic review and meta-analysis of observational studies. *BMJ*. 2011;342:d35. doi:10.1136/bmj.d35.

Yin J, Xing H, Ye J. Efficacy of berberine in patients with Type 2 diabetes. *Metabolism*. 2008;57(5):712–717. doi:10.1016/j.metabol.2008.01.013.

Yin J, Ye J, Jia W. Effects and mechanisms of berberine in diabetes treatment. *Acta Pharm Sin B*. 2012;2(4):327–334. doi:10.1016/j.apsb.2012.06.003.

Yin K, Agrawal D. Vitamin D and inflammatory disease. *J Inflamm Res*. 2014;7:69–87. doi:10.2147/JIR.S63898.

Yue L, Zhang Y, Liu D-B, Liu H-Y, Hou W-G, Dong Y-S. Curcumin attenuates diabetic neuropathic pain by downregulating TNF-a in a rat model. *Int J Med Sci*. 2013;10(4):337–381. http://www.medsci.org/v10p0377.htm.

Yuting R, Sun J, He J, Chen F, Chen R, Chen H. Effect of probiotics on glycemic control: A systematic review and meta-analysis of randomized, controlled trials. *PLOS ONE*, 2015;10(7):e0132121. doi:10.1371/journal.pone.0132121.

Zhang D-W, Fu M, Gao S-H, Liu J-L. Curcumin and diabetes: A systematic review. *Evid Based Complement Alternat Med*. 2013;doi:10.1155/2013/636053.

Zhang Y, Leung DY, Richers BN, et al. Vitamin D inhibits monocyte/macrophage proinflammatory cytokine production by targeting MAPK phosphatase-1. *J Immunol*. 2012;188(5):2127–2135. doi:10.4049/jimmunol.1102412.

Zhang Y, Zhang H. Microbiota associated with Type 2 diabetes and its related complications. *Food Sci Hum Wellness*. 2013;2(3–4):167–172. doi:10.1016/j.fshw.2013.09.002.

Zhong Y, Deng Y, Chen Y, Chuang PY, He JC. Therapeutic use of traditional Chinese herbal medications for chronic kidney diseases. *Kidney Int*. 2013;84(6):1108–1118. doi:10.1038/ki.2013.276.

Zhu Y, Zhang XL, Zhu BF, Ding YN. Effect of antioxidant N-acetylcysteine on diabetic retinopathy and expression of VEGF and ICAM-1 from retinal blood vessels of diabetic rats. *Mol Biol Rep*. 2012;39(4):3727–3735. doi:10.1007/s11033-011-1148-9.

Index

Page numbers in *italics* refer to photographs and figures; page numbers followed by *t* refer to tables.

About the Author

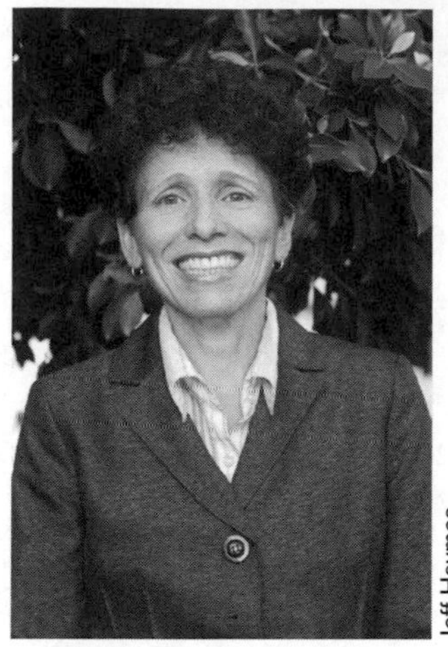

Jeff Haymes

Dr. Mona Morstein is a naturopathic physician with a medical practice focused on integrative diabetes treatment. Her clinic, Arizona Integrative Medical Solutions, is located in Tempe, Arizona, where she sees patients of all ages and genders for acute and chronic conditions. An expert on prediabetes and diabetes, she is a frequent lecturer at conferences and webinars, the founder and executive director of The Low Carb Diabetes Association, and the creator of the comprehensive diabetic supplement Diamend. Dr. Morstein is also a member of the Arizona Diabetes Coalition.

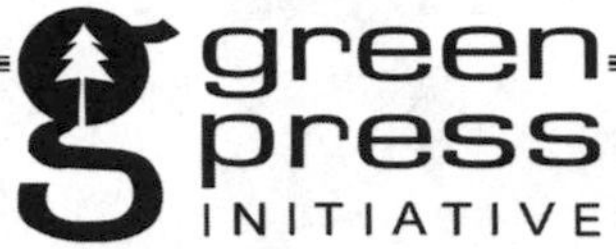

Chelsea Green Publishing is committed to preserving ancient forests and natural resources. We elected to print this title on 100-percent postconsumer recycled paper, processed chlorine-free. As a result, for this printing, we have saved:

96 Trees (40' tall and 6-8" diameter)
44 Million BTUs of Total Energy
8,311 Pounds of Greenhouse Gases
45,076 Gallons of Wastewater
3,018 Pounds of Solid Waste

Chelsea Green Publishing made this paper choice because we and our printer, Thomson-Shore, Inc., are members of the Green Press Initiative, a nonprofit program dedicated to supporting authors, publishers, and suppliers in their efforts to reduce their use of fiber obtained from endangered forests. For more information, visit: www.greenpressinitiative.org.

Environmental impact estimates were made using the Environmental Defense Paper Calculator. For more information visit: www.papercalculator.org.

the politics and practice of sustainable living

CHELSEA GREEN PUBLISHING

Chelsea Green Publishing sees books as tools for effecting cultural change and seeks to empower citizens to participate in reclaiming our global commons and become its impassioned stewards. If you enjoyed *Master Your Diabetes*, please consider these other great books related to health and wellness.

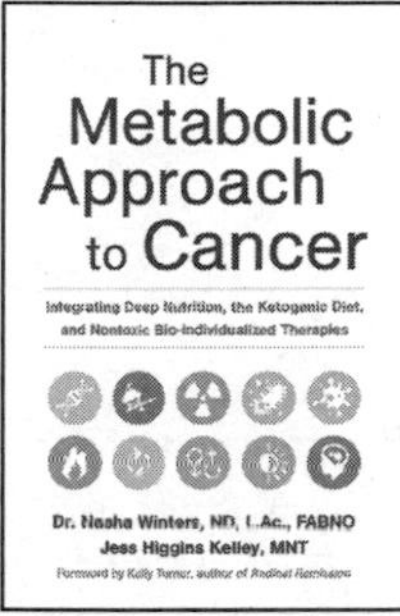

THE METABOLIC APPROACH TO CANCER
Integrating Deep Nutrition, the Ketogenic Diet, and Nontoxic Bio-Individualized Therapies
DR. NASHA WINTERS and JESS HIGGINS KELLEY
9781603586863
Hardcover • $29.95

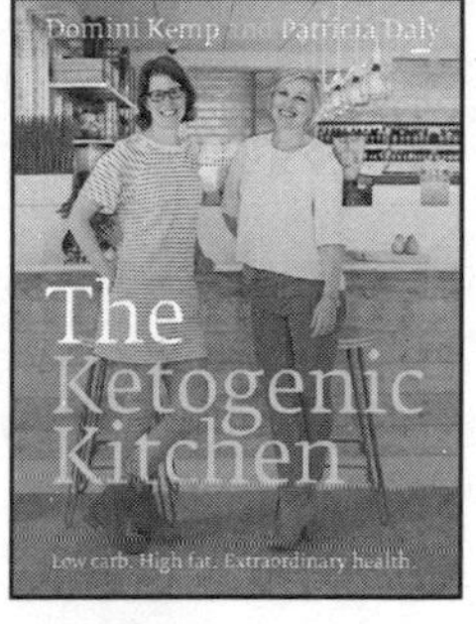

THE KETOGENIC KITCHEN
Low carb. High fat. Extraordinary health.
DOMINI KEMP and PATRICIA DALY
9781603586924
Paperback • $29.95

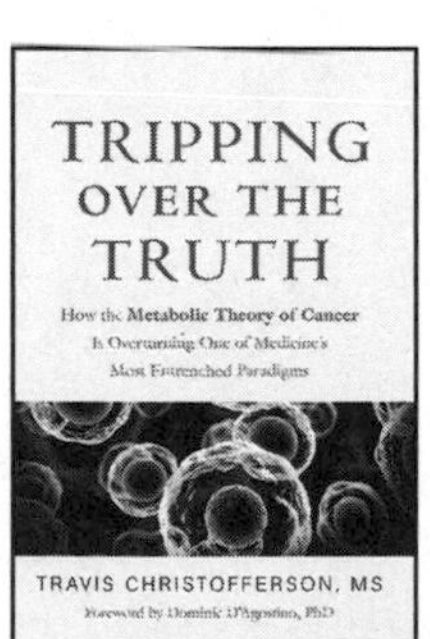

TRIPPING OVER THE TRUTH
How the Metabolic Theory of Cancer Is Overturning One of Medicine's Most Entrenched Paradigms
TRAVIS CHRISTOFFERSON, MS
9781603587297
Hardcover • $24.95

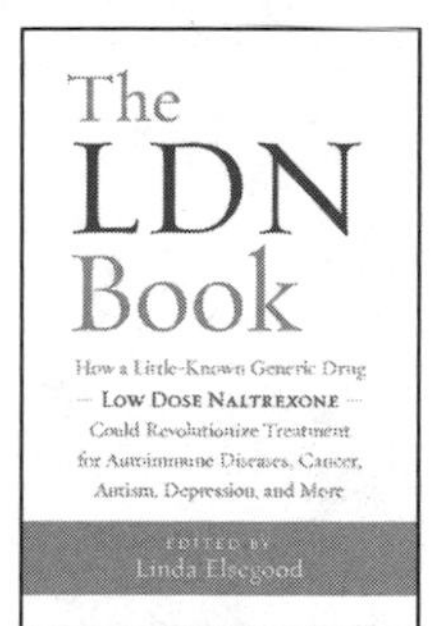

THE LDN BOOK
How a Little-Known Generic Drug — Low Dose Naltrexone — Could Revolutionize Treatment for Autoimmune Diseases, Cancer, Autism, Depression, and More
Edited by LINDA ELSEGOOD
9781603586641
Paperback • $27.99

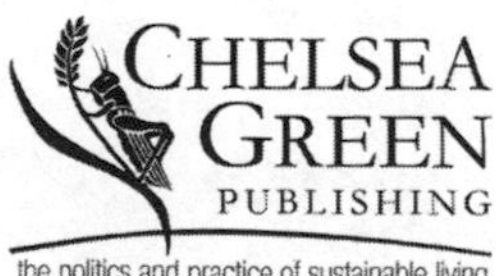

For more information or to request a catalog, visit **www.chelseagreen.com** or call toll-free **(800) 639-4099**.